Pneumonologie – Pneumonology

Official Organ of the Gesellschaft für Lungen- und Atmungsforschung

Pneumonologie – Pneumonology publishes original papers on all aspects of diseases of the bronchi and lungs and cognate subjects. Such work should be concerned mainly with clinical, physiopathological and epidemiological studies, although case reports, short communications and technical notes can be accepted if they are of particular interest. Review articles are solicited by the editors.

50 reprints of each paper are supplied free of charge; additional copies may be ordered at cost price. No page charges.

It is a fundamental condition that submitted manuscripts have not been, and will not simultaneously be submitted or published elsewhere. With the acceptance of a manuscript for publication, the publishers acquire full and exclusive copyright for all languages and countries. Unless special permission has been granted by the publishers, no photographic reproductions, microform or any other reproductions of a similar nature may be made of the journal of individual contributions contained therein or of extracts therefrom.

The use of registered names, trademarks, etc. in this publication does not imply, even in the absence of a specific statement, that such names are exempt from the relevant protective laws and regulations and therefore free for general use.

Subscription information. Volume 153 (4 Issues) will appear in 1976. The publishers reserve the right to issue additional volumes during the calendar year. Information about obtaining back volumes available upon request. **All Contries (Except North America).** Subscription rate: DM 128,–, plus postage and handling. Orders can either be placed with your bookdealer or sent directly to: Springer-Verlag. Heidelberger Platz 3, D-1000 Berlin 33. **North America.** Subscription rate $ 56.60, including postage and handling. Subscriptions are entered with prepayment only. Orders should be addressed to: Springer-Verlag New York Inc., 175 Fifth Avenue, New York, N.Y. 10010.

Manuscripts in duplicate (they should not exceed 20 manuscript pages) may be submitted to any of the following:

Prof. Dr. A. Bouhuys, Yale University
Lung Research Center, 333 Cedar Street
New Haven, Connecticut 06510, USA

Prof. Dr. K. H. Kilburn, University of
Missouri-Columbia, Department of Medicine
Division of Pulmonary and Environmental
Medicine, Columbia, Missouri 65201, USA

Prof. Dr. M. Scherrer, Medizinische Klinik
der Universität, Inselspital, Pneumologische
Abteilung, CH-3010 Bern, Switzerland

Prof. Dr. F. Trendelenburg, Department
Pneumonologie, Universitätskliniken,
D-6650 Homburg/Saar, Federal Republic
of Germany

Prof. Dr. W. T. Ulmer, Medizinische Abteilung des Silikose-Forschungsinstitutes
der Bergbau-Berufsgenossenschaft,
Hunscheidtstraße 12, D-4630 Bochum,
Federal Republic of Germany

ISBN 978-3-662-23364-1   ISBN 978-3-662-25411-0 (eBook)
DOI 10.1007/978-3-662-25411-0

Responsible for Advertisements:
L. Siegel, Kurfürstendamm 237, D-1000 Berlin 15, Tel. (0 30) 8 82 10 31, Telex 01-85 411

INHALT/CONTENTS

SUPPLEMENT 1976

**Leistungsbegrenzung von seiten der Lunge
Band 5 Verhandlungen der Gesellschaft für Lungen- und Atmungsforschung
Tagung 5./6. Dezember 1976
Herausgegeben von W. T. Ulmer, Bochum**

S. Kunke, V. Schulz, W. Erdmann, K. H. Schnabel: A System of PaO2 Continuously Controlled Ventilation   229

K. Diether, W. K. R. Barnikol: Über die klinische Anwendbarkeit der Methode des Totluftplateaus zur Messung des anatomischen Totraumes   233

M. Reinert, D. Heise, W. Mall, F. Trendelenburg: Zum Problem der herzsynchronen Partialdruckschwankungen von Atemgasen   241

A. Bouhuys: Experimental Studies on Airway Smooth Muscle Responses   249

K. Lanser, E. Kaukel, V. Sill: Reflektorische und lokal-irridativ induzierte Bronchokonstriktion   253

E. Vastag, K. Vass, L. Nagy: Bronchoconstriction Reflex in Bronchial Asthma   259

J. Iravani, G. N. Melville, H.-G. Richter: Mucus Production Influenced by Drugs: An Electron Microscopic Study   267

J. Ahrens: Theophylline Blood Levels with Theophylline Ethylene Diamine   275

P. Wyličil, M. Beil, E. Herrmann: Die Analyse belastungsabhängiger Störungen der Atemmechanik mit Ergo-Bodyplethysmographie   279

J. Piiper, F. Adaro: Importance of Stratificational Inhomogenity for Pulmonary Gas Exchange   285

Pneumonologie Suppl. 1976, 1-9
© by Springer-Verlag 1976

Comperative Aspects of Respiration and Circulation in Mammals

Heinz Bartels

Institut für Physiologie, Medizinische Hochschule Hannover

Abstract. Adaptational mechanisms concerning the higher metabolic rate in small mammals compared to big ones are discussed. The alveolar gas exchange area is relatively larger in small mammals, because the individual alveoli are smaller. The capillarization of muscle tissue is higher in small mammals like mice and small bats. Ventilation and cardiac index increase in correlation to metabolic rate. Blood oxygen affinity is lower in small mammals supporting oxygen delivery into tissue. From the point of view of comparative respiratory and circulatory physiology man has all the biological advantages to be "average".

Key words: Alveoli - Capillarization - Gas diffusion - Cardiac index - Ventilation - Oxygen affinity - Bohr effect - Altitude - 2,3-diphosphoglycerate - Cytochrome oxidase - Camel - Llama - Elephant - Bat - Mouse

---

The board of the Society of Lungen- und Atmungsforschung decided last year to confront its members with the aspects of comparative physiology of respiration and circulation, because it was thought it might sometimes be necessary to remember that man is only one page in the large book of nature.

This seems to be also in good agreement with the topic of our meeting this year, because the main point of this discussion will deal with the fact that small animals consume more oxygen per unit of tissue than large animals. We will try to understand how nature solved this problem although the anatomical similarity in a relatively uniform class like the mammals is most remarkable. Figure 1 illustrates the problem, if we look at the metabolic rate of the elephant on the one hand and that of the shrew on the other. The shrew has almost a hundredfold higher oxygen consumption per kg and min compared to the elephant.

In order to understand how nature met these very different metabolic needs we have to consider morphologic and functional adaptations.

A. Morphological adaptations may concern: (1) the lung volume, (2) the alveolar gas exchange area, (3) the diffusion distance from alveolar gas into capillary blood of the lung, (4) the heart's adjustment to required

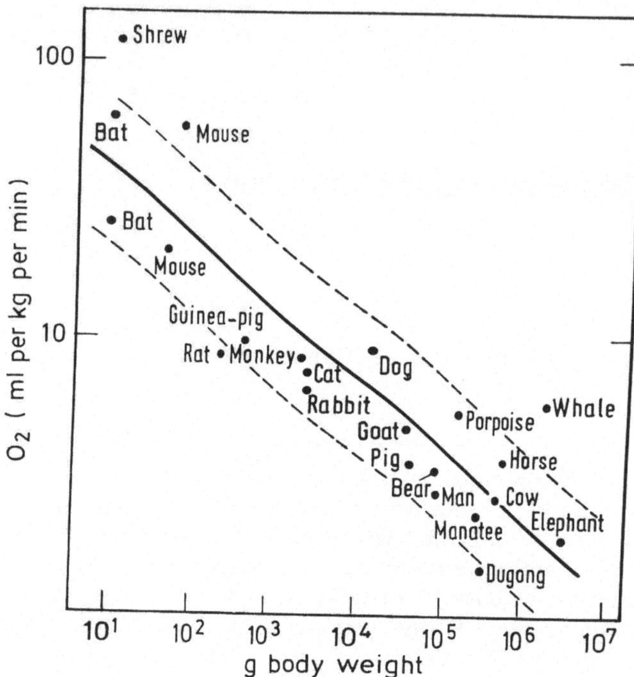

Fig. 1. Metabolic rate (ml O_2 per kg per min) as function of body weight (After Bartels, 1964)

cardiac output, and (5) the capillarization of the tissue with respect to the exchange are between blood and tissue.

1. The lung volume is, as Figure 2 shows, obviously not correlated to metabolic rate but to body weight representing on the average 8 volume percent of the total body volume.

2. The alveolar gas exchange on the other hand is very well adapted to higher metabolic rates (Fig. 3). The higher the metabolic rate, the smaller the alveolar diameter, thus increasing the exchange area markedly. Fick's diffusion equation in the simplified form shows that exchange area (A) is directly proportional to the exchanged amount of gas ($\dot{V}_{O2}$) per time unit, other factors (diffusion constant D and distance d, gas concentration difference $C_1 - C_2$) being constant:

$$\dot{V}_{O2} = D \frac{A}{d} (C_1 - C_2).$$

3. The diffusion distance is not yet reported to be reduced in smaller mammals.

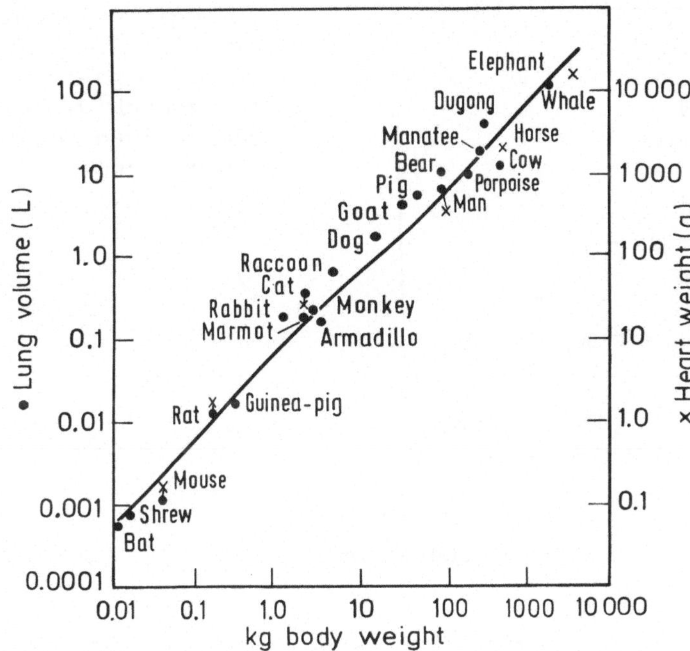

Fig. 2. Logarithmic plot of lung volume as function of body weight (After Tenney and Remmers, 1963)

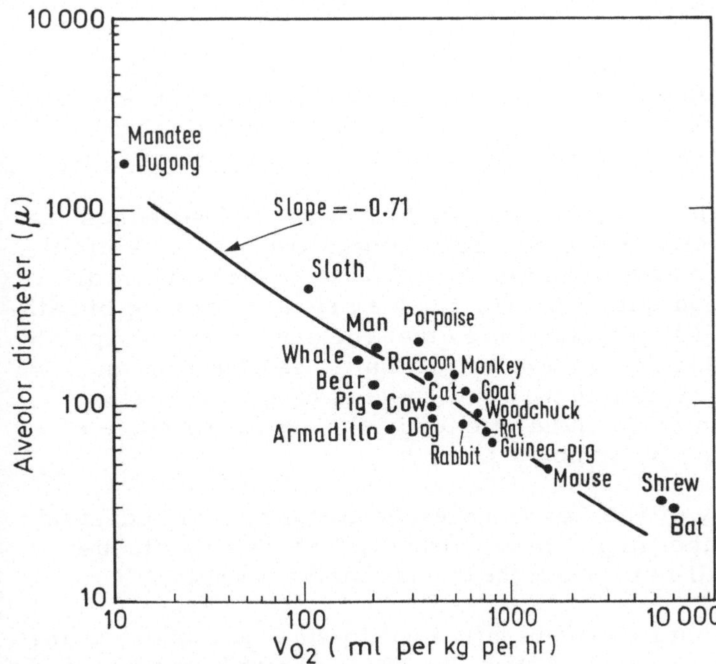

Fig. 3. Mean alveolar diameter as function of metabolic rate (After Tenney and Remmers, 1963)

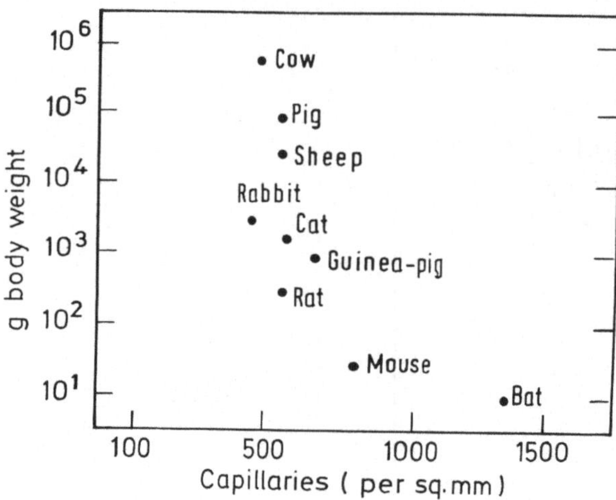

Fig. 4. Body weight as function of capillaries per sq mm in gastrocnemius muscle (After Schmidt-Nielsen and Pennycuik, 1961)

4. The heart size is, like the lung volume, on the average not correlated to metabolic rate.

5. The capillarization of muscular tissue shows adaptation only in quite small animals, like mice and small bats (Fig. 4).

B. Functional adaptations should be related to (1) ventilation, (2) diffusion, (3) perfusion, (4) gas transport in blood, and (5) activities of metabolic enzymes in tissues.

1. Ventilation. There is no complete information on alveolar or total ventilation over a sufficient wide weight range in mammals, but breathing frequences are known (Fig. 5) and show an inverse correlation to body weight, suggesting that animals with a high metabolic rate have a higher pulmonary ventilation.

It is interesting that in large animals with low breathing frequences the functional residual capacity is proportionally larger than in small animals, thus avoiding an increase of alveolar and arterial oxygen and carbon dioxide pressure fluctuation during breathing. The net energy cost of breathing can be calculated and it is quite obvious that the small mammal spends more energy for breathing per kg body weight than does a large animal. But as the metabolic rate is higher in the small species compared to larger ones, small and large animals spend practically the same percentage of their total metabolism for breathing.

2. Diffusion capacity of the lung is increased by the relative increase of the exchange area in the lung. The same should be true at the tissue level, for mice and small bats due to the higher capillary density.

3. Perfusion of the lung should be increased in small animals to transport the exchanged gases. Figure 5 shows the higher heart frequences and Figure 6 the increased cardiac index (ml blood per min and kg body weight) supporting our reasoning.

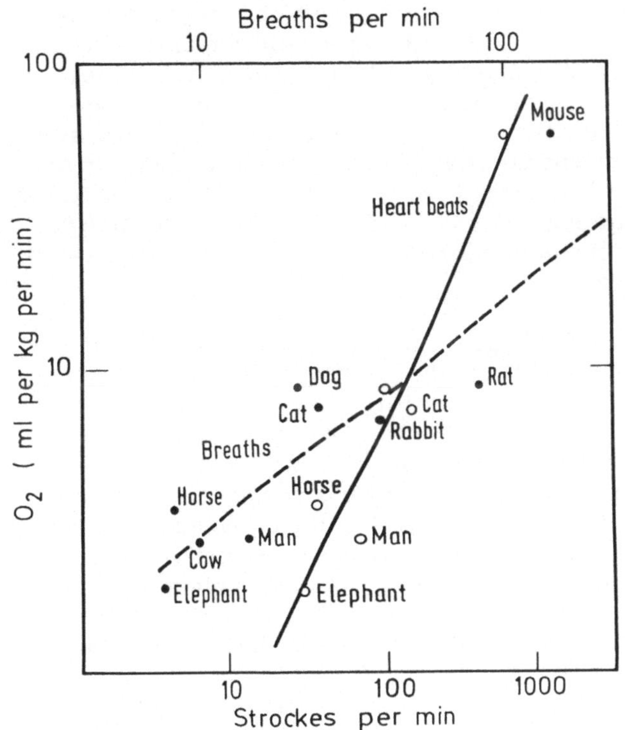

Fig. 5. Metabolic rate as function of **frequencies** of respiration and heart rate, respectively (After Bartels, 1964)

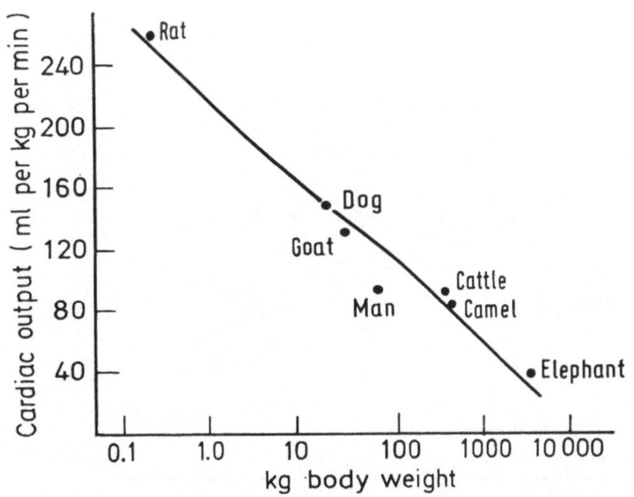

Fig. 6. Cardiac index as function of body weight (After Bartels, 1966)

4. Oxygen transport in blood can be enhanced by increasing (a) the hemoglobin concentration, the uptake and unloading capacity (expressed by) (b) oxygen affinity, and (c) the Bohr effect.

6

a) Hemoglobin concentration is not well correlated to body weight, but there is a small tendency toward an inverse correlation to body weight. An increase of hematocrit above 50% would increase blood viscosity and therefore need increased heart work. In a quite specialized mammalian family, the tylopodae (camels and llamas), a relatively high hemoglobin concentration is present together with a low hematocrit due to the exceptionally high hemoglobin concentration of 45% in the ovalocytes. This special shape of red cells may perhaps facilitate heart work by a lower viscosity and enable these species to live under high altitude conditions, which is true for llamas but also for camels living up to 4500 m of altitude in Afghanistan. These properties persist in tylopodae, when living on sea level, probably due to their genetic basis.

b) Oxygen affinity shows a fairly good correlation to body weight (Fig. 7) suggesting that mammals with a high metabolic rate need a high unloading tension for sufficient oxygen supply into their tissues. Special ecologic conditions, like diving and high altitude also seem to be related to the oxygen affinity. Small rodents native to high altitude have higher oxygen affinities (guinea pig) compared to their low land relatives of approximately the same body weight. The same is true for bird species. The Tibetan goose is reported to fly up to 10,000 m crossing the Himalayas in fall and spring. Though the heme group of the hemoglobin molecule is the same in all species so far considered, there are different, now fairly well-known mechanisms, which establish different oxygen affinities in mammals

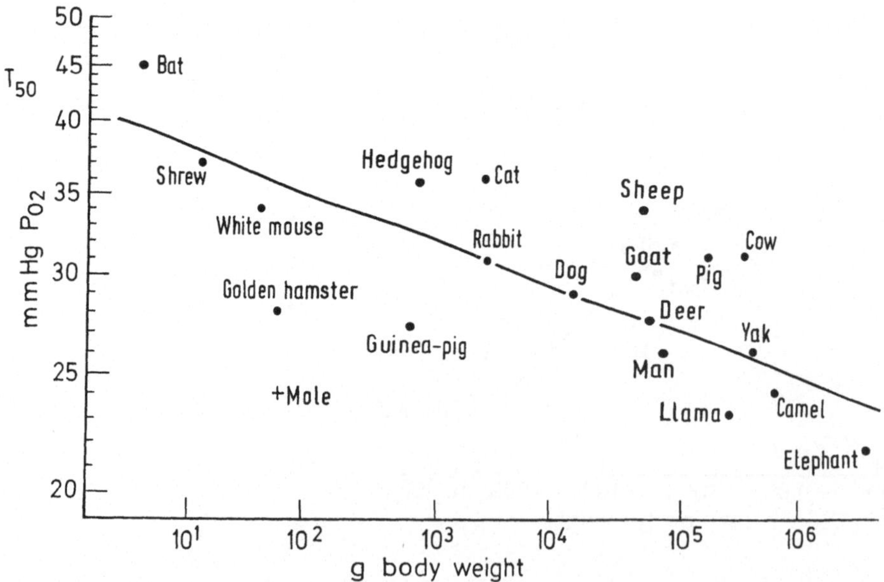

Fig. 7. Half-saturation oxygen tension (blood pH 7.4, 37°C) as function of body weight

and birds. The affinity of the hemoglobin itself can differ by different amino acid sequences leading finally to altered quaternary structures and thus giving rise to different allosteric effects on the oxygen binding sites. Furthermore cofactors, especially 2,3 diphosphoglycerate (2,3-DPG) in many but not all mammals, and inositole penta or hexaphosphate (IHP) in birds, can decrease an intrinsically high oxygen affinity of hemoglobins. A comparison between man and llama (Ll. guanaco) as well as between the gray and the Tibetan goose (Petschow et al., 1975) indicates (Table 1) that the cofactor 2,3-DPG itself decreases the affinity in both mammals, but in the birds the avian cofactor IHP must have a more pronounced effect on the hemoglobin's affinity of the Tibetan goose compared to its effect on the affinity of hemoglobin of the grey goose.

c) The Bohr effect was found in hemoglobin solution to be very well correlated inversely to body weight, suggesting an enhanced oxygen delivery into tissue (Fig. 8). This correlation of the Bohr effect is less convincing when estimated in blood and it is blood after all, which runs in our vessels and not hemoglobin solutions.

5. Cytochrome oxidase activity and cytochrome-C concentration were found higher in tissues of small mammals thus enabling them to meet their higher metabolic demands.
   These considerations may lead to the conclusion that smaller mammals than the Etruscan shrew have no chance of survival because to be smaller would mean to need even more food per g and feeding more than 24 h a day.

Table 1. Half-saturation oxygen pressure of stripped hemoglobin and blood, 2,3 diphosphoglycerat and inositole pentaphosphate - hemoglobin quotient, respectively, in different species (After Petschow et al., 1975)

Species	HbO_2 1/2 Sat. pressure (P_{50}) mmHg		$\dfrac{[DPG]}{[Hb]}$	$\dfrac{[IP_5]}{[Hb]}$
	Hb	blood		
Man	12	27	1.1	-
L. guanacoe	15	23	0.57	-
Ansa ansa	6	42	-	0.80
Ansa indiaca	5	28	-	0.87

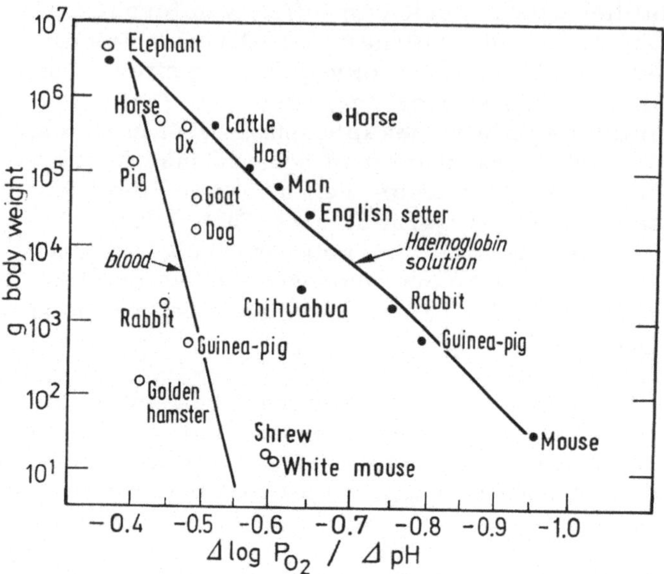

$$\Delta \log P_{O_2} \, / \, \Delta \, pH$$

Fig. 8. Body weight as function of the Bohr effect in hemoglobin solutions and blood (After Bartels, 1964)

The same may be true for bigger land mammals than the elephant, because under the present conditions for food supply in the wilderness of Africa the elephant feeds almost 24 h a day due to the high absolute amount of food this creature needs. Very small mammals expending more energy for feeding than the shrews are the small bats like myotis myotis because they feed during flight. They can survive with a body weight of only 6 g in spite of a high metabolic rate, because their body temperature drops from 38°C during flight to an environment temperature of around 20°C at rest, thus saving a great amount of energy otherwise not available.

Finally one should come to a balanced view of the position of man in this frame. There is no reason for misanthropic or hubric ideas. Man is a really average creature as we have seen from our discussion. He is of average size, his oxygen consumption is on an average level, and this seems to be his great advantage for survival as species. He is not the fastest runner, but he is fairly good at running, he is not the best climber, but he can climb and he is by far not the best swimmer or diver, but he can swin and even dive. Due to his highly developed brain he can thus technically compensate for certain lacks in any field.

REFERENCES

1. Bartels, H.: Comparative physiology of oxygen transport in mammals
   Lancet 1964, 599-604

2. Bartels, H. : Some aspects of circulatory and respiratory functions in mammals. Amer. Heart J. 72, 1-6 (1966)
3. Petschow, D. , Baumann, R. , Würdinger, I. , Bauer, C. : Comparative studies of hemoglobin from lowland and highland mammals and birds. Pflügers Arch. (in press)
4. Schmidt-Nielsen, K. , Pennycuik, P. : Capillary density in mammals in relation to body size and oxygen consumption. J. appl. Physiol. 200, 746 (1961)
5. Tenney, S. M. , Remmers, J. E. : Comparative quantitative morphology of the mammalian lung: diffusing area. Nature (Lond.) 197, 54 (1963)

Professor Dr. Heinz Bartels
Institut für Physiologie
Medizinische Hochschule Hannover
Karl Wiechert Allee 9
3000 Hannover 61

DISCUSSION

E. Kehler, Bleckede: Is there an analogous difference between the inhabitants of the lowland and the Indian of the Andes, who is adapted to heights, as there is between the normal gray goose and the Ansa indiaca, which flies over the Himalayas?

H. Bartels, Hannover: The concentration of 2, 3-diphosphoglycerate is slightly lower in the blood of the inhabitant of the lowland.

Pneumonologie Suppl. 1976, 11-16

Respiration as a Limiting Factor for Working Capacity

Gunnar Grimby

Department of Rehabilitation Medicine I, Sahlgren's Hospital, Göteborg, Sweden

Diseases of the cardiorespiratory system often considerably limit the physical work performance. However, to what extent is the respiratory system a limiting factor for exercise tolerance without manifest respiratory disease? What factors should be taken into consideration?

In a population sample of 54-years-old Swedish men, about a third had dyspnea during exercise according to a questionnaire (Wilhelmsen et al., 1974). There was a significant relationship between smoking habits and dyspnea, but also independent of smoking, there was a relationship between dyspnea and ventilation capacity measured as the forced expiratory volume in 1 sec corrected for anthropometric variables (FEV_1 index). The FEV_1 index correlated with several expressions of physical work capacity, also independent of smoking habits. This finding may indicate that at high work levels - in middle-aged men - the perception of dyspnea may contribute to the limitation of exercise and in that way also to the degree of physical activity and training. The finding that those with a low FEV_1 index stopped at the same perceived exertion as those with a high FEV_1 index, although with lower maximal heart rate also points in the same direction.

The question then arises how various factors in the respiratory function can limit exercise tolerance. The different aspects of the respiratory function to be analyzed are:

Pump capacity
 Alveolar ventilation
 Flow-volume relationship
 Work of breathing

Diffusion capacity

Sensation of dyspnea

Measurements of the arterial carbon dioxide tension demonstrate whether the alveolar ventilation is adequate for the metabolic situation or not. According to several reports in the literature, CO_2 tension is fairly constant at moderate work loads and decreases with heavy exercise. For data on healthy middle-aged men see, e.g., Bjure et al. (1971). These authors did not find any definite change in arterial oxygen saturation or tension with increasing work loads, but an increasing alveolo-arterial oxygen difference. The transfer factor increased with increasing oxygen uptake and no leveling off of the values could be demonstrated. These results indicate that even at heavy exercise the capacity for gas exchange is sufficient, although there is an increased burden on the respiratory system, as indicated by the increased alveolo-arterial oxygen difference.

The sensation of dyspnea should be sought in mechanical factors connected with the increased work of breathing at alveolar hyperventilation during heavy exercise. The precise nature of dyspnea is insufficiently understood and consists probably of several factors. The "pump function" of the respiratory system can be analyzed in several ways. One is in the flow-volume representation. At rest, only a minor fraction of the potential volume and flow changes are used, and even at heavy exercise during expiration, the maximal expiratory flow-volume (MEFV) curve is usually not reached in sedentary young men (see Grimby, 1968). In very well-trained young subjects with a higher ventilation at maximal exercise, the MEFV curve may actually be reached at maximal work load (Fig. 1) (Grimby et al., 1971). With age the MEFV curve becomes more curvilinear (Mead et al., 1967, and others) and the possibility for the flow-volume curve obtained during exercise to reach the MEFV curve increases. The person may have to make nearly maximal inspirations in order to use the "highest part" of the MEFV curve, and thus a burden is placed also on the inspiratory muscles. In patients with chronic bronchitis, the MEFV curve may be reached at rest or in moderate exercise (Grimby and Stiksa, 1970; Potter et al., 1971). This may be associated with an increase of the thorax in

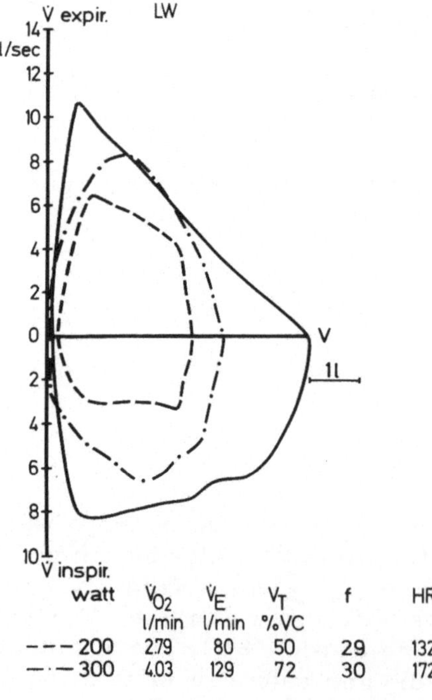

Fig. 1. Maximal expiratory and inspiratory flow (V̇)-volume (V) curves in one well-trained man (L. W.), aged 28 years, together with flow-volume curves at submaximal (200 W) and maximal (300 W) exercise

	watt	V̇$_{O_2}$	V̇$_E$	V$_T$	f	HR
		l/min	l/min	%VC		
- - -	200	2.79	80	50	29	132
— · —	300	4.03	129	72	30	172

inspiratory direction both at the end of inspiration and expiration (Grimby et al. , 1973).

Over most part of the vital capacity there exists a transpulmonary pressure, beyond which increases in pressure do not produce an increase in expiratory flow. Thus, if the transpulmonary pressure exceeds that pressure, ventilation can be termed inefficient (Olafsson and Hyatt, 1969), as the work of breathing increases without any increase in flow. In healthy males, Olafsson and Hyatt (1969) did not find that the transpulmonary pressures to any appreciable extent exceeded the flow-limiting pressures. In very well-trained men with higher maximal ventilation at exhaustive exercise, the same is true, even if somewhat higher maximal transpulmonary pressures are reached during breathing (Fig. 2) (Grimby et al. , 1971). In patients with obstructive lung disease, somewhat varying results have been reported. Potter et al. (1971) found transpulmonary pressures in excess of the flow-limiting pressures, indicating that the ventilation became mechanically inefficient. The transpulmonary pressure at which expiratory flow becomes limited is furthermore reduced in patients with chronic airways obstruction. However, according to Leaver and Pride (1971) an adjustment in the respiratory muscle force during heavy exercise usually occurs, so that pressures in excess of the flow-limiting pressure, and, thus, also "inefficient ventilation" is avoided.

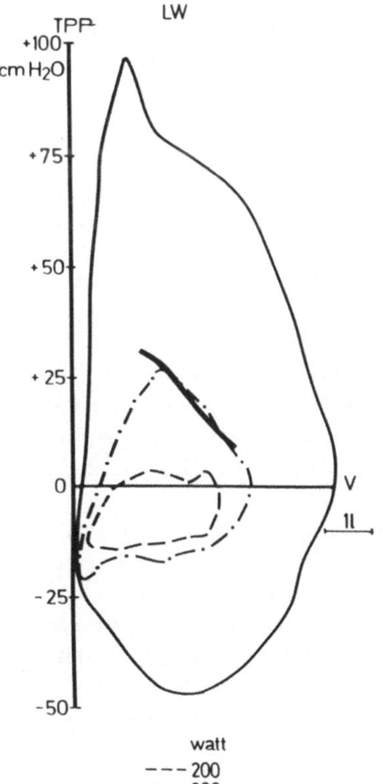

Fig. 2. Relationship between transpulmonary pressure (TPP) and volume for subject L. W. in Figure 1 at forced expiratory and inspiratory vital capacity maneuvers, and at submaximal (200 W) and maximal (300 W) exercise. Short thick line connects points of pressure, where flow limitation appeared (lowest pressure at which maximal flow was achieved at fixed lung volume)

However, the total work of breathing is not only determined by the volume and the transpulmonary pressure variations as defined from the Campbell diagram, but also from any amount of work added by the work to distort the thoracoabdominal configuration. This part of the actual total work of breathing has not been taken into account in earlier studies, but has through the analysis of Goldman et al. (1976) been shown to account for up to 20-25% of the total work of breathing. In that analysis, the assumption is made that the chest wall can be divided into two parts, the rib cage and the diaphragm-abdomen. As the relative motion of these two parts during breathing deviates from the relationship at the relaxed state of corresponding lung volumes, an extra amount of energy is needed. The deviation from the relaxed configuration of the chest wall also indicates that an inappropriate relationship between length and tension in the chest wall structures is achieved which according to Howell and Campbell (1966) may be connected with the sensation of dyspnea.

The pulmonary ventilation may as postulated by Riley (1960) reach a point, where any further increase in oxygen uptake by an increased ventilation will be used by the respiratory muscles. At that degree "maximum efficient ventilation" is reached. It must, however, be observed that ventilation and oxygen uptake as such may not be at their maxima. Using data from the literature on the oxygen cost of breathing, Riley (1960) published a diagram as shown in Fig. 3. Even if those figures are very approximate, among other reasons because of those pointed out by Goldman et al. (1976), it seems as if a ventilation of 100-120 l/min may be critical in this respect. At high ventilation an anaerobic process may also start to provide the additional energy required to further increase the ventilation.

A possibility to evaluate the degree of exertion and dyspnea is to use different rating scales (Borg, 1970). During exercise the subject has to grade his perceived exertion according to a scale from 6 to 20 with verbal expression as a guide: 7 very, very light; 9 very light; 11 fairly light; 13 somewhat hard; 15 hard; 17 very hard; 19 very, very hard. The perceived degree of breathlessness can be rated in a similar way with a scale from 1 to 16: 1 none; 3 quite negliable; 5 very light; 7 rather light; 9 neither light nor heavy; 11 heavy; 13 very heavy; 15 very, very heavy. At least in subjects with a fairly maintained ventilatory capacity there is good correlation between these two forms of perceived sensations, which may indicate that breathlessness constitutes a major factor for the general feeling of fatigue. These types of rating scales also open a possibility for evaluating, whether a particular sensation subjectively limits the physical performance.

In conclusion, an adequate gas exchange is achieved also with strenous exercise in healthy man. A burden is, however, placed on the respiratory system by hyperventilation. The transpulmonary pressures produced seem normally to be within its efficient range. An increased work of breathing is, however, caused by distorsion of the chest wall from the relaxed thoracoabdominal configuration. Furthermore, the increase in work of breathing at an increased ventilation may use all the extra oxygen

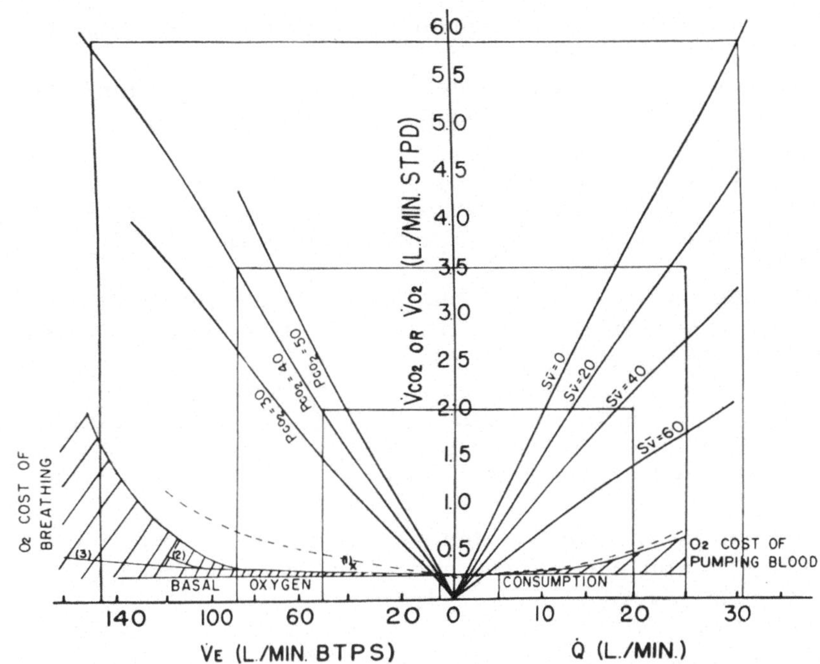

Fig. 3. Relationships between gas exchange, ventilation, and blood flow. Cross-hatched areas represent oxygen cost of breathing (left) and oxygen cost of pumping blood (right).

Solid curve forming upper boundary of cross-hatched area (left) has shape similar to cost-of-breathing curves from literature and is a compromise, representing as well as possible the cost of breathing of average man. Broken curves (left and right) indicate sum of basal oxygen consumption, oxygen cost of breathing, and oxygen cost of pumping blood.

Isopleths represent alveolar or arterial PCO_2 (left) and mixed venous blood oxygen saturation (right).

Horizontal and vertical lines represent simultaneous relationships at different levels of exercise (from Riley, 1960)

uptake, so that ventilation becomes inefficient from the total point of view, or there may be an increasing amount of anaerobic metabolism in the respiratory muscles.

Dyspnea is connected with mechanical factors, the detailed nature of which is unclear.

REFERENCES

Bjure, J., Grimby, G., Nilsson, N.J.: Pulmonary gas exchange during submaximal and maximal exercise in healthy middle-aged men. In: Pulmonary diffusing capacity on exercise. (M. Scherrer Ed.) pp. 107-131. Bern-Stuttgart-Vienna: Hans Huber 1971

Borg, G. : Perceived exertion as an indicator of somatic stress. Scand. J. Rehab. Med. 2, 92-98 (1970)

Goldman, M. , Grimby, G. , Mead, J. : Mechanical work of breathing derived from rib cage and abdominal volume-pressure partitioning. J. Appl. Physiol. in press (1976)

Grimby, G. : Respiration in exercise. Med. Sci. Sport. 1, 9-14 (1969)

Grimby, G. , Stiksa, J. : Flow-volume curves and breathing patterns during exercise in patients with obstructive lung disease. Scand. J. Clin. Lab. Invest. 25, 303-313 (1970)

Grimby, G. , Elgefors, B. , Oxhöj, H. : Ventilatory levels and chest wall mechanics during exercise in obstructive lung disease. Scand. J. Resp. Dis. 54, 45-52 (1973)

Grimby, G. , Saltin, B. , Wilhelmsen, L. : Pulmonal flow-volume and pressure-volume relationship during submaximal and maximal exercise in young well-trained men. Bull. Physio-path. Resp. 7, 157-168 (1971)

Howell, J. B. L. , Campbell, E. J. M. In: Breathlessness. Oxford: Blackwell 1966

Leaver, D. G. , Pride, N. B. : Flow-volume curves and expiratory pressures during exercise on patients with chronic airways obstruction. Scand. J. Resp. Dis. Suppl. 77, 23-27 (1971)

Mead, J. , Turner, J. M. , Macklem, P. T. , Little, J. A. : Significance of the relationship between lung recoil and maximum expiratory flow. J. Appl. Physiol. 22, 95-108 (1967)

Olafsson, S. , Hyatt, R. E. : Ventilatory mechanics and expiratory flow limitation during exercise in normal subjects. J. Clin. Invest. 48, 546-573 (1969)

Potter, W. A. , Olafsson, S. , Hyatt, R. E. : Ventilatory mechanics and expiratory flow limitation during exercise in patients with obstructive lung disease. J. Clin Invest. 50, 910-919 (1971)

Riley, R. : Pulmonary function in relation to exercise. In: Science and medicine of exercise and sports. New York: Harper and Brothers 1960

Wilhelmsen, L. , Tibblin, G. , Aurell, M. , Bjure, J. , Ekström-Jodal, B. , Grimby, G. : Ventilatory function and work performance in a representative sample of 803 men aged 54 years. Chest 66, 506-510 (1974)

Dr. Gunnar Grimby
Department of Rehabilitation
Medicine I
Sahlgren's Hospital
S-413 45 Göteborg, Sweden

Pneumonologie Suppl. 1976, 17-26
© by Springer-Verlag 1976

Die Lunge als leistungsbegrenzender Faktor bei Patienten: Blutgase

H. Matthys

Ärztlicher Direktor der Abteilung Pulmologie, Zentrum Innere Medizin
Universitätsklinik Freiburg i. Br.

The Lung as a Limiting Factor for Physical Exercise in Patients:
Blood Gases

Summary. Respiration is a feed back system controling mainly arterial
O_2, CO_2 partial pressures and pH to maintain the O_2 and CO_2 gas transfer
according to the metabolic needs of the body. The arterial O_2 partial pressure is rarely the primary factor which limits the working capacity of patients at sea level. This may be due to the fact, that the controled variables
of the respiratory system are maintained within tolerable limits as long as
possible. Therefore mechanics of breathing, hemodynamics, O_2 capacity
of the blood and muscular fatigue are more often exercise limiting factors
than the tonometric function of the lung to achieve the necessary O_2-trans-
port. This can be prooved on patients by repeating the maximal tolerable
work load with 100% oxygen breathing providing all the necessary data we
need to apply "Ficks principle" to calculate cardiac output.

Zusammenfassung. Die humoralen Regelgrößen der Atmung sind
O_2-CO_2-Partialdruck und pH, um die O_2-Aufnahme und CO_2-Abgabe unseres
Körpers sicherzustellen. Der arterielle O_2-Partialdruck ist selten der
primär leistungslimitierende Faktor bei Patienten mit Lungenkrankheiten,
sofern keine exogenen Hypoxiebedingungen vorliegen. Bei einer kybernetischen Betrachtungsweise der Atemfunktion ist dies nicht erstaunlich, sind
doch die arteriellen Blutgase Regelgrößen, welche der Körper unter allen
Bedingungen im Normbereich zu halten versucht. Die Äquilibrationsfunktion
der Lunge als den O_2-Transport limitierenden Faktor kann durch Atmung
von 100% O_2 überprüft werden, falls wir uns alle Meßdaten beschaffen, welche
wir für die Anwendung des Fickschen Prinzips zur Herzzeitvolumenbestim-
mung sowieso benötigen.

Der Regelkreis der Atmung dient primär der Sicherstellung der lebens-
notwendigen O_2-Versorgung und der Ausscheidung des quantitativ wichtigsten
Stoffwechselendprodukts CO_2. Die Menge O_2, welche den Körpergeweben

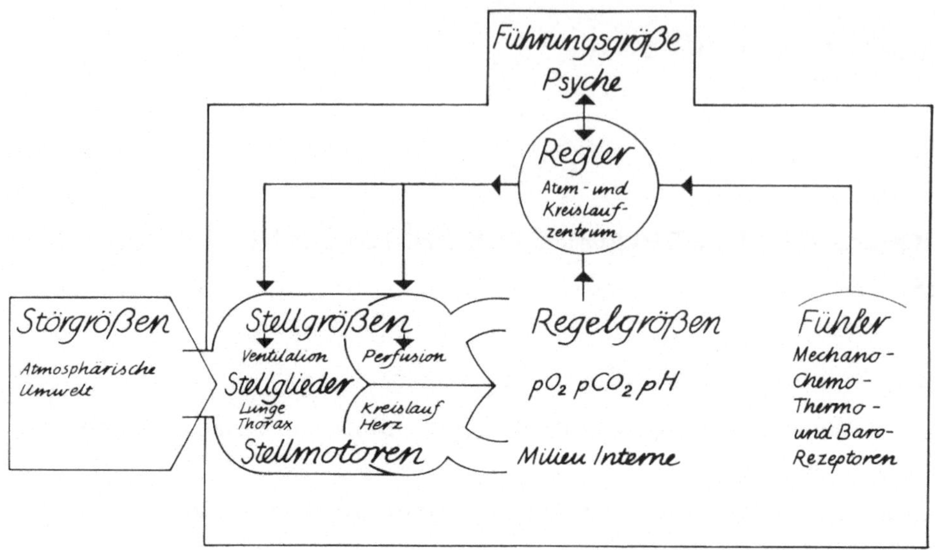

Abb. 1. Regelkreis der Atmung

zur Verfügung gestellt wird, hängt entscheidend vom pulmonalen Gasaustausch, dem Herzzeitvolumen und seiner regionalen Verteilung, der Hämoglobinkonzentration, sowie seiner Bindungsfähigkeit für O_2 ab. Die CO_2-Ausscheidung wird praktisch nur durch die alveoläre Ventilation limitiert (Roughton 1964).

REGELKREIS DER ATMUNG (Abb. 1)

Die humoralen Regelgrößen der Atmung sind O_2-Partialdruck (pO_2) CO_2-Partialdruck (pCO_2) und H^+-Ionenkonzentration (pH). Durch vielfältige Fühler (Chemo-, Mechano-, Thermo- und Barorezeptoren) sowie durch direkte Aktion der Führungs- und Regelgrößen auf das Atem- und Kreislaufzentrum (Regler) wird eine Homöostase der arteriellen Blutgas- und Säure-Basenverhältnisse angestrebt. Die Stellgrößen Ventilation und Perfusion sind durch den alveolokapillären Gasaustauschraum verbunden. Die Atemmechanik und die Hämodynamik kosten den Organismus für die Konvektion von Luft (Ventilation) und Blut (Perfusion) mechanische Arbeit, welche dem Körper durch Wärme verloren geht. Andererseits garantiert die für Ventilation und Perfusion notwendige Bewegungsenergie auch gleichzeitig die Aufrechterhaltung von Patialdruckdifferenzen, welche für die passive Diffusion von Gasen zwischen Alveolen, Blut und Körpergeweben unabdingbar sind. Damit sind die Blutgaspartialdrucke die entscheidenden Prüfgrößen zur Beurteilung des kypernetischen Systems, welches wir unter dem Begriff Regelkreis der Atmung subsummieren.

Sind die arteriellen Blutgaspartialdrucke in Ruhe im Normbereich liegend, bedeutet dies lediglich, dem Regelkreis ist eine normgerechte arteriellen CO_2-Partialdruckerniedrigung führt, eine normale alveolo-arterielle O_2-Differenz vorausgesetzt, zu einer O_2-Partialdruckerhöhung. Das Gleiche wäre von der nicht Stellglied bedingten Hypoventilation zu sagen. Auch hier ist die Aquilibrationsfunktion der Lunge z. B. bei einer Schlafmittelintoxikation zumindest nicht primär gestört. Dabei ist der arterielle O_2-Partialdruck lediglich entsprechend dem Anstieg des arteriellen CO_2-Partialdrucks aufgrund einer globalen alveolären Hypoventilation, bei im Normbereich liegender alveolo-arterieller O_2-Differenz erniedrigt.

Ist bei erniedrigtem CO_2 - der arterielle O_2-Partialdruck im Sollbereich oder vermindert, so entspricht die Äquilibrationsfunktion der Lunge ebensowenig der Norm wie bei einer reinen arteriellen Hypoxie mit Normokapnie. Diesen drei Blutgaskonstellationen liegt eine Erkrankung der mechanischen Stellglieder Thorax - Lunge und/oder Herz - Kreislauf zugrunde. Wir fassen diese Störungen im Bereiche der Stellglieder, die noch zu keinem abnormen Anstieg des arteriellen CO_2-Partialdrucks führen unter dem Begriff "respiratorische Partialinsuffizienz" zusammen, d. h. es besteht in keinem Fall eine ventilatorische CO_2-Abgabeinsuffizienz.

Ist hingegen die Homöostase des arteriellen CO_2-Partialdrucks als Folge einer Stellglied bedingten Insuffizienz nicht mehr möglich, beobachten wir bei Luftatmung stets eine schwere arterielle Hypoxie. Unabhängig von Sitz und Ursache der Atemstörung (Stellglied d. h. mechanisch und/oder nicht Stellglied d. h. steuerungsbedingt), fassen wir die Blutgaskonstellationen arterielle Hypoxie und Hyperkapnie unter dem Begriff "respiratorische Globalinsuffizienz" zusammen.

Sind die beschriebenen Blutgaskonstellationen bereits in Ruhe nachweisbar, sprechen wir von einer manifesten, werden sie erst bei körperlicher Belastung offenbar, von einer latenten Atemfunktionsstörung. Geht die Atemfunktionsstörung mit gegenüber den Sollwerten pathologischen Blutgaskonstellationen einher (2 - 6) verwenden wir den Oberbegriff der "respiratorischen Insuffizienz". Die emotionelle und höhenbedingte Hyperventilation fällt somit nicht unter den Begriff der respiratorischen Insuffizienz, ein erhöhter kardialer rechts - links Shunt hingegen schon.

Wie wir wissen kann eine manifeste Atemfunktionsstörung bei körperlicher Belastung in eine quantitativ und qualitativ andere Blutgaspartialdruckkonstellation übergehen. Das Verhalten der arteriellen und venösen Blutgaskonstellationen in Ruhe und bei körperlicher Belastung, erlaubt uns daher, wenn auch mit Einschränkungen, auf die Schwere und die Pathogenese des zugrundeliegenden Mechanismus rückzuschließen.

O_2-TRANSPORTSTÖRUNGEN DES BLUTES

CO_2-Transportstörungen des Blutes sind klinisch irrelevant, wir können uns daher auf den O_2-Transport allein konzentrieren. (Abb. 2)

Nebst einer ungenügenden äquilibrations- oder steuerungsbedingten Funktion der Lunge können bekanntlich noch andere Ursachen zu einem verminderten O_2-Gehalt des Blutes führen. Einen verminderten O_2-Gehalt

Homöostase entsprechend den atmosphärischen Umweltbedingungen gelungen. Ist dies auch bis zur maximalen Sollwertbelastung möglich, können
wir eine funktionell relevante Krankheit im Bereiche des Regelkreises der
Atmung ausschließen. Bekanntlich ist die körperliche Leistungsfähigkeit
gesunder Trainierter und Untrainierter nicht durch die Lungenfunktion im
engeren Sinne sondern durch die Muskulatur und das O_2-Transportvermögen
des Kreislaufs ($\dot{Q}$ x CaO_2) limitiert (Åstrand und Rodahl, 1970).

Für die Beurteilung der Lunge als leistungsbegrenzender Faktor:
Blutgase bei Patienten, genügt es daher die O_2 und CO_2 Partaildrucke im
arteriellen und venösen Blut entsprechend den atmosphärischen Bedingungen
allein zu beachten.

EINTEILUNG DER ATEMFUNKTIONSSTÖRUNGEN

Folgende sechs blutgasanalytische Kombinationen stehen uns zur Klassifizierung der "äusseren" Atemfunktionsstörungen bei Luftatmung zur Verfügung (Tabelle I).

Dabei sind nur vier Lungenfunktionsstörungen im engeren Sinne (2 - 5),
d. h. Stellglied bedingte Blutgaskonstellationen, während die zwei anderen
(1 + 6) nicht Stellglied bedingt d. h. Störungen im Bereiche der Steuerungsorgane sind.

Die nicht Stellglied bedingte Hyperventilation beinhaltet, die Äquilibrationsfunktion der Lunge entspricht der Norm. Mit anderen Worten die Ursache der Hyperventilation (= arterielle Hypokapnie) ist im Bereich des
"Milieu interne" (z. B. Schwangerschaft, metabolische Azidose etc.),
des "Milieu externe" (z. B. exogene Hypoxie) der Fühler- und Regelorgane
oder der Führungsgröße Psyche zu suchen. Quantitative bedeutet dies, die

Tabelle 1. Die 6 möglichen arteriellen Blutgaskonstellationen, welche eine
Atemfunktionsstörung anzeigen. n = im Normbereich liegend, ↑ gegenüber der Norm erhöht, ↓ gegenüber der Norm erniedrigt

	P_{aO2}	P_{aCO2}	Atemfunktionsstörungen	
1)	↑	↓	nicht stellgliedbedingte Hyperventilation	
2)	n	↓	stellgliedbedingte Hyperventilation	
3)	↓	n	Stellgliedbedingte Hypoxie	respiratorische Partialinsuffizienz
4)	↓	↓	stellgliedbedingte Hyperventilation	
5)	↓↓	↑	stellgliedbedingte Hypoventilation	respiratorische Globalinsuffizienz
6)	↓	↑	nicht stellgliedbedingte Hypoventilation	

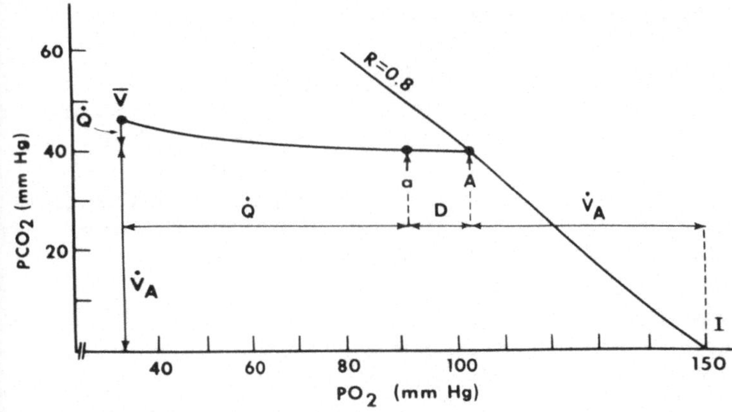

Abb. 2. O_2- und CO_2-Partialdruckdiagramm. Es zeigt die relative Bedeutung der alveolaren Ventilation ($\dot{V}_A$) und der Lungendurchblutung ($\dot{Q}$) für den Transport von O_2 und CO_2. Der O_2-Partialdruck fällt durch Mischung von Inspirationsluft (I) mit Alveolarluft (A) entsprechend dem respiratorischen Quotienten (R) ab. Die alveolo-arterielle O_2-Differenz (A-a)D spiegelt die ungenügende Äquilibrationsfunktion der Lunge für O_2 wieder. Letztere ist für CO_2 praktisch Null und die CO_2-Ausscheidung ist im Gegensatz zur O_2-Aufnahme lediglich eine Funktion der alveolaren Ventilation ($\dot{V}_A$)

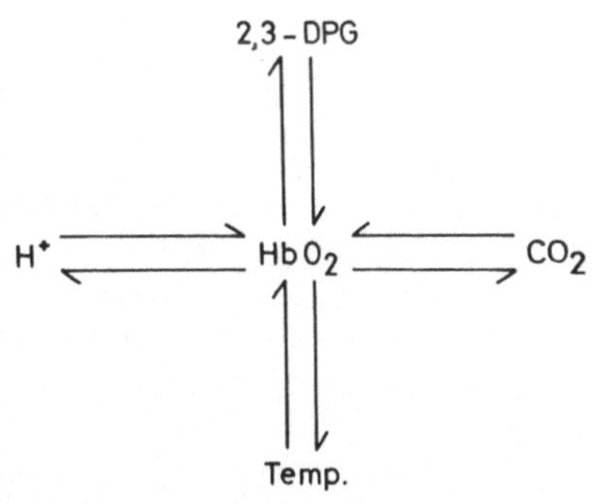

Abb. 3. Die vier Hauptliganden, welche das O_2-Bindungsvermögen des Hämoglobins wesentlich beeinflussen und damit den die Lage der O_2-Dissoziationskurve charakterisierenden Halbsättigungsdruck (P_{50}). 2,3-DPG = 2,3-Diphosphoglycerat

des Blutes bezeichnen wir unabhängig von der O_2-Sättigung und dem O_2-Partialdruck als Hypoxämie. Bei gegebenem Partialdruck ist der O_2-Gehalt des Blutes eine Funktion der O_2-bindenden Hämoglobinkonzentration und deren O_2-Affinität.

Die O_2-Affinität des Hämoglobins wird im wesentlichen von vier Faktoren entscheidend beeinflußt. (Abb. 3)

H^+-Ionenkonzentration-, 2,3-DPG-, CO_2- und Temperaturerhöhung vermindern die Affinität des Hämoglobins für O_2 und führen zu einer

Rechtsverschiebung der O_2-Dissoziationskurve sowie des ihre Lage beschreibenden P_{50}.

Dabei ist der sog. Bohr-Effekt in vivo der bedeutendste, da die H^+-Ionenkonzentration auch die 2,3-DPG-Synthese der Erythrocyten entscheidend beeinflußt (Benesch et al., 1969). Andere organische und anorganische Phosphate spielen nur eine untergeordnete Rolle (Duhm, 1971, Weber et al., 1971). Hormone (Cortisol, Aldosteron etc.) und Medikamente z.B. Dipyridamol (Matthys et al. 1973) beeinflussen z.T. ebenfalls über die oben beschriebenen Mechanismen das O_2-Bindungsvermögen des Hämoglobins (Robert, 1975, Foex, 1975).

Nebst der O_2-Bindungskinetik des Hämoglobins ist der absolute Gehalt an O_2-transportfähigem Hämoglobin für den O_2-Gehalt des Blutes oft allein entscheidend. Vermindertes (Anämie), inaktives (z.B. Meth- und Sulfhämoglobine), abnormes (Hämoglobinopathien) und blockiertes (CO-Hämoglobin) Hämoglobin schränken die körperliche Leistungsfähigkeit bei Patienten mit und ohne Lungenfunktionsstörungen ein. Nebst der O_2-Partialdruckmessung für die Beurteilung der Atemfunktionsstörungen ist daher die direkte O_2-Gehaltsmessung für die Beurteilung der Blutgastransportstörungen stets erforderlich. Wegen der ebenfalls notwendigen Kenntnis der O_2-Aufnahme für die Leistungsfähigkeitsbeurteilung zwingt sich die Messung des Herzzeitvolumens nach "Fick" geradezu auf. Die O_2-Transportfähigkeit des Kreislaufes berechnet sich wie folgt:

$$CaO_2 \times \dot{Q} = CaO_2 \times \dot{V}O_2/(CaO_2 - C\bar{v}O_2) = \dot{V}O_2/(1 - C\bar{v}O_2/CaO_2)$$

O_2-ABGABE ANS GEWEBE

Die O_2-Abgabe aus dem Blut ans Gewebe ist im wesentlichen durch die lokalen Perfusions- und Metabolisationsverhältnisse gegeben. Sie geschieht wie in der Lunge aufgrund der örtlichen Partialdruckdifferenzen. Die Mitochondrien halten ihren Betrieb noch bei einem O_2-Partialdruck von 1 mm Hg aufrecht. Bei einem endkapillären O_2-Partialdruck von 5 - 1O mm Hg arbeitet die Skelettmuskulatur noch aerob (Stainsby und Otis, 1964). Für den Herzmuskel gelten bekanntlich noch tiefere Werte.

Eine linksverschobene O_2-Dissoziationskurve ist nicht nur für den Embryo Fötus und Höhenadaptierten von Vorteil sondern auch für die arbeitende Muskulatur, welche sich ihre O_2-Reserve in Form der linksverschobenen Myoglobin-O_2-Dissoziationskurve hält, die erst bei einem Partialdruck von 40 mm Hg O_2 abgibt. Was dem Myoblogin recht ist sollte dem Hämoglobin des Patienten mit respiratorischer Insuffizienz billig sein (Bürkmann et al. 1971)

Abb. 4. zeigt, daß bei einem endkapillären O_2-Partialdruck von 5 - 10 mm Hg die Lage der O_2-Dissoziationskurve quantitativ für die O_2-Versorgung des Gewebes, eine normale O_2-Abgabekinetik voraussetzt, keine Rolle mehr spielt. Hingegen bringt eine Linksverschiebung der

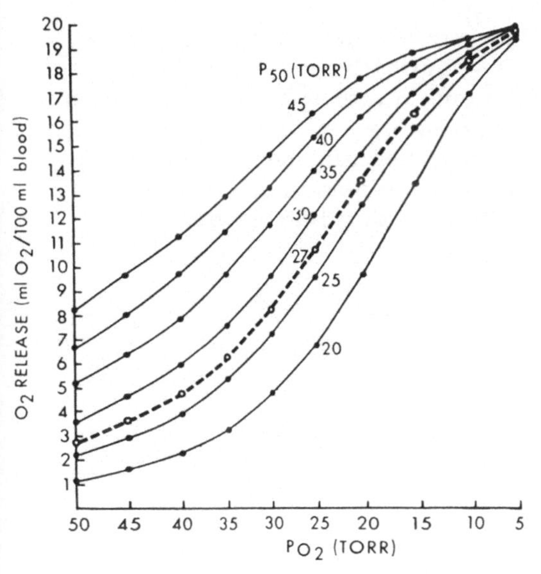

Abb. 4. Änderung der O_2-Abgabekapazität (O_2-release) als Funktion des O_2-Partialdrucks (P_{O2}) und des standardisierten Halbsättigungspartialdrucks (P_{50}), unter Annahme eines Hämoglobingehaltes des Blutes von 15g%, pH = 7,4, 2,3-DPG = 14 nM/gHb, CO_2-Partialdruck = 40 mmHg (Torr), Temperatur = 37°C

O_2-Dissoziationskurve bei Lungenkranken entscheidende Vorteile für die O_2-Transportkapazität des Blutes.

Nun zur Frage, wann ist die tonometrische Funktion der Lunge bei Patienten blutgasbedingt leistungsbegrenzend?

Bei allen Patienten mit einer respiratorischen Globalinsuffizienz ist die Stellgröße Ventilation primär leistungslimitierend. Bei allen Patienten mit einer respiratorischen Partialinsuffizienz ist die Stellgröße Perfusion, wenn auch nicht in allen Fällen, primär leistungslimitierend. Gelingt es durch O_2-Atmung die körperliche Leistungsfähigkeit und damit das O_2-Transportvermögen des Kreislaufs zu steigern, resp. die gleiche körperliche Leistung mit einem geringeren haemodynamischen Aufwand zu vollbringen ist die respiratorische Partialinsuffizienz leistungsbegrenzender Faktor. Wir führen daher bei allen Patienten mit entsprechender Fragestellung die individuell maximale Belastungsstufe im steady state mit gegenüber der Norm erniedrigtem zentralvenösem und arteriellem O_2-Partialdruck ($P_{\bar{v}O2}$, P_{aO2}) auch mit Atmung von 100% O_2 durch. Tabelle 2 zeigt die 3 Möglichkeiten des Verhaltens des zentralvenösen leitungslimitierenden O_2-Partialdrucks bei Vorliegen einer respiratorischen Partialinsuffizienz unter O_2-Atmung. Je größer die körperliche Belastung je repräsentativer wird der zentralvenöse O_2-Partialdruck für die O_2-Versorung der arbeitenden Skelettmuskulatur (Abb. 5). Ändert sich bei gleicher körperlicher Belastung der zentralvenöse O_2-Partialdruck unter O_2-Atmung nicht ($\sim$), so liegt ein rechts-links shunt im Kleinkreislauf vor. Steigt der zentralnervöse O_2-Partialdruck unter O_2-Atmung hingegen wie der arterielle an ($\uparrow$) ohne das Hämaglobin normal zu sättigen ($<$n S_{O2}) so liegt ebenfalls eine leistungslimitierende O_2-Äquilibrationsstörung der Lunge vor. Das Gleiche

Tabelle 2. Die respiratorische Partialinsuffizienz mit einem gegenüber der Norm erniedrigten zentralvenösen O_2-Partialdruck ($P_{\bar{v}O_2}$) macht eine blutgasbedingte Leistungslimitation durch eine ungenügende Äquilibrationsfunktion der Lunge wahrscheinlich. Durch Atmung von 100% O_2 kann die blutgasbedingte Leistungslimitation der Lunge bei gleicher körperlicher Belastung wie unter Luftatmung nachgewiesen respektive ausgeschlossen werden. nS_{O_2} = normale arterielle O_2-Sättigung des Hämoglobins

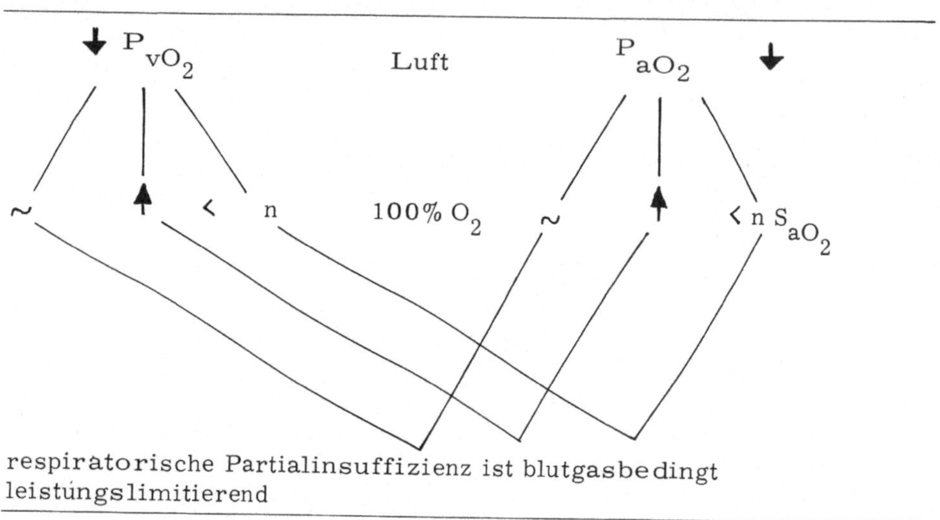

gilt für ein Ansteigen des zentralvenösen- und arteriellen O_2-Partialdrucks unter O_2-Atmung in den Norm-(n) oder Supranormbereich für Luftatmung. In allen anderen Fällen von respiratorischer Partialinsuffizienz mit subnormalem zentralvenösem O_2-Partialdruck ist nicht die Äquilibrationsfunktion der Lunge leistungslimitierend, sondern die O_2-Kapazität des Hämoglobins respektive O_2-Transportkapazität des Kreislaufs ($Q \times C_{aO_2}$), sowie steuerungsbedingte Faktoren im Regelkreis der Atmung. Daher versäumen wir es auch nie die Patienten nach ihren subjektiven leistungslimitierenden Eindrücken wie z.B. Schmerzen, Dyspnoe etc. zu fragen.

Wir sind immer wieder erstaunt, wie selten die arterielle Hypoxie ($P_{aO_2}\downarrow$) mit und ohne Hypoxämie ($C_{aO_2}\downarrow$) bei Patienten leistungslimitierend ist. Im Gegensatz zu Normalpersonen unter exogenen Hypoxiebedingungen, kann bei Patienten in Meereshöhe die körperliche Leistungsfähigkeit durch O_2-Atmung akut selten gesteigert werden.

Atemmechanik, Hämodynamik und verminderte O_2-Kapazität des Hämoglobins führen naturgemäß öfters zu den afferenten Impulsen, welche die körperliche Leistungsfähigkeit von Patienten begrenzen. Bei einer kybernetischen Betrachtungsweise der Atemfunktion ist diese Feststellung auch nicht besonders erstaunlich, sind doch die arteriellen Blutgase R e g e l - g r ö ß e n, welche der Organismus unter allen Bedingungen nach Möglichkeit im Normbereich zu halten versucht.

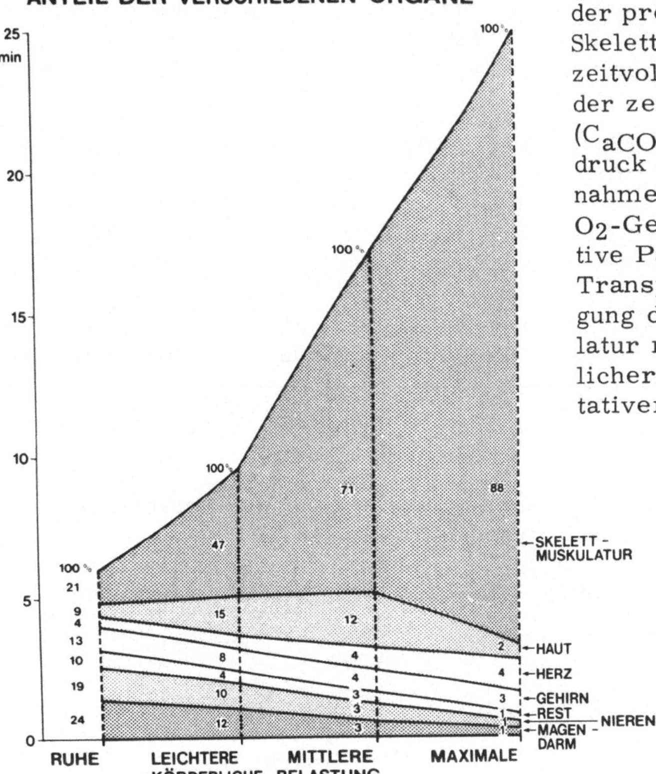

Abb. 5. Mit zunehmender körperlicher Belastung nimmt der prozentuale Anteil der Skelettmuskulatur am Herzzeitvolumen zu. Daher wird der zentralvenöse O_2-Gehalt (C_{aCO2}) respektive Partialdruck bei gegebener O_2-Aufnahme ($\dot{V}_{O2}$) arteriellem O_2-Gehalt (C_{aO_2}) respektive Partialdruck für den O_2-Transport und die O_2-Versorgung der arbeitenden Muskulatur mit steigender körperlicher Belastung repräsentativer

LITERATUR

Astrand, P. O. , Rodahl, K. : Textbook of Work Physiology, New.York: McGraw Hill 1970

Benesch, R. E. , Benesch, R. , Yu, C. I. : The exygenation of hemoglobin in the presence of 2, 3-diphosphoglycerate. Effect of temperature , pH, ionic strenght and hemoglobin concentration. Biochem. 8, 2567 (1969)

Bürkmann, I. , Behn, P. , Herold, B. , Rosenkranz, U. : Zum Verlauf der O_2-Dissoziationskurve bei Gesunden sowie bei Kranken mit angeborenem zyanotischem Herzfehler bzw. chronischem obstruktivem Lungenemphysem. Respiration 28, 36 (1971)

Duhm, J. : Effects of 2, 3 DPG and other organic compunds on oxygen affinity and intracellular pH of human erythrocytes. Pflügers Arch. ges. Physiol. 326, 341 (1971)

Foex, P. : Le rôle de las P_{50} en réanimation. Bull. Physiopath. resp. 11 637 (1975)

Matthys, H. , Rühle, K. H. , Schilling, M. , Freitag, M. , Konietzko, N. ,
Schlehe, H. , Kleeberg, U. : Einfluß von akuter Höhenexposition und
Dipyridamol auf das O_2. Bindungsvermögen des Hömoglobins von
Normalpersonen. Schweiz. med. Wschr. 103, 1288 (1973)
Robert, M. : Affinité de l' hémoglobine pour l' oxygène. Bull. Physiopath.
resp. 11, 79 (1975)

Roughton, F. J. W. : Transport of Oxygen and carbon dioxide. In: Handbook
of Physiology, Sec. 3 Respiration Vol. I p. 767. Washington, D. C. :
American Physiology Society 1964
Stainsby, W. N. , Otis, A. B. : Blood flow, blood oxygen tension, Oxygen
uptake and Oxygen transport in skeletal muscle. Amer. Physiol. 206,
858 (1964)
Weber, R. , Kleeberg, U. , Rühle, K. H. , Matthys, H. : pH-unabhängige
Verschiebungen der O_2-Dissoziationskurve vor und nach Hämodialyse.
Schweiz. med. Wschr. 101, 1795 (1971)

Terminologie

Terms for respiratory clinical physiology and syndromes: Nomenclature
and definitions. Bull. Physiopath. resp. 11, 937 (1975)
Deutsche Übersetzung: Internationale Nomenklatur für die Pathophysiologie
und Klinik der Atmungskrankheiten. Literas Medicinales Thomae 1975

Prof. Dr. med. H. Mattys
Einsteinweg 1
7900 Ulm-Jungingen

Pneumonologie Suppl. 1976, 27-39
© by Springer-Verlag 1976

Der Lungenkreislauf als leistungsbegrenzender Faktor bei Patienten

R. Keller, C. Kopp, W. Zutter, J. Mlczoch und H. Herzog

Abteilung für Atmungskrankheiten des Departmentes für Innere Medizin, Kantonsspital Basel

Pulmonary Circulation as a Limiting Factor in Physical Work Capacity

---

Abstract. The relationship between heart rate and different ergometric work loads is often used as a simple method to estimate systemic and pulmonary cardiovascular function. However in several patients with additional bronchopulmonary diseases the actual physical work capacity may rather be limited by respiratory than cardiogenic factors. Thus right heart catheterization still provides the most accurate evaluation of pulmonary circulation and right heart function. The technique used for catheterization should always enable the measurement of pulmonary "wedge pressure" to separate active from passive forms of hypertension. Furthermore the most important values of pulmonary circulation in normal individuals are presented as a function of age.
The knowledge of the pulmonary hemodynamics is of actual clinical importance in the preoperative evaluation of patients undergoing thoracic surgery. According to previous investigations in a further series it has been demonstrated that patients with normal preoperative function at rest and during moderate exercise also had normal hemodanimics after pneumonectomy; whereas a preexisting pulmonary hypertension as a rule exceeded markedly after operation. An extensive investigation of the pulmonary circulation should include the differentiation into irreversible and reflex-induced, reversible components of a pulmonary hypertension with regard to some important clinical implications.
In fact an obvious limitation of physical work capacity by an impaired pulmonary circulation is merely present in severe pulmonary hypertension with acute or decompensated right heart failure; in contrast to most patients with stable and chronic cor pulmonale which first are limited by an abnormal work of breathing with marked exertional dyspnoe and respiratory insufficiency.

Key words: Pulmonary hypertension - Physical work capacity - Right heart catheterization - Haemodynamics after lung resection

Zusammenfassung. Von den einfacheren Methoden zur Beurteilung des Lungenkreislaufs hat sich unter anderem die Bestimmung der Herzfrequenz unter verschiedenen Belastungsstufen bewährt. Bei Patienten mit Erkrankungen der Atmungsorgane wird indessen die Belastbarkeit nicht selten durch die respiratorische Insuffizienz vorzeitig eingeschränkt, bevor eine kardiovaskuläre Störung am inadäquaten Anstieg der Pulsfrequenz erkennbar wird. Für eine differenzierte Beurteilung des Lungenkreislaufs eignet sich deshalb besser die Untersuchung der Verhältnisse durch den Rechtsherzkatheter in Ruhe und unter einer leichten Belastungsstufe am Ergo meter. Die Meßtechnik sollte unbedingt auch die Bestimmung des pulmonalkapillären Verschlußdruckes ermöglichen, damit die klinisch bedeutsamen Formen der aktiven, passiven und hyperdynamen Hypertension differenziert werden können. Bei der Beurteilung muß ferner die Altersabhängigkeit der Druckwerte beim Gesunden mitberücksichtigt werden.

Von besonderer praktischer Bedeutung ist die Kenntnis der pulmonalen Hämodynamik bei der präoperativen Abklärung von Patienten vor einer thoraxchirurgischen Resektionsbehandlung. Bisher hat sich jedenfalls gezeigt, daß bei präoperativ normaler Hämodynamik in Ruhe und unter leichter Belastung auch nach einer Pneumonektomie keine relevanten Funktionsstörungen auftreten werden; im Gegensatz zu den Patienten mit vorbestehender pulmonaler Hypertonie, wo jede Lungenresektion den Hochdruck erheblich verstärkte. Bei gutachterlichen Fragen empfiehlt sich eine kurzfristige Sauerstoffatmung, um fixierte von funktionellen Widerstandserhöhungen im Lungenkreislauf abgrenzen zu können.

Eine manifeste Beeinträchtigung des täglich geforderten Leistungsvermögens durch eine abnorme Funktion des Lungenkreislaufs ist praktisch nur bei schwerer pulmonaler Hypertonie mit Zeichen der Herzinsuffizienz gegeben. Bei den normalerweise zur Untersuchung gelangenden Patienten wird die physische Aktivität primär meist durch respiratorische Störungen begrenzt, so daß der kardialen Komponente vorwiegend theoretisches Interesse zukommt.

Eine Leistungsbegrenzung durch Veränderungen im Lungenkreislauf ist vor allem bei Patienten mit pulmonaler Hypertonie und abnormer Belastung des rechten Ventrikels zu erwarten. Das Ausmaß der kardialbedingten Leistungsminderung wurde bisher vielfach auf relativ einfache Art anhand der Pulsfrequenz unter verschiedenen Belastungsstufen am Ergometer gemessen. Beim Gesunden ergibt sich dabei eine seit längerem bekannte, praktisch lineare Beziehung zwischen Herzfrequenz und Belastungswert [32], wobei sich für die vergleichende Ergometrie aus praktischen Gründen vor allem die folgenden Stufen bewährt haben (Abb. 1)
1.   Herzfrequenz in Ruhe
2.   Herzfrequenz bei 30% der maximalen Belastungskapazität, welche nach Astrand [2] der physischen Anforderung eines normalen Tagesablaufs entspricht, oder aber mit den eigenen Worten des Autors die Voraussetzung bedeutet "to be able to enjoy life and to be efficient in most jobs".

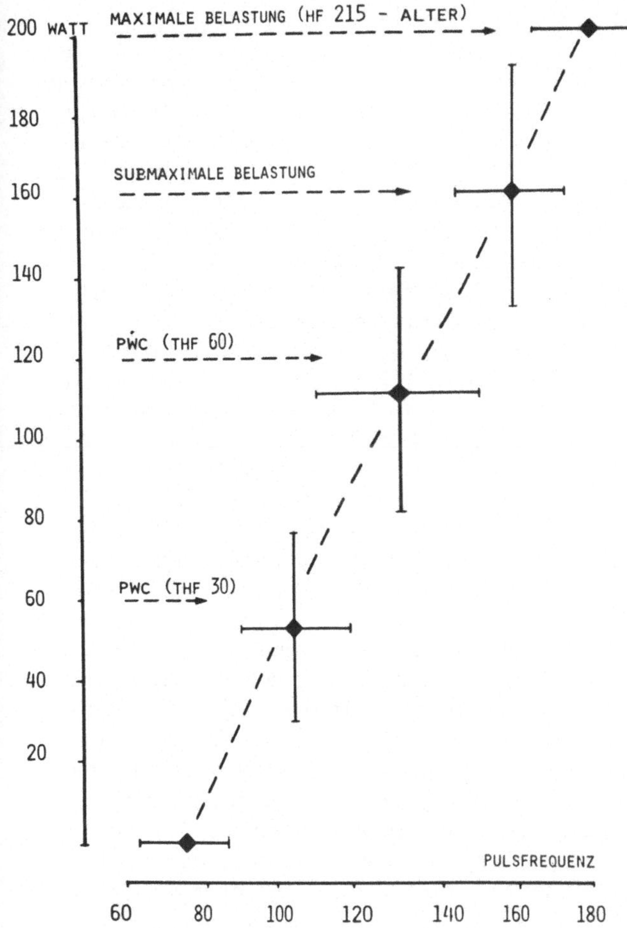

Abb. 1. Lineare Beziehung zwischen Belastung und Pulsfrequenz bei 78 lungen- und kreislaufgesunden Patienten (36 $\pm$ 14 Jahre)

3. Belastungsstufe mit Steigerung der Herzfrequenz um 60% der maximal möglichen Steigerungskapazität, welche auch nach dem Vorschlag der Weltgesundheits-Organisation vielerorts als die "physical work capacity" bei der Rehabilitation des Herzinfarktes bezeichnt wird [8].

4. Herzfrequenz bei 80-90% der maximalen Belastungskapazität entsprechend auch dem Begriff der submaximalen Belastung oder der "physical work capacity" im engeren Sinne [3, 10].

5. Die maximale Belastung schließlich bedeutet das Erreichen der maximalen Sauerstofftransportkapazität mit Übergang zum obligat anaeroben Stoffwechsel, wobei der Belastungswert selbst neben individuellen Schwankungen auch von Alter, Größe und Geschlecht abhängig ist. Die zugehörige Herzfrequenz darf nach übereinstimmenden Angaben aus der bisherigen Literatur durch die Zahl 215 minus das Alter

des Probanden angegeben werden [22, 28, 1] .

Eine gegenüber diesem Nomogramm inadäquat hohe Herzfrequenz deutet in der Regel auf das Vorliegen einer Herzkreislaufstörung hin - allerdings ohne nähere Differenzierung derselben - wobei besonders in den höheren Belastungsstufen die vorerst noch lineare Beziehung der beiden Größen zueinander oftmals verlassen wird [18, 29]. Damit wären zur Ermittlung der effektiven Leistungsminderung mit dieser Methode stets maximale Belastungsversuche notwendig, welche indessen bei herzkranken Patienten eine nicht unerhebliche Gefährdung darstellen, wogegen Patienten mit Erkrankungen der Atmungsorgane höhere Belastungsstufen wegen frühzeitig einsetzender Dyspnoe meist gar nicht erreichen können. Bei niedrigeren Belastungen sind die Abweichungen der Herzfrequenz beim Kranken oftmals zu gering, so daß dadurch keine sichere Beurteilung der Arbeitskapazität möglich ist. Außerdem wird die Herzfrequenz neben relativ breiten individuellen Schwankungen heute nicht selten auch durch medikamentöse Einflüsse wie Digitalis oder Betarezeptorenblocker verfälscht. Auch andere, einfache und wenig invasive Untersuchungsmethoden, welche sich zur Beurteilung des Lungenkreislaufs anbieten, wie beispielsweise das Thoraxröntgenbild, das Elektrokardiogramm, diverse pathologische Auskultationsbefunde am Herzen, etc. [11, 27, 31] sind in der Regel nur für eine summarische , qualitative Beurteilung brauchbar.

Die zuverlässigste Untersuchungsmethode zur Abklärung der Verhältnisse im Lungenkreislauf ist weiterhin die Bestimmung der Hämodynamik mittels Rechtsherzkatheter. Sie ist in den letzten Jahren durch die Einführung sogenannter Einschwemmkatheter wesentlich vereinfacht worden, indem nun gegenüber der konventionellen Technik die Passage durch den Ventrikel erleichtert und für die Untersuchung selbst nicht mehr unbedingt eine kostspielige Durchleuchtungs-Apparatur benötigt wird [15, 21, 30]. Besonders bewährt hat sich hierfür der Swan-Ganz-Katheter, der sich mühelos über einen Führungsschaft in die Cubitalvene einführen läßt, wodurch eine Venae sectio vermieden und gute Venen für allfällige spätere Kontrolluntersuchungen erhalten bleiben. Zur routinemäßigen Untersuchung gehören Messungen der Drücke im rechten Vorhof, im Ventrikel, in der Pulmonalarterie sowie bei geblähtem endständigem Ballon im Lungenkapillargebiet. Das Herzzeitvolumen wird normalerweise nach dem Fick' schen Prinzip ermittelt, da Sauerstoffaufnahme und zentralvenöse Sauerstoffsättigung ohnehin noch für die Berechnung anderer wichtiger Meßgrößen benötigt werden. Die Untersuchung sollte in Ruhe sowie nach Möglichkeit auch unter einer leichten Belastung von 40-60 Watt, entsprechend der oben erwähnten minimalen physical work capacitiy für die Bewältigung eines normalen Tagesablaufs durchgeführt werden. Erst dadurch ergibt sich eine umfassende und befriedigende Beurteilung des Lungenkreislaufs, wo auch die Ursachen einer gestörten Hämodynamik nach dem Gesichtspunkt der verschiedenartigen pathophysiologischen Mechanismen differenziert werden können [4, 6]:

1. Die aktive pulmonale Hypertonie infolge erhöhter Gefäßwiderstände
   im arteriolären, präkapillären Bereich, wie man sie bei primären

Lungengefäßerkrankungen, bei diffusem Lungenparenchymverlust oder aber als reversible funktionelle Vasokonstriktion bei alveolärer Hypoxie und Hypoventilation beobachten kann.

2. Die passive pulmonale Hypertonie als Folge eines erhöhten Druckes im postkapillären Bereich der Lungenvenen, zumeist verursacht durch eine abnorme linksventrikuläre Funktion mit erhöhtem enddiastolischem Füllungsdruck; differentialdiagnostisch sind davon vor allem Mitral-vitien, Vorhofstumoren oder vaskuläre Obstruktionen im Bereich der einmündenden Lungenvenen abzugrenzen.

3. Die hyperdyname pulmonale Hypertonie beruht auf einer übermäßigen Steigerung des Herzzeitvolumens wie man es beispielsweise bei aus-geprägter Anämie, Hyperthyreosen, Links-Rechts-Shunts etc. beob-achten kann. Damit der Pulmonalisdruck allein dadurch in einen pa-thologischen Bereich steigt, muß allerdings das Herzzeitvolumen um mindestens das Dreifache der Norm erhöht sein.

Für diese differenzierte Art der Funktionsdiagnostik ist stets die Kenntnis des pulmonal-kapillären Verschlußdruckes, bzw. des daraus ab-geleiteten linksaurikulären Mitteldruckes unerläßlich, der bei der üblichen Technik der Einschwemmkatheter nach dem Modell von Grandjean [15] in der Regel nicht gemessen werden kann. Man behilft sich bei jener Methode gelegentlich mit der Bestimmung des diastolischen Pulmonalisdruckes, welcher beim Gesunden auch weitgehend dem kapillären Verschlußdruck entspricht. Bei Patienten mit pulmonaler Hypertonie ist die Koinizdenz aller-dings nur bei der passiven Form vorhanden [5, 26], wogegen bei aktiver Hypertonie sowohl in Ruhe wie unter Belastung derart große Diskrepanzen auftreten, daß eine zuverlässige Beurteilung der linksventrikulären Funk-tion aufgrund des diastolischen Pulmonalisdruckes illusorisch ist (Abb. 2).

Schließlich ist für die Beurteilung der Hämodynamik im Lungenkreislauf auch die Kenntnis der Normalwerte beim Gesunden erforderlich. Seit längerem ist eine gewisse Altersabhängigkeit verschiedener Druckwerte bekannt [16] eine Beobachtung, welche auch bei unseren eigenen Unter-suchungen an einem größeren Kollektiv klinisch herz- und lungengesunder Probanden sowohl in Ruhe wie besonders ausgeprägt unter Belastung be-stätigt werden konnte (Tabelle 1). Überhaupt wird vielerorts dem Arbeits-versuch zur Beurteilung der Hämodynamik noch zu wenig Bedeutung bei-gemessen. Zwar besteht statistisch eine eindeutige Korrelation zwischen dem Pulmoalarteriendruck in Ruhe und demjenigen unter Belastung (vgl. Abb. 3); individuell finden sich indessen recht erhebliche Diskrepanzen, welche besonders bei der erheblichen Zahl latenter Hypertonien augen-fällig sind. Bei der Bewertung der pulmonalen Hypertonie sollte dem Be-lastungswert deshalb selektivere Bedeutung beigemessen werden. Noch bes-ser diskriminierend wären zweifellos mehrere Belastungsstufen bis zur Be-stimmung der maximalen oder submaximalen Belastbarkeit. Erneut muß auch hier die Gefährdung des Patienten sowie die zeitliche Belastung des Untersuchers berücksichtigt werden, so daß man sich in der Regel mit den Messungen in Ruhe und unter einer mittleren Belastungsstufe begnügen wird.

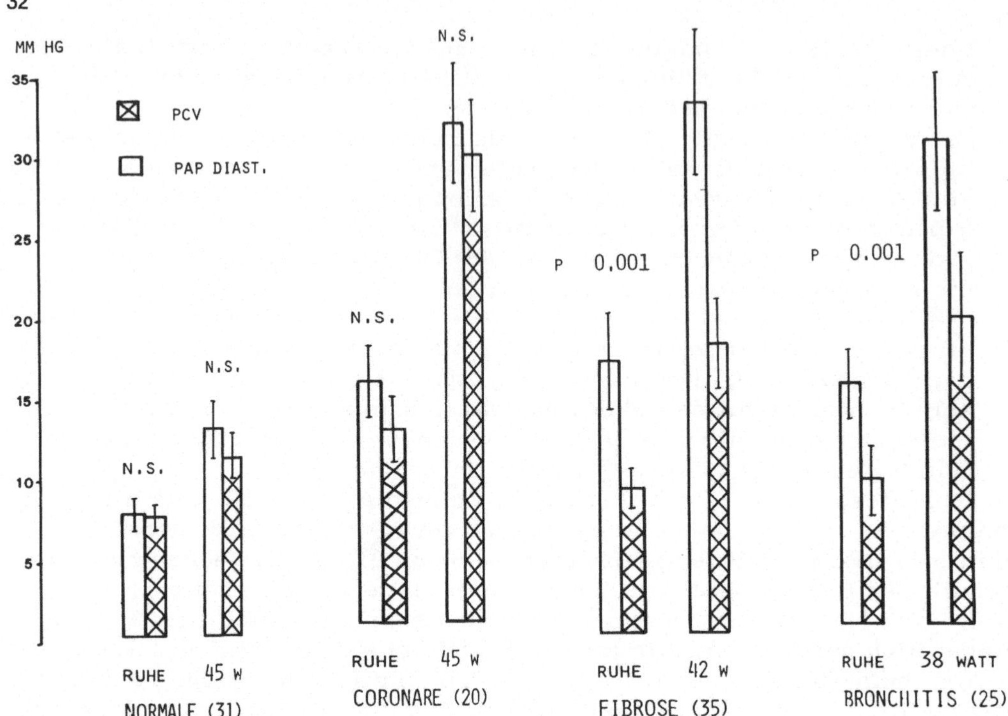

Abb. 2. Vergleich zwischen diastolischem Pulmonalarteriendruck und kapillärem Verschlußdruck in Ruhe und unter Belastung bei Gesunden, und bei Patienten mit pulmonaler Hypertonie. Vergleichbare Meßwerte finden sich nur bei den gesunden Probanden sowie bei den Patienten mit passiver pulmonaler Hypertonie (z. B. koronare Herzkrankheit)

Eine offenkundige und praktische Bedeutung hat die Untersuchung der Hämodynamik bei der Abklärung der Operabilität von Lungenresektionen, um zu verhindern, daß postoperativ ein unmittelbar bedrohliches oder später sukzessive invalidisierendes Cor pulmonale resultiert [12, 19, 23, 33]. Bei der Frage nach dem Ausmaß der noch zulässigen Resektionsbehandlung sind vor allem die postoperativen Druckströmungsbeziehungen im Lungenkreislauf zu berücksichtigen, wie sie im Modellversuch am Tier als auch beim Menschen von Brofman und Mitarb. [7] sowie von Epstein und Mitarb. [13] ausführlich untersucht wurden (Abb. 4). Daraus ist ersichtlich, daß vorgängig normaler Hämodynamik eine Erhöhung des Herzzeitvolumens um das Doppelte, entsprechend einer Pneumonketomie mit Reduktion der Lungengefäßbahn um die Hälfte nur eine Steigerung des Pulmo-

Tabelle 1. Mittelwerte und Standardabweichung hämodynamischer Messungen im Lungenkreislauf in Ruhe und unter leichter Belastung bei 127 klinisch lungen- und kreislaufgesunden Probanden, nach Altersklassen getrennt (Drücke in mmHg)

Alter / Anzahl	26± 3 N = 43		34 ± 3 N = 24		44 ± 3 N = 31		53 ± 2 N = 13		64 ± 3 N = 16	
Belastung	0	47 ±6	0	43 ±7	0	47 ±6	0	46 ±5	47 0	47 ±6
re Vorhof (RAP mittel)	2.4 ± 2.1	2.6 ±2.4	2.8 ± 2.1	2.8 ±2.5	2.8 ± 1.6	3.0 ±2.0	3.0 ± 1.7	4.3 ±3.0	4.0 ± 2.1	7.3 ± 4.2
Pulmonalis (PAP mittel)	12.0 ± 3.0	17.5 ±4.5	12.7 ± 2.7	19.8 ±4.2	13.0 ± 3.0	20.3 ±4.6	13.3 ± 3.2	24.3 ±5.5	16.4 ± 3.1	32.8 ± 8.9
Kap. Verschluß (PCV mittel)	7.4 ± 2.4	9.9 ±4.1	7.1 ± 2.2	10.3 ±3.4	6.9 ± 1.9	11.0 ±2.9	6.1 ± 3.0	12.3 ±4.4	8.6 ± 2.2	18.1 ± 7.2
Kard. Index (CI) L/min/m^2	4.6 ± 1.5	6.9 ±2.1	4.5 ± 1.5	7.0 ±1.9	4.5 ± 1.5	7.0 ±3.0	3.8 ± 1.0	6.0 ±1.5	3.6 ± 0.7	6.1 ± 1.3
praekap. Gefäßwiderstand (PVR) mmHg/L/min	0.7 ± 0.3	0.7 ±0.2	0.8 ± 0.4	0.8 ±0.4	0.9 ± 0.4	0.8 ±0.4	1.1 ± 0.4	1.1 ±0.4	1.3 ± 0.4	1.4 ± 0.5

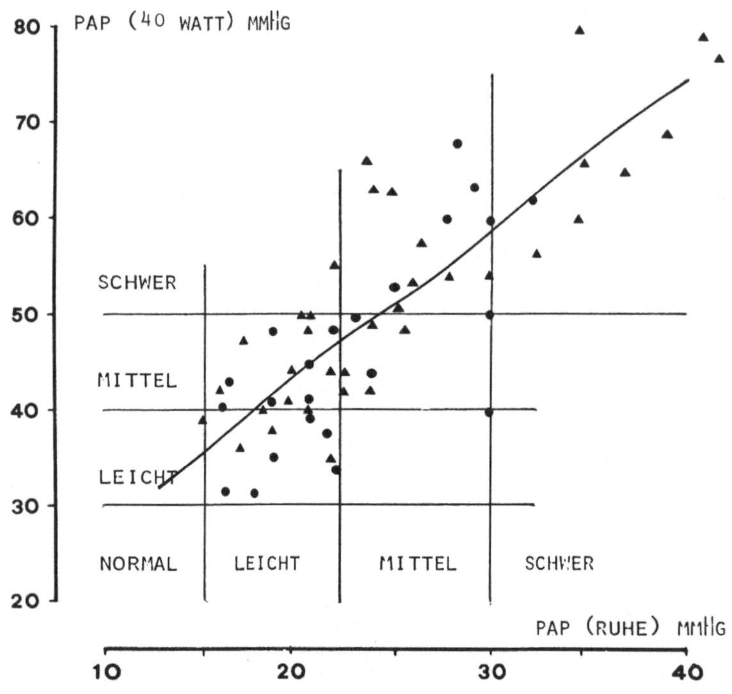

Abb. 3. Beziehung des mittl. Pulmonal-Arteriendruckes in Ruhe und bei Belastung bei 60 Patienten mit chronischem Cor pulmonaris

nalisdruckes um 20-50% zur Folge hätte; anders bei einem Patientenkollektiv mit Lungenfibrose und chronischem Cor pulmonale, wo der Druck theoretisch auf über 300% des Ausgangswertes ansteigen müßte. Klinische und experimentelle hämodynamische Untersuchung vor und nach Lungenresektion [19, 20] bestätigen diese theoretischen Überlegungen. Auch unsere eigenen postoperativen Kontrollen etwa 12 Monate nach erfolgter Pneumonektomie belegen, daß bei präoperativ normaler Hämodynamik auch postoperativ normale Verhältnisse vorliegen werden, wogegen bei abnormen präoperativen Funktionen postoperativ eine erhebliche pulmonale Belastungshypertonie zu erwarten ist (Abb. 5). Vor einer ausgedehnten Lungenresektion sollte deshalb grundsätzlich eine normale Hämodynamik im Lungenkreislauf mit normalem Pulmonalisdruck und normalem Gefäßwiderstand auch unter Belastung gefordert werden. In Zweifelsfällen kann die Untersuchung während unilateraler Pulmonalis-Okklusion der zu operierenden Seite mittels eines speziellen Ballon-Katheters [12] zur Simulierung der postoperativen Verhältnisse erforderlich sein.

Eine weitere praktische Bedeutung hat die Beurteilung der Hämodynamik bei Lungenkrankheiten mit potentiell reversibler, reflektorisch bedingter

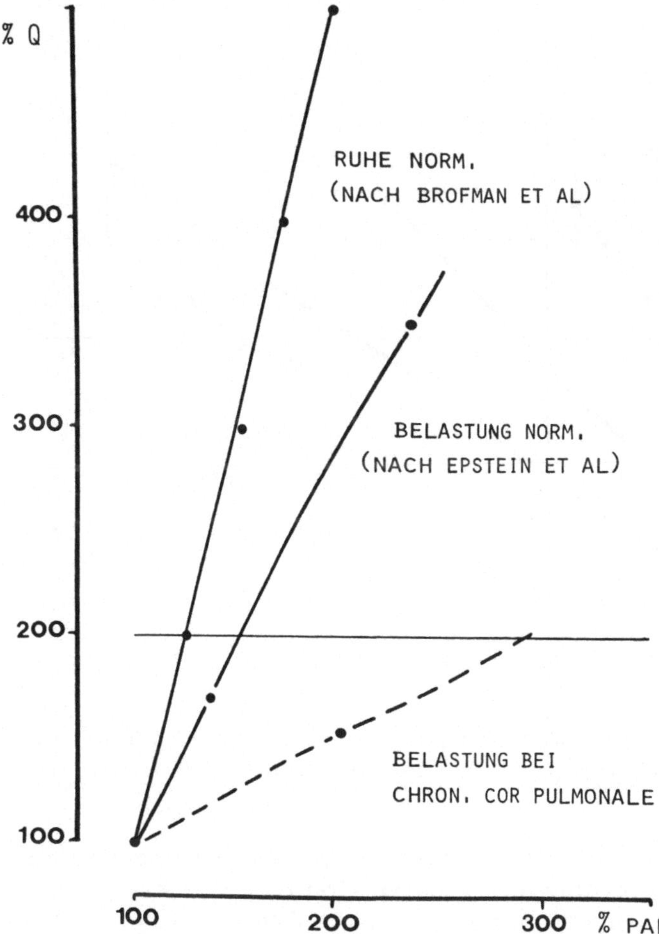

Abb. 4. Die Druck-Strömungs-Relation im Lungenkreislauf

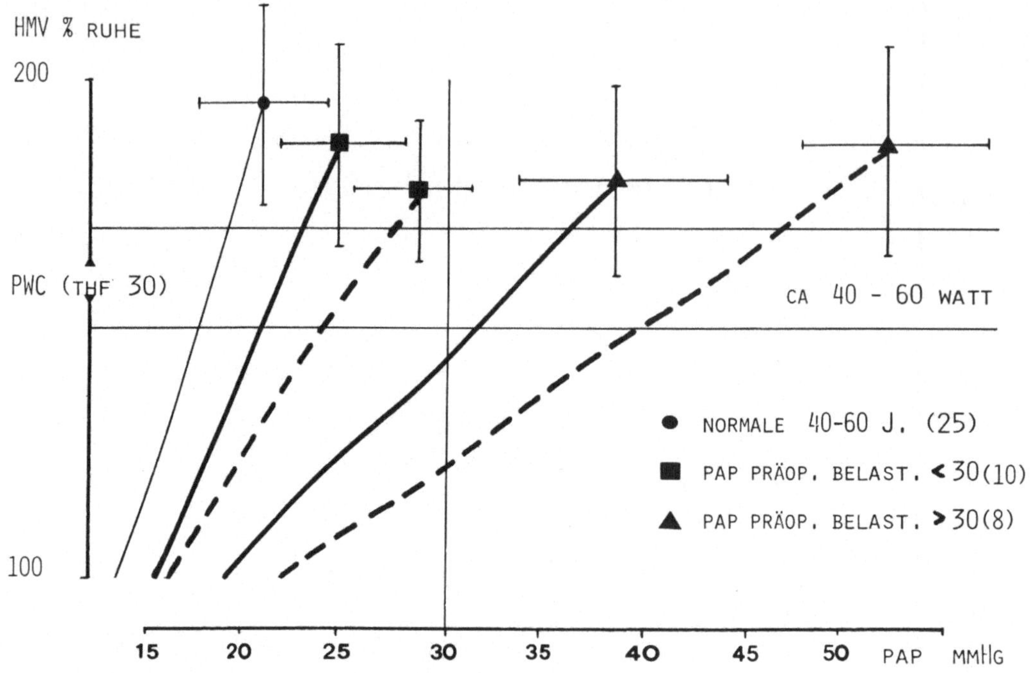

Abb. 5. Druck-Strömungsrelation im Lungenkreislauf beim Gesunden und bei Patienten vor (—) und nach (----) Pneumonektomie

pulmonaler Hypertonie erlangt. Die durch alveoläre Hypoxie und Minderbelüftung verursachte arterioläre Vasokonstriktion im Lungenkreislauf kann durch Erhöhen der inspiratorischen Sauerstoffkonzentration beseitigt werden, ein Effekt, wie er erstmals von Euler und Liljestrand [14] beschrieben und später in verschiedenartigen Versuchsanordnungen reproduziert und bestätigt werden konnte [9, 17, 24, 25]. Auch die von uns untersuchten Patienten mit chronischer global-respiratorischer Insuffizienz ließen einen signifikanten Abfall des Pulmonalisdruckes unter reiner Sauerstoffatmung erkennen (Abb. 6). In einigen Fällen handelte es sich allerdings nicht nur um eine Abnahme des präkapillären Gefäßwiderstandes, sondern um einen gleichzeitigen Abfall auch des kapillären Verschlußdruckes. Möglicherweise handelte es sich hierbei um die Folge einer verbesserten Myokardfunktion mit Rückbildung des enddiastolischen Füllungsdruckes durch die verbesserte Oxygenation des coronaren Blutes. Besonders in gutachterlichen Fragen dürfte der Anteil der potentiell reversiblen Funktionsstörung am Ausmaß der pulmonalen Hypertonie von erheblichem Interesse sein, um definitive von behandlungfähigen Schädigungen abgrenzen zu können.

   Eine objektive Leistungsbegrenzung durch pathologische Veränderungen im Lungenkreislauf liegt grundsätzlich nur dann vor, wenn entweder bereits in Ruhe oder aber im Bereiche einer submaximal liegenden Be-

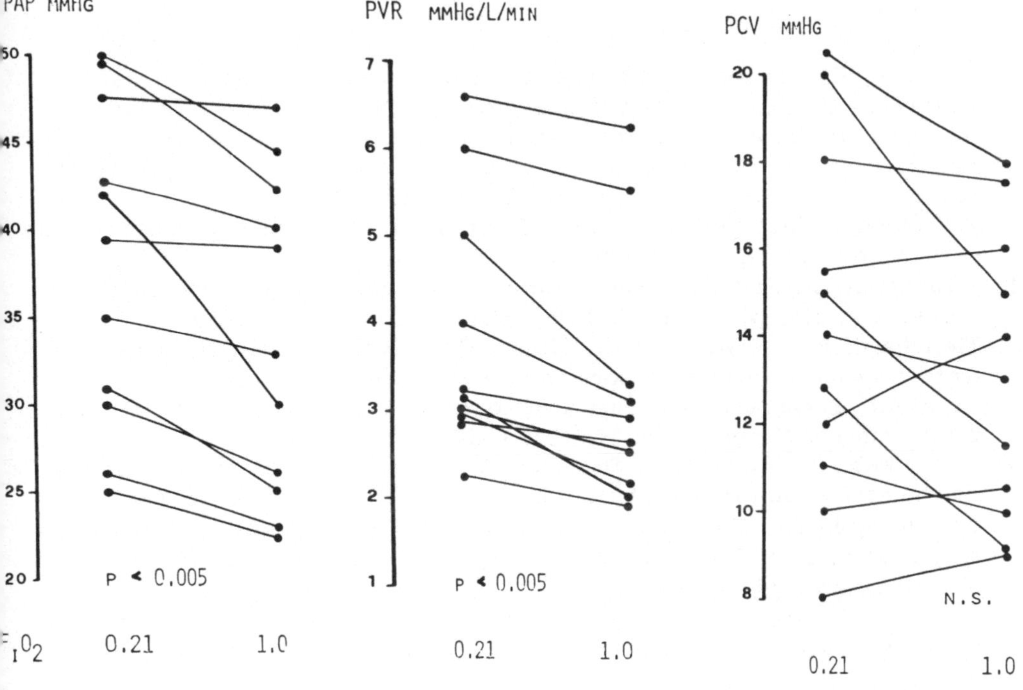

Abb. 6. Einfluß einer reinen Sauerstoffatmung auf die Hämodynamik bei Patienten mit global-respiratorischer Insuffizienz: Signifikante Abnahme des mittleren Pulmonalarteriendruckes und des präkapillären Gefäßwiderstandes; unterschiedliches nicht gerichtetes Verhalten des kapillären Verschluß-druckes (siehe auch Text)

lastungsstufe eine nach Braunwald definierte Herzinsuffizienz [6] mit unge-nügender Sauerstofftransportkapazität nachweisbar wird. Bei den üblicher-weise zur hämodynamischen Abklärung vorgesehenen Patienten tritt diese Situation in der Regel erst bei hohen Belastungstufen auf, welche aus den oben bereits mehrfach erwähnten Gründen in der routinemäßigen Abklärung nicht zu empfehlen sind. Mit Ausnahme von akuten, intensiv pflegebedürf-tigen Patienten im kardiogenen Schock wegen. akutem oder dekompensiertem Cor pulmonale ist die Leistungsbegrenzung durch Veränderungen im Lungen-kreislauf bis zu einer mittleren Belastungsstufe eine Seltenheit. Anderseits bedeutet der Nachweis einer fixierten und chronischen pulmonalen Hypertonie bei einem Patienten die unweigerliche Entwicklung in ein chronisches Cor pulmonale, so daß aus präventiv-medizinischen Aspekten die verlangte Arbeitskapazität dieser Patienten eingeschränkt werden sollte.

LITERATUR

1. Astrand, I.: Aerobic work capacity in men and women with special
   reference to age. Acta physiol. Scand. 49 (Suppl. 169) 11, (1960)
2. Astrand, P.O.: Methods for measurements of physical fitness in population studies in Malmborg. In: Coranary heart disease and physical
   fitnes, p. 193-198. Copenhagen: Munksgaard 1971
3. Benestad, A.M.: Determination of physical work capacity and exercise
   tolerance in cardiac patients. Acta med. Scand. 183, 521 (1968)
4. Bluont, S.G., Grover, R.F.: Pulmonary hypertension. In: The Heart,
   Hurst E.J. Ed. p. 1248-1264 New York: McGraw Hill 1974
5. Bouchard, R.J., Gault, J.H., Ross, J.: Evaluation of pulmonary
   arterial enddiastolic pressure as an estimate of left ventricular enddiastolic pressure in patients with normal and abnormal left ventricular
   performance. Circulation 44, 1072 (1971)
6. Braunwald, E, Ross, J., Sonnenblick, E.H.: Mechanisms of contraction
   of the normal and failing heart. Boston: Little, Brown & Co 1968
7. Brofman, B.L., Charms, B.L., Kohn, P.M., Elder, J., Newman,
   R., Rizika, M.: Unilateral pulmonary artery occlusion in man. J.
   Thorac. Surg. 34, 2o6 (1957)
8. Bruce, R.A., Hornstein, T.R.: Exercise stress testing in evaluation
   of patients with ischaemic heart disease. Progr. cardivasc. Dis. 11,
   371 (1969)
9. Bühlmann, A., Schaub, F., Luchsinger P.: Die Hämodynamik des
   Lungenkreislaufs während Ruhe und körperlicher Arbeit beim Gesunden
   und bei den verschiedenen Formen der pulmonalen Hypertonie. Schweiz.
   med. Wschr. 85, 253 (1955)
10. Bühlmann, A., Gattiker, H.: Herzzeitvolumen, Schlagvolumen und
    physische Arbeitskapazität. Schweiz. med. Wschr. 94, 443 (1964)
11. Burckhardt, D.: Diagnostik des chronischen Cor pulmonale.
    Eern/Stuttart: Hans Huber 1971
12. Daum, S., Herzog, H., Goerg, R., Spillmann, B., Burckhardt, D.:
    Beurteilung der Lungenoperabilität vom Standpunkt der Hämodynamik
    im kleinen Kreislauf. Pneumologie 144, 266 (1971)
13. Epstein, S.E., Beiser, G.D., Stampfer, M., Robinson, B.F.,
    Braunwald, E.: Characterization of the circulatory response to
    maximal upright exercise in normal subjects and patients with heart
    disease. Circulation 35, 1049 (1967)
14. Euler von, U.S., Liljestrand G.: Observations on the pulmonary
    arterial blood pressure in the cat. Acta physiol. Scand. 12, 301 (1946)
15. Grandjean, T.: Une microtechnique du cathétérisme cardiaque droit
    practicable au lit du malade sans contrôle radioscopique. Cardiologia
    (Basel) 51, 184 (1967)
16. Granath, A., Jonsson, B., Strandell, T.: Circulation in healthy old
    men studied by right heart catheterization at rest and during exercise
    in supine and sitting position. Acta med. Scand. 176, 425 (1964)
17. Harvey, R.M., Enson, Y., Ferrer, I.: A reconsideration of the origins
    of pulmonary hypertension. Chest 59, 82 (1971)

18. Hofman, H., Golling, F.R., Meier, E., Günthner, W.: Ergometrische Diagnostik des beginnenden Cor pulmonale bei obstruktiver Lungenerkrankung. Med. Klin. 65, 1784 (1970)

19. Jezek, V.: Pulmonary haemodynamics in bronchogenic cancer before and after lung resection. Progr. Resp. Res. 5, 237 (1970)

20. Kammler, E., Gude, A.W., Engineer, S., Ulmer, W.T., Weller, W.: Über den Einfluß lungenverkleinernder Operationen auf den Gasaustausch, die Hämodynamik des kleinen Kreislaufs und die Atemmechanik. Respiration 29, 289 (1972)

21. Klempt, H.W., Bachour, G., Most, E., Bender, F.: Druckmessung im kleinen Kreislauf mit Ballon-Einschwemmkatheter. Med. Klin. 68, 585 (1973)

22. König, K., Messin, R.: Methods of evaluating the physical work activity. Acta cardiol (Suppl.) 14, 30 (1970)

23. Mlczoch, J., Zutter, W., Keller, R., Herzog, H.: Influence of lung resection on pulmonary circulation and lung function at rest and on exercise. Respiration 32, 424 (1975)

24. Motley, H.J., Cournand, A., Werkö, L., Himmelstein, A., Dresdale, D.: Influence of short periods of induced anoxia upon pulmonary pressure in man. Amer. J. Physiol. 105, 315 (1947)

25. Reichel, G., Weller, W., Reif, E.: Der Einfluss der alveolären Hypoventilation auf den Kreislauf und das Herz. Med. Thorac. 23, 197 (1966)

26. Saubermann, A., Burkart, F.: Der diastolische Pulmonalisdruck zur Beurteilung des linksaurikulären Mitteldruckes. Schweiz. med. Wschr. 101, 599 (1971)

27. Schüren, K.P., Hüttemann, U.: Effect of respiratory and haemodynamic abnormalities on the electrocardiogram in chronic obstructive lung disease. Respiration 30, 234 (1973)

28. Schweizer, W., Burkart, F., Glaus, L., Nissen, C., Widmer, L.: The Basle longitudinal study. Scand. J. clin. lab. Invest. (inpress)

29. Spiro, S.G., Hahn, H.L., Edwards, R.H.T., Pride, N.B.: An analysis of the physiological strain of submaximal exercise in patients with chronic obstructive bronchitis. Thorax 30, 415 (1975)

30. Swan, H.J.C., Ganz, W., Forrester, J., Marcus, H., Diamond, G., Chonette, D.: Catheterization of the heart in man with use of a flow-directed ballon-tipped catheter. New Eng. J. Med. 283, 447 (1970)

31. Tandon, M.K.: Correlations of electrocardiographic features with airway obstruction in chronic bronchitis. Chest 63, 146 (1973)

32. Taylor, H.L., Wang, Y., Rowell, L., Blomquist, G.: The standardization and interpretation of submaximal and maximal tests of working capacity. Pediatrics 32, 703 (1963)

33. Widimsky, J., Stanek, V., Hurych, J.: Die Lungenzirkulation während der Arbeit bei den Patienten nach der Pneumonektomie. Beitr. Klin. Tuberk. 141, 109 (1968)

Priv. Doz. Dr. med. R. Keller
Kantonsspital
CH-5000 Aarau

Pneumonologie Suppl. 1976, 41-60

Leistungsbegrenzung durch Störungen der Atemmechanik

M. Beil

Institut für Lungenfunktionsforschung, Bochum, in Verbindung mit der
Westfälischen Wilhelms-Universität, Münster
(Chefarzt: Professor Dr. W. T. Ulmer)

Altered Mechanics of Breathing Responsible for Exercise Limitation

Abstract. Altered mechanics of breathing can limit exercise by: The
expiratory flow limitation mechanism, the intrinsic airway resistance
and/or the static behaviour of the lung and the chest wall. The adaptation
of these parameters to exercise was studied in 11 patients with chronic
obstructive lung disease and in 6 normal persons for control.
1. At rest, 7 patients (B-group) showed a high intrinsic resistance during
   spontaneous breathing and during a slow vital-capacity (VC) maneuver
   with a pronounced inverse dependence from the actual lung volume, a
   low VC, and a normal or a little reduced lung elasticity. 4 patients
   (E-group) had during spontaneous breathing none or only a little increase of
   the intrinsic resistance and during a slow VC maneuver a less pronounced
   dependence of this resistance from the lung volume, a only little reduction
   of VC, and a marked decrease of the lung elasticity.
2. All patients (B-group < E-group) had a marked decrease of the critical
   dynamic pleura-pressures (P_{max}) in the isovolume-pressure-flow-
   diagram and therefore a premature limitation of the maximal expiratory
   flow ($\dot{V}_{max}$) by an increase of airway compressibility.
3. During exercise (200 watts) the normal persons did not reach P_{max} and
   $\dot{V}_{max}$ of the ventilated lung volume. During exercise (50 or 100 watts)
   7 B-patients and 2 E-patients exceeded P_{max} and 7 B-patients and
   3 E-patients reached V_{max}.
4. During exercise the B-group presented an increased mean expiratory
   airway resistance by means of the high ineffective pressures developed
   after flow limitation had occured. This was not so marked in the E-group.
5. During exercise the end-expiratory lung volume increased (B-group
   < E-group) as partial compensation of both of the lung volume related
   premature flow limitation and increased intrinsic resistance. This mechanism of compensation is limited by the amount of the VC and/or the static forces of the lung and chest wall.
6. The adaptation to exercise requires a less respiratory power, when
   P_{max} is higher, VC is larger, the lung and chest wall elasticity is
   lower and/or the intrinsic obstruction is smaller, than when the inverse
   is the case.

K e y   w o r d s : Mechanics of breathing - Exercise limitation - Flow
limitation - Chronic obstructive lung disease

Z u s a m m e n f a s s u n g . Für die Leistungsbegrenzung bei Störungen der
Atemtechnik sind der Limitierungsmechanismus des exspiratorischen
Flows, der endobronchiale Strömungswiderstand und/oder die statische
Lungen-/Thoraxwandcharakteristik von Bedeutung. Die Adaptation dieser Parameter an die Bedingungen der Belastungsventilation wurde bei
11 Patienten mit chronisch obstruktiver Lungenerkrankung im Vergleich
zu 6 Normalpersonen untersucht.

1. In Ruhe hatten 7 Patienten (B-Gruppe) bei Spontanatmung und langsamer
   Atmung der Vitalkapazität (VC) eine hohe endobronchiale Resistance mit
   ausgeprägter inverser Abhängigkeit vom aktuellen Lungenvolumen, eine
   stark erniedrigte VC und eine leichte oder fehlende Verminderung der
   Lungenelastizität. 4 Patienten (E-Gruppe) zeigten bei Spontanatmung
   keine oder nur eine leicht erhöhte endobronchiale Resistance, bei langsamer Atmung der VC eine weniger ausgeprägte Abhängigkeit der
   Resistance vom aktuellen Lungenvolumen, eine leicht erniedrigte VC
   und eine stark verminderte Lungenelastizität.
2. Im Isovolume-Pressure-Flow-Diagramm hatten alle Patienten (B-Grup-
   pe< E-Gruppe) bei zunehmender Forcierung der Ausatmung eine deutliche Erniedrigung der kritischen dynamischen Pleuradrucke (P_{max})
   und damit eine vorzeitige Limitierung des maximalen exspiratorischen
   Flows (V_{max}) durch erhöhte Atemwegskompressibilität.
3. Unter einer 200-Watt-Belastung wurde bei keiner Normalperson im
   Bereich des ventilierten Lungenvolumens während der Exspiration
   P_{max} oder $\dot{V}_{max}$ erreicht. Unter einer 50- oder 100-Watt-Belastung
   überschritten alle 7 B- und 2 E-Patienten P_{max}. Der exspiratorische
   $\dot{V}_{max}$ wurde bei allen 7 B- und bei 3- E-Patienten erreicht.
4. Der exspiratorische Bronchialwiderstand stieg, vorwiegend zu Lasten
   eines überschießenden Druckaufbau, nach erfolgter Flow Limitierung
   unter Belastung im Mittel bei der B-Gruppe deutlich stärker an als
   bei der E-Gruppe.
5. Im Sinne einer Teilkompensation der jeweils volumenabhängigen vor-
   zeitigen Flow Limitierung und endobronchialen Resistanceerhöhung
   resultierte unter Belastung bei den Patienten (B-Gruppe< E-Gruppe)
   eine Verschiebung des endexspiratorischen Volumenniveaus zur Inspiration. Dieser Kompensationsmechanismus wird durch die Größe
   der VC und/oder die statische Retraktion der Lunge und des Thorax begrenzt.
6. Die atemmechanische Adaptation an eine Belastung erfordert eine
   kleinere Atemleistung, wenn P_{max} höher, die VC größer, die Lungen/
   Thoraxelastizität niedriger und/oder die endobronchiale Obstruktion
   geringer ausfällt als bei umgekehrter Konstellation.

)ie Fähigkeit des Organismus, körperliche, d.h. im engeren Sinne muskuläre
Leistungen zu erbringen, wird unter physiologischen Bedingungen nicht
durch Faktoren der Atemmechanik und der ihren Gesetzen folgenden Venti-
ation begrenzt. Die schon bei submaximaler Belastung im Vergleich zur
O_2-Aufnahme vorhandene relative Hyperventilation und die nach Erreichen
der aeroben Leistungsgrenze, also mit Plateaubildung der Sauerstoffaufnahme
noch mögliche Ventilationssteigerung, zeigen, daß die Ventilationsreserven
im sogenannten "breaking point" nicht erschöpft sind (Asmussen, 1964;
Ouellet et al., 1969). Ein Gesunder nutzt in Abhängigkeit vom Trainingszustand in der Regel nicht mehr als 70% der maximalen willkürlichen Ventilation (Cotes, 1968), wobei der Atemgrenzwert unter Belastung eher noch
höher anzusetzen ist als in Ruhe (Ouellet et al., 1969).

Eine theoretische Grenze der Ventilationskapazität, die erreicht wird,
wenn der Zuwachs des Sauerstoffbedarfs der Atemmuskulatur die Änderung
der Sauerstoffaufnahme durch Steigerung der Ventilation übersteigt, spielt
bei Normalpersonen keine Rolle für die Begrenzung ihrer körperlichen Leistungsbreite (Riley, 1960; Otis, 1964; Jonson, 1971).

Abgesehen vom globalen Umfang der Ventilationsreserven zeigen die
einzelnen Teilgrößen der Atemmechanik einen unterschiedlichen Spielraum
ihrer Anpassungsfähigkeit für die Herausforderungen der Belastungsventilation. Auch wenn die physiologischen Grenzen beim Gesunden unter Belastung nicht erreicht werden, so können sie doch bei bestimmten Atemmanövern oder im Rahmen des Hustenmechanismus in Erscheinung treten.
Die Adaptation der atemmechanischen Einzelgrößen und ihrer Wechselbeziehungen an die Bedingungen der Belastungsatmung läßt beim Gesunden
mit Einschränkung eine Tendenz zur Optimierung des Energieumsatzes
bzw. zur Minimalisierung der Atemarbeit erkennen. Das gilt namentlich
für die Regulation der Atemmittellage (Cotes, 1968; Yamashiro, et al.,
1975), der Atemfrequenz (Otis, 1954; Mead, 1960; Yamashiro et al.,
1975), der Atemzeitquotienten (Yamashiro et al., 1975) des Bronchialmuskeltonus (Widdicombe und Nadel, 1963) und des Alveolarraum-/Tot-
raumverhältnisses (Widdicombe und Nadel, 1963; Yamashiro et al., 1975).

Das schwächste Glied im dynamischen, atemmechanischen System mit
dem geringsten Adaptationsspielraum ist der exspiratorische Flow. Wie
sich an Hand von Isovolume-Pressure-Flow-Diagrammen (IVPF) zeigen
läßt (Abb. 1), erreicht bei forcierter Ausatmung der Flow im unteren und
mittleren Bereich der Vitalkapazität (VC) (bis ca. 70%) mit Zunahme des
transpulmonalen Druckes, also mit Zunahme der Muskelanstrengung, für
jedes Lungenvolumen unter Abflachung des Flow-Anstieges ein Maximum.
Trotz weiterer Drucksteigerung resultiert kein weiterer Flow-Anstieg,
sondern ein hier etwas idealisiertes Flow-Plateau. Der kritische Flow,
d.h. der Flow des Plateaus, wird bei kleinem Lungenvolumen durch einen
kleineren kritischen Druck (P_{max}) hervorgerufen als bei einem größeren
Lungenvolumen. Das zugehörige maximale exspiratorische Flow-Volume-
Diagramm (MEFV) beschreibt über den entsprechenden Bereich der VC
den Verlauf des anstrengungsunabhängigen kritischen Flows.

Ohne hier auf spezielle Modellvorstellungen von Fry (1958), Fry und
Hyatt (1960), Mead et al. (1967) ("Equal-pressure-point"-Konzept) oder
Pride et al. (1967) ("Starling-Resistor"-Konzept) im einzelnen einzugehen,

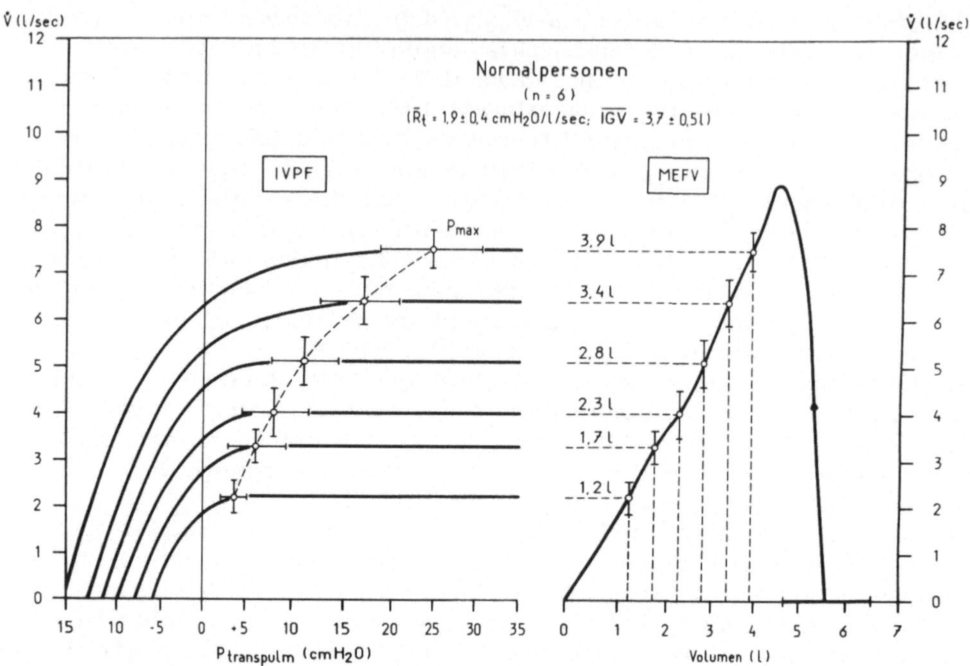

Abb. 1. Mittleres Isovolume-Pressure-Flow-Diagramm (IVPF) für 1, 2 bis 3, 9 l Lungenvolumen (= 20 - 70% VC) und mittleres Maximal-Expiratory-Flow-Diagramm (MEFV) bei 6 Normalpersonen. -Ordinate: Flow ($\dot{V}$), Abszisse: Transpulmonaldruck Ptranspulm) bzw. Volumen. P_{max}: Mittlerer Transpulmonaldruck, bei dem Flow-Limitierung erfolgt.

kann festgestellt werden, daß die Flow-Limitierung bei forcierter Exspiration durch eine dynamische Kompression intrathorakaler Luftwege zustandekommt. Für Lokalisation, Ausdehnung und Querschnittsänderung des dynamisch komprimierten, flow-limitierenden Segments sind neben den bereits erwähnten Faktoren - Pleuradruck und Lungenvolumen - die elastische Lungenretraktion, der intrinsic Bronchialwiderstand im distal anschließenden Segment (sog. Upstream-Segment) und die Bronchial- bzw. Trachealwand-compliance potentiell von Bedeutung (Macklem und Wilson, 1965; Macklem et al., 1965; Macklem und Mead, 1967; Mead et al., 1967; Pride et al., 1967; Bouhuys, 1974; Jones et al., 1975). Die Bronchialwandcompliance zeigt wiederum Abhängigkeiten vom anatomischen Wandaufbau, also z.B. vom Knorpelbesatz, vom Bronchialmuskeltonus, von der Lungenelastizität einschließlich ihrer regionalen Unterschiede, von Oberflächenkräften im Bereich des Bronchialepithels und von eventuellen Wandläsionen.

Da die Verteilung der verschiedenen Einflußgrößen inhomogen ist und da z. T. physikalische, z. T. nervale Wechselbeziehungen bestehen, ist der reale Ablauf der Flow-Limitierung vor allem unter pathologischen Bedingungen ein instabiler und zeitabhängiger Vorgang (Fry, 1958; Bouhuys und Jonson, 1967; Mead et al., 1967, Takishima et al., 1967). Die er-

fahrungsgemäß große Meßwertstreuung im Flow-Plateaubereich der IVPF-
Kurven weist darauf hin (Bouhuys und Jonson, 1967).

Die Verbindungslinie der für jedes Lungenvolumen spezifischen kritischen
Maximaldrucke schneidet im Druck-Volumen-Diagramm auf der Exspirations-
seite aus der Fläche der maximal möglichen dynamischen Atemarbeit den
wesentlich kleineren Bereich der maximal verfügbaren effektiven exspiratorischen Atemarbeit heraus (Hyatt und Flath, 1966). Die durch die Kraft-
Geschwindigkeitsbeziehung der Atemmuskulatur determinierte maximale
dynamische Atemarbeit (Agostoni und Fenn, 1960) deckt sich inspiratorisch
über den ganzen Umfang, exspiratorisch nur im oberen Anteil der VC mit
der effektiven Atemarbeit. Die Differenzfläche umschreibt das maximale
Ausmaß der ventilationsineffektiven Atemarbeit, die überwiegend als Gas-
kompressionsarbeit verlorengeht, aber im Rahmen des Hustenmechanismus
auch eine physiologische Bedeutung hat (Mead et al., 1967).

Eine exspiratorische Flow-Limitierung findet bei Normalpersonen nur
bei forcierten Atemmanövern oder beim Hustenstoß statt. Unter extremen
Belastungen werden zwar auch positive Transpulmonaldrucke bis + 10 cm
H_2O registriert (Olafsen und Hyatt, 1969), jedoch bleiben sie für den dann
ventilierten Bereich der VC unterhalb des kritischen Transpulmonaldruckes.

In einer eigenen Untersuchungsreihe wurden 6 Normalpersonen bis 200
Watt belastet (Abb. 2). Die jeweils höchsten exspiratorischen Pleuradrucke
(höchster gemessener Wert bei plus 3 cm H_2O) wurden entsprechend dem
zugehörigen aktuellen Lungenvolumen aufgetragen. Die dem jeweils gleichen
Lungenvolumen zugehörigen mittleren kritischen Maximaldrucke (P_{max})
werden bei weitem nicht erreicht; entsprechend treten keine kritischen exspiratorischen Flows auf (Beispiel: Proband H.M.). Es resultiert unter Belastung eine nur leichte, nicht signifikante Anhebung des endexspiratorischen
Volumenniveaus. In- und exspiratorischer Flow nehmen etwa gleich stark
zu bei Wahrung eines Atemzeitverhältnisses von 1 : 1.

Da für ein bestimmtes Lungenvolumen die elastitische Lungenretraktion
als konstant anzusehen ist, können die genannten dynamischen Beziehungen
zwischen Volumen, Flow und Transpulmonaldruck bei Korrektur der
statischen Druckkomponente und unter Annahme einiger Vereinfachungen
auch auf die Isovolume-Alveolardruck-Flow-Beziehungen übertragen werden
(Mead und Whittenberger, 1953; Bouhuys und Jonson, 1967). Sofern der
Alveolardruck nicht direkt gemessen wird, betreffen die Vereinfachungen
die Vernachlässigung der Inertance der Luft und des Gewebes, den viskösen Gewebswiderstand, die Inflations-/Deflationshysterese des statischen
Druck-Volumen-Diagramms und die Effekte eventuell vorhandener in- und
exspiratorisch gefesselter Luft. Der Reziprokwert der Steigung in jedem
Punkt der IVPF-Kurve stellt dann für jedes Lungenvolumen den momentanen
Strömungswiderstand (R_1 bzw. R_{aw}) dar.

Der Bronchialwiderstand zeigt über den gesamten Flow-Bereich eine
Volumenabhängigkeit (Briscoe et al., 1958; Macklem und Wilson, 1965;
Macklem und Mead, 1967; DuBois, 1969; Vastag et al., 1972), also auch
im Bereich der niedrigen Flows der Spontanatmung, wo er bei der ganz-
körperplethysmographischen Routinemessung bestimmt wird. Bei konstantem
Volumen wächst der Bronchialwiderstand mit Größerwerden des Flows;

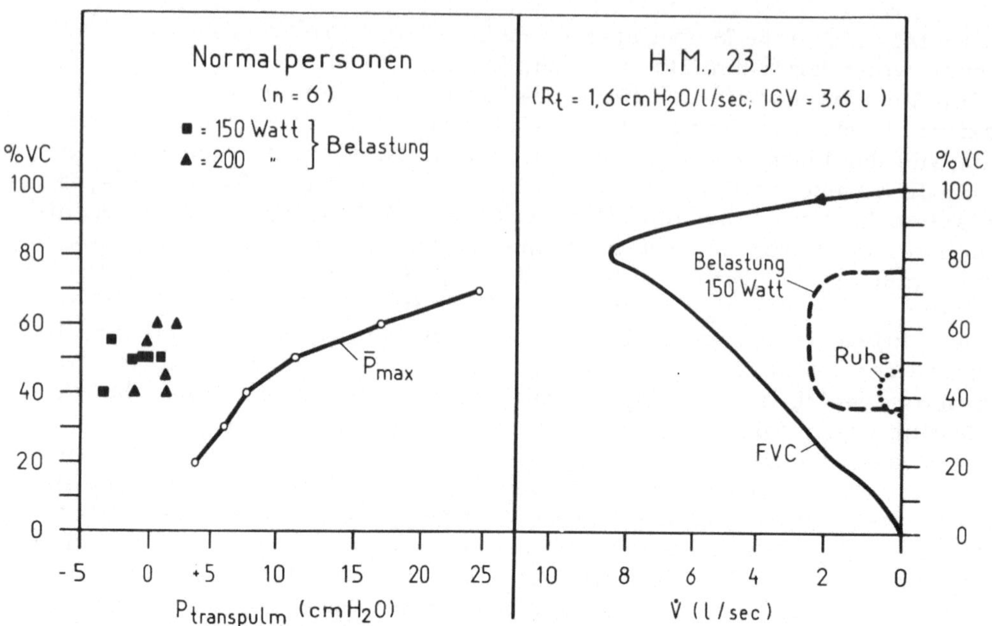

Abb. 2. Links: Höchster exspiratorischer Transpulmonaldruck ($P_{traspulm}$) unter Belastung (150 und 200 Watt) als Funktion des Lungenvolumens (% VC) im Vergleich zum mittleren Transpulmonaldruck (Pmax), bei dem Flow-Limitierung erfolgt (6 Normalpersonen). Rechts: Einzelbeispiel (H. M.) einer exspiratorischen Flow-Volume-Kurve in Ruhe, unter Belastung (150 Watt) und bei maximal forcierter Ausatmung (FVC).

diese Beziehung zwischen Resistance und Flow kann zunächst empirisch mit der bekannten Rohrer' schen Formel (1915) ($P_A = K_1 \dot{V} + K_2 \dot{V}^2$ bzw. $R = K_1 + K_2 \dot{V}$) beschrieben werden (Mead et al., 1967; Bouhuys und Jonson, 1967). Mit Einsetzen der dynamischen Kompression steigt der Bronchialwiderstand ungleich stärker an, um nach Überschreiten des kritischen Transpulmonaldrucks, also im Bereich des Flow-Plateaus, in den Grenzen der dynamischen Muskeleigenschaften gegebenenfalls extreme Werte anzunehmen (Bouhuys, 1974). Es ist unter diesen Umständen sinnvoll, im Hinblick auf die Anpassungsmöglichkeit an einen erhöhten Ventilationsbedarf die Bronchialwiderstandserhöhung durch endobronchiale Querschnittsänderung des Bronchialsystems oder Veränderung der Strömungseigenschaften der Luft von der Resistanceerhöhung durch dynamische Kompression abzutrennen. Bei der ersten Form führt, wenn auch wegen verschiedener Energieverluste nicht im Sinne einer einfachen linearen Beziehung, eine Steigerung des transbronchialen Druckgradienten zu einer Zunahme des Flows; sie erlaubt also grundsätzlich eine Ventilationssteigerung über den Flow. Bei der zweiten Form führt, da jenseits des kritischen Transpulmonaldruckes, ein Anstieg des Druckgradienten zu keiner Flow-Änderung. Diese Form erlaubt, trotz geleisteter Atemarbeit, grundsätzlich keine Ventilations-

steigerung über den Flow. Übergänge ergeben sich, wenn im Rahmen der
Steigerung des Druckgefälles zur Überwindung einer endobronchialen Obstruktion der kritische Transpulmonaldruck überschritten wird. Ulmer et
al. (1966) fanden z.B. bei Stenoseversuchen positive Pleuradrucke während
Spontanatmung in Ruhe bis $\pm$ 16 cm H_2O.

Die überschießende, ventilationsineffektive Druckschwankung im Bereich
des limitierten Flows geht größtenteils als Gaskompression verloren, ein
kleiner Teil führt bekanntlich zur Anhebung der kinetischen Energie der
Strömung im limitierenden Segment (Hustenmechanismus). Bei phasen-
bezogener Registrierung kommt es zur Phasenverschiebung zwischen Flow
und Alveolardruck, so daß am Koordinatenschreiber eine sogenannte Kippkurve resultiert (Matthys et al., 1972), wobei der Effekt der gleichzeitigen
Lungenvolumenänderung mit eingeht.

Bei unserem Normalkollektiv wurden die Mittelwerte des exspiratorischen
Bronchialwiderstandes als Funktion des aktuellen Lungenvolumes (die Zahlen
an den Kurven bedeuten: Volumen in % der VC) für verschiedene Atemmanöver und für eine Belastung von 200 Watt dargestellt (Abb. 3). Als orien-
tierendes Maß für den Eintritt des Flow-Limitierungsmechanismus bzw.
für das Auftreten von Bronchialwiderständen, die zu Lasten der dynamischen
Kompression gehen, wurde der aus dem kritischen Druck und dem zugehörigen kritischen Flow der IVPF-Kurven errechnete Bronchialwiderstand
für das jeweils zugehörige Lungenvolumen als R' -Kurve aufgetragen. Oberhalb von R' geht die Resistanceerhöhung zu Lasten der Atemwegskompression, unterhalb zu Lasten einer endobronchialen Querschnittsänderung des
Bronchialbaumes oder veränderter Strömungseigenschaften der Luft.

Zur Methodik muß hierbei gesagt werden, daß die Belastungs- und R' -
Resistance als "lung-resistance" (R_l) aus dem Transpulmonaldruck bestimmt wurde (Mead und Whittenberger, 1953), während die Messung der
übrigen Resistancewerte als "airway resistance" (R_{aw}) ganzkörperplethysmographisch erfolgte. Aufgrund dieser methodischen Unterschiede sollen
vergleichende Ergebnisse vorwiegend als qualitativ verstanden werden.

Der hyperbolische Kurvenverlauf bei dem langsamen Deflationsmanöver
(VC) entspricht der schon erwähnten inversen Abhängigkeit des Bronchialwiderstandes vom Lungenvolumen (Briscoe et al., 1958; Macklem und
Wilson, 1965; Macklem und Mead, 1967; Bouhuys und Jonson, 1967;
Vastag et al., 1972). Etwas unterhalb eines Volumens von 25% VC steigt
der Bronchialwiderstand sehr steil an und überschreitet die R' -Linie.
Es kann angenommen werden, daß hier der Flow-Limitierungsmechanismus
in Kraft getreten ist. Da im gleichen VC-Bereich bei unseren Normalpersonen (Alter 30 $\pm$ 12 Jahre) der Verschluß der kleinen kaudalen Luftwege be-
ginnt, liegt es nahe, einen Zusammenhang zwischen dem hier gezeigten Kreu-
zungspunkt und dem fremdgasanalytischen closing point zu sehen. Islam und
Ulmer (1974) haben auf diesen Zusammenhang hingewiesen. Bei der von An-
fang an forcierten Deflation (FVC-Manöver) wird erwartungsgemäß die R' -
Linie zwischen 60 und 70% VC überschritten. Unter der 200 Watt-Belastung
resultiert, jetzt unter einem anderen Blickwinkel als im vorhin gezeigten
Druck-Volumen- und Flow-Volumendiagramm, keine Flow-Limitierung.

Unter den pathophysiologischen Bedingungen einer obstruktiven oder re-

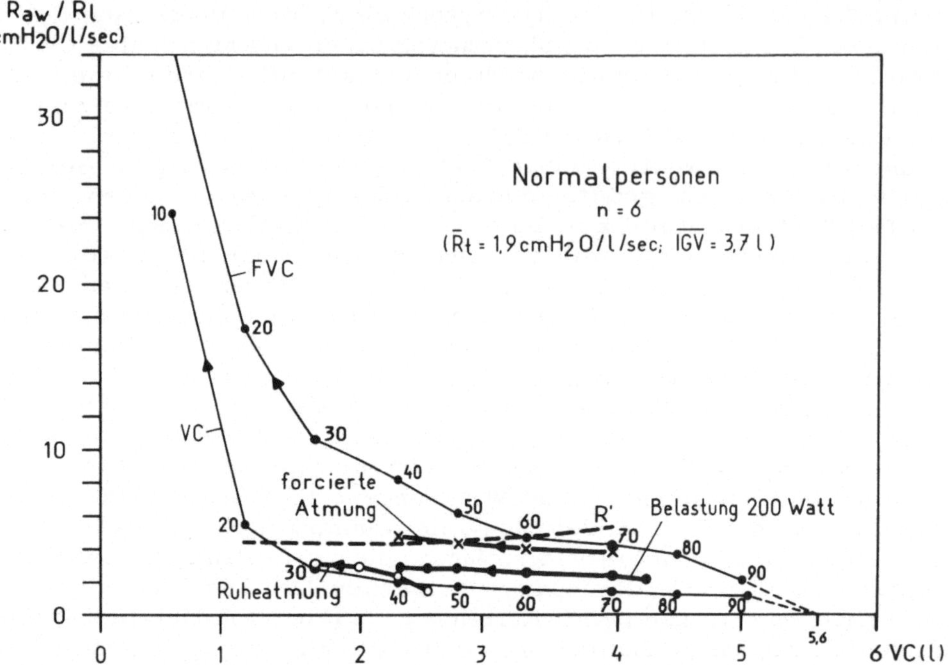

Abb. 3. Exspiratorischer Bronchialwiderstand (R_{aw} bzw. R_1) als Funktion des Lungenvolumens (VC, 1) bei langsamem Vitalkapazitätsmanöver (VC, Zahlen = % VC) bei maximal forciertem Vitalkapazitätsmanöver (FVC), bei Ruheatmung, bei forcierter Atmung (Atemgrenzmanöver) und bei Belastung (200 Watt). Mittelwerte von 6 Normalpersonen. R' : Bronchialwiderstand bei Eintritt des Flow-Limitierungsmechanismus.

restriktiven Ventilationsstörung ist der Anpassungsvorgang an einen erhöhten Ventilationsbedarf generell durch eine ungünstigere Energiebilanz gekennzeichnet. Die Anpassungsfähigkeit der einzelnen Teilgrößen der Atemtechnik ist von der primär vorgegebenen Steigerungsmöglichkeit, vom Schädigungsgrad und vom Vorhandensein von Kompensationsmechanismen abhängig.

Die Gruppe der obstruktiven Lungenerkrankungen umfaßt, je nach Reversibilität, Lokalisation und Umfang der Obstruktion sowie je nach Grad der Inflation und des Elastizitätsverlustes neben reinen Funktionstypen alle möglichen funktionellen Kombinationen; gemeinsam, wenn auch in unterschiedlichem Ausmaß, ist die vorzeitige Limitierung des exspiratorischen Flows. Von den eingangs erwähnten Größen, die Einfluß auf den Vorgang der dynamischen Kompression nehmen, bekommen der erhöhte endobronchiale Strömungswiderstand, die reduzierte Lungenretraktion und/oder die erhöhte Bronchialwandcompliance unter Berücksichtigung des Bronchialmuskeltonus entscheidende Bedeutung.

Zur Demonstration des Adaptationsvorgangs bei forcierten Atemmanövern
und bei körperlicher Belastung untersuchten wir ein, vor allem im Hinblick
auf die Mitarbeit, selektiertes Patientenkollektiv (n = 11) mit chronisch
obstruktiver Lungenerkrankung, das nach einfachen funktionellen Kriterien
in eine sogenannte "Bronchitisgruppe" (B-Gruppe) und in eine sogenannte
"Emphysemgruppe" (E-Gruppe) unterteilt wurde (Tabelle 1). Maßgebend
für die Zuteilung zur B-Gruppe war eine Resistanceerhöhung bei Ruheatmung,
also eine Obstruktion der großen Luftwege (Bouhuys, 1974) mit einem resist-
anceangepaßten Inflationsgrad (Beil und Ulmer, 1975); maßgebend für die
Zuteilung zur Emphysemgruppe war eine starke Erhöhung des endexspiratorischen Thoraxgasvolumens (IGV) ohne oder mit nur geringer Erhöhung
der Resistance bei Ruheatmung, also ohne wesentliche endobronchiale Obstruktion der großen Luftwege. Die Gruppenbezeichnungen, die Parallelen
zu verschiedenen anderen Klassifizierungen aufweisen, die sich z. T. ganz
anderer Merkmale bedienen, sollen nur in Anführungszeichen verstanden
werden. Alter und Broca-Index waren nicht signifikant verschieden. Beide
Gruppen hatten eine Verminderung der elastischen Lungenretraktion, die

Tabelle 1. Lungenfunktionsbefunde der 3 untersuchten Kollektive: Mittelwerte und Standardabweichung; Mittelwertsvergleich der beiden Patientengruppen im t-Test. Sollwerte nach K.H. Rühle (1974); (VC = Vitalkapazität,
IGV = intrathorakales Gasvolumen, TLC = Totalkapazität, R_t = Totalresistance, R_{us} = upstream resistance, P_{st} = statischer Transpulmonaldruck,
p = Irrtumswahrscheinlichkeit, n. s. = nicht signifikant).

	Normalpersonen n = 6	Bronchitisgruppe n = 7	Emphysemgruppe n = 4	B-/E-Gruppe p
Alter (Jahre)	31 ± 12	63 ± 10	65 ± 8	n. s.
Broca - Index	93 ± 10	96 ± 7	93 ± 15	n. s.
VC (l) %Soll	5,6 ± 0,9 98 ± 11	2,9 ± 0,5 59 ± 5	4,3 ± 0,7 86 ± 10	<0,001
IGV (l) %Soll	3,7 ± 0,5 101 ± 11	5,6 ± 1,1 153 ± 26	6,6 ± 1,1 169 ± 21	n. s.
TLC (l) %Soll	7,5 ± 1,1 102 ± 5	7,6 ± 1,1 112 ± 15	9,4 ± 1,2 128 ± 17	n. s.
R_t (cmH_2O/l/sec)	1,9 ± 0,4	7,1 ± 2,9	3,6 ± 0,3	< 0,05
R_{us} bei V = 1,7 l (cmH_2O/l/sec)	2,6 ± 0,8	10,3 · 2,0	6,0 ± 0,4	< 0,01
P_{st} bei V = 1,7 l (cmH_2O)	-8,4 ± 2,2	-6,5 ± 1,3	-3,9 ± 1,1	< 0,01

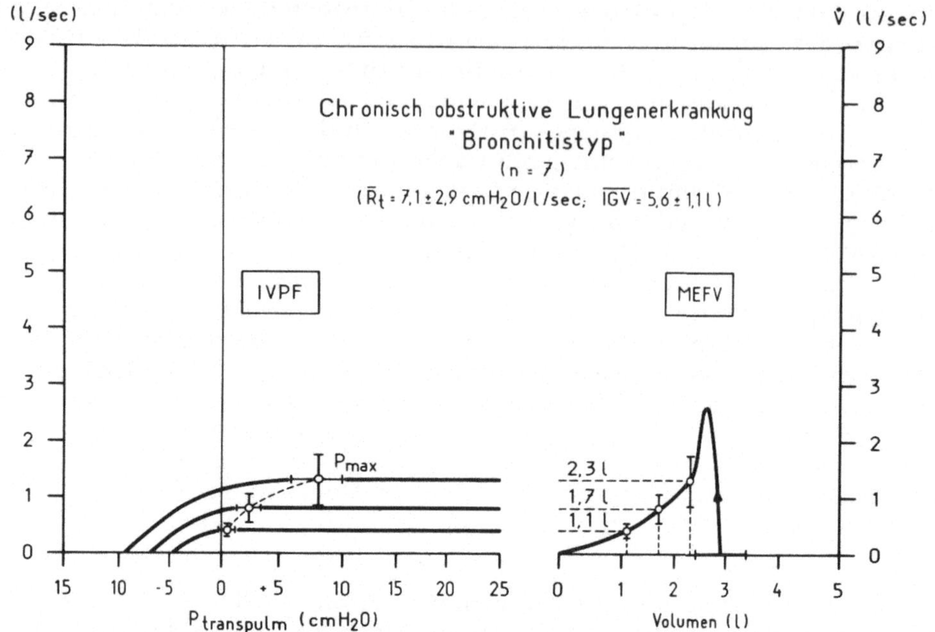

Abb. 4. Mittleres Isovolume-Pressure-Flow-Diagramm (IVPF) für 1,1 bis 2,3 l Lungenvolumen (= 40 - 80% VC) und mittleres Maximal-Expiratory-Flow-Volume-Diagramm (MEFV) bei 7 Patienten vom "Bronchitistyp" (siehe Text); weitere Erklärungen siehe Abb. 1

E-Gruppe jedoch stärker als die B-Gruppe. Beide Gruppen hatten eine Obstruktion der kleinen Luftwege, ausgedrückt als "upstream resistance" (Mead et al., 1967), die B-Gruppe jedoch stärker als die E-Gruppe; beide Gruppen hatten eine erniedrigte VC, die B-Gruppe jedoch stärker als die E-Gruppe. Der hier signifikante Unterschied bei der VC steht in Übereinstimmung mit Befunden von Burrows et al. (1964) und Duffel et al. (1970), scheint jedoch nicht generell obligatorisch zu sein (Filley et al., 1968, Hüttemann und Schüren, 1972).

Es ist offensichtlich, daß durch die hier vorgenommene Einteilung die beiden wesentlichen Pathomechanismen, die Einfluß auf die exspiratorische Flow-Limitierung nehmen - nämlich die endobronchiale Obstruktion und die Verminderung der elastischen Retraktionskraft -, nur schwerpunktsmäßig getrennt werden.

Die IVPF- und MEFV-Kurven in Abb. 4 sind für das Patientenkollektiv im gleichen Maßstab wie bei der Normalgruppe dargestellt. Das jeweilige Lungenvolumen der IVPF-Kurven der B-Gruppe entspricht dem der untersten drei Kurven bei den Normalpersonen. Der statische Transpulmonaldruck (bei Flow = 0) ist gegenüber normal weniger negativ. Die Steigung der Kurven zeigt bereits im Bereich der kleinen Flows (Ruheatmung) eine Verminderung entsprechend der ganzkörperplethysmographisch gemessenen Resistanceerhöhung, die zur Gruppenzuteilung führte. Die kritischen Pleuradrucke (P$_{max}$) liegen in einer deutlich kleineren Größenordnung als beim

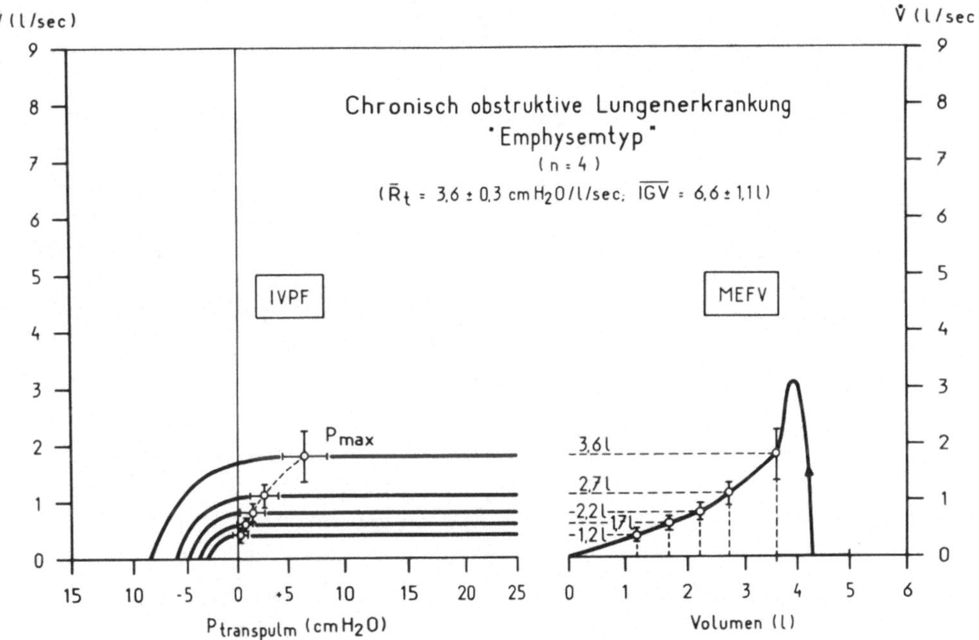

Abb. 5. Mittleres Isovolume-Pressure-Flow-Diagramm (IVPF) für 1, 2 bis 3, 6 l Lungenvolumen (= 30 - 80% VC) und mittleres Maximal-Expiratory-Flow-Volume-Diagramm (MEFV) bei 4 Patienten vom "Emphysemtyp" (siehe Text); weitere Erklärungen siehe Abb. 1

Normalkollektiv, nachdem deutlich niedrigere kritische Flows erreicht wurden. Diese Verlagerung der kritischen Drucke, wie sie auch von Pride et al. (1967), Potter et al. (1971) und Leaver und Pride (1971) mitgeteilt wird, belegt die leichtere Kompressibilität der intrathorakalen Luftwege.

Bei der E-Gruppe (Abb. 5) stimmt das jeweilige Lungenvolumen der eingezeichneten 5 IVPF-Kurven mit den ersten 5 Kurven des Normalkollektivs überein. Die elastische Lungenretraktion ($P_{transpulm}$ bei Flow = 0) ist bei gleichem Lungenvolumen noch geringer als bei der B-Gruppe. Die Kurvensteigung bei den niedrigen Flows entspricht größenordnungsmäßig der ganzkörperperplethysmographisch gemessenen Resistance über den Ruheatmungsbereich, die definitionsgemäß nicht oder nur leicht erhöht war. Die kritischen Pleuradrucke, bei denen eine dynamische Kompression erfolgt, finden sich auch hier bereits bei leicht positiven Werten, die bei gleichem Lungenvolumen eher noch weniger positiv sind als bei der B-Gruppe. Die Unterschiede im Verlauf der IVPF-Kurven bei B- und E-Patienten stimmen mit den Ergebnissen von Duffel et al. (1970) überein.

Unter Belastung (Abb. 6), die bei 50 Watt begonnen und, falls kein Belastungsabbruch erfolgte, nach 4 Minuten auf 100 Watt gesteigert wurde, überschritt der exspiratorische Pleuradruck bei allen 7 Patienten der B-Gruppe und bei 2 Patienten der E-Gruppe (nicht nur an der Mittelwertskurve) den kritischen Transpulmonaldruck (P_{max}). Das entspricht Ergeb-

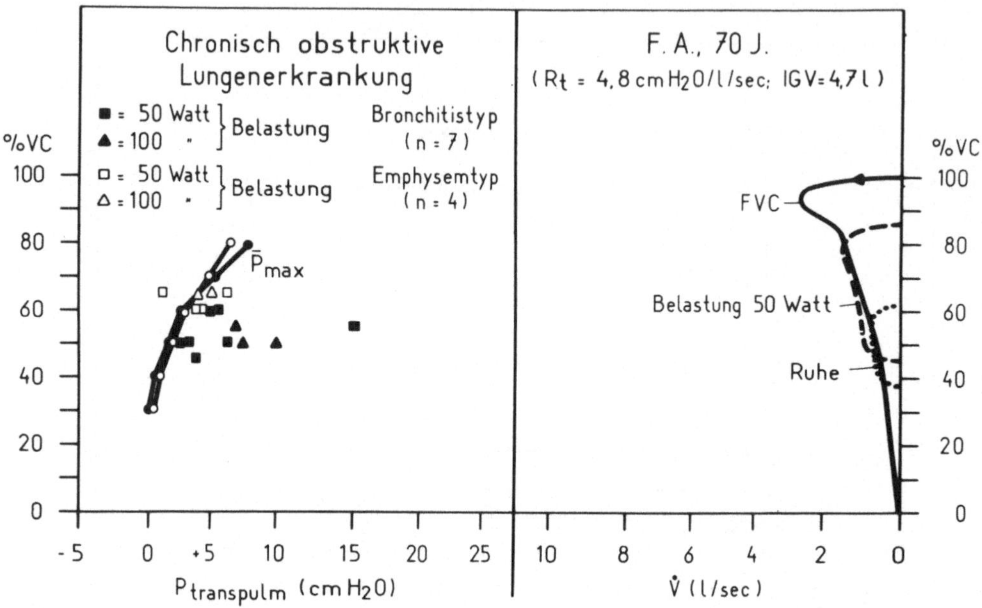

Abb. 6. Links: Höchster exspiratorischer Transpulmonaldruck (P$_{transpulm}$) unter Belastung (50 und 100 Watt) als Funktion des Lungenvolumens (% VC) im Vergleich zum mittleren Transpulmonaldruck (P$_{max}$), bei dem Flow-Limitierung erfolgt (7 Patienten vom "Bronchitistyp" und 4 Patienten vom "Emphysemtyp"). - Rechts: Einzelbeispiel (F.A.) einer exspiratorischen Flow-Volume-Kurve in Ruhe, unter Belastung (50 Watt) und bei maximal forcierter Ausatmung (FCV)

nissen von Potter et al. (1971) sowie Leaver und Pride (1971), bei denen aber keine Gruppierung der Patienten vorgenommen wurde. Am Beispiel F.A. ist erkennbar, daß die Atemmittellage deutlicher als bei den Normalpersonen unter Vergrößerung des endexspiratorischen Thoraxgasvolumen nach der Inspirationsseite verschoben wurde, eine Beobachtung, die auch Grimby und Stiksa (1970) sowie Potter et al. (1971) gemacht haben. Es fällt außerdem auf, daß der exspiratorische Flow nicht nur in einem weiten Bereich die MEFV-Kurve tangiert, sondern bei 5 Patienten der B-Gruppe und bei einem Patient der E-Gruppe unter Belastung überschreitet. Ausgeprägt ist diese Überschreitung allerdings nur bei 4 Patienten der B-Gruppe. Dieses Phänomen wird ebenfalls von Grimby und Stiksa (1970), Leaver und Pride (1971) sowie von Potter et al. (1971) beschrieben. Die wahrscheinlichste Erklärung ist eine Abhängigkeit des Flows von der sogenannten "flow history". Nach Takishima et al. (1967) ergibt sich solche Zeitabhängigkeit des Flows bei großer Inhomogenität der Zeitkonstanten parallel geschalteter Lungeneinheiten; es kommt dann für ein bestimmtes Lungenvolumen zu einem relativ höheren Maximal-Flow, wenn der vorausgehende Flow niedriger war, als wenn ein höherer Flow vorausgeht.

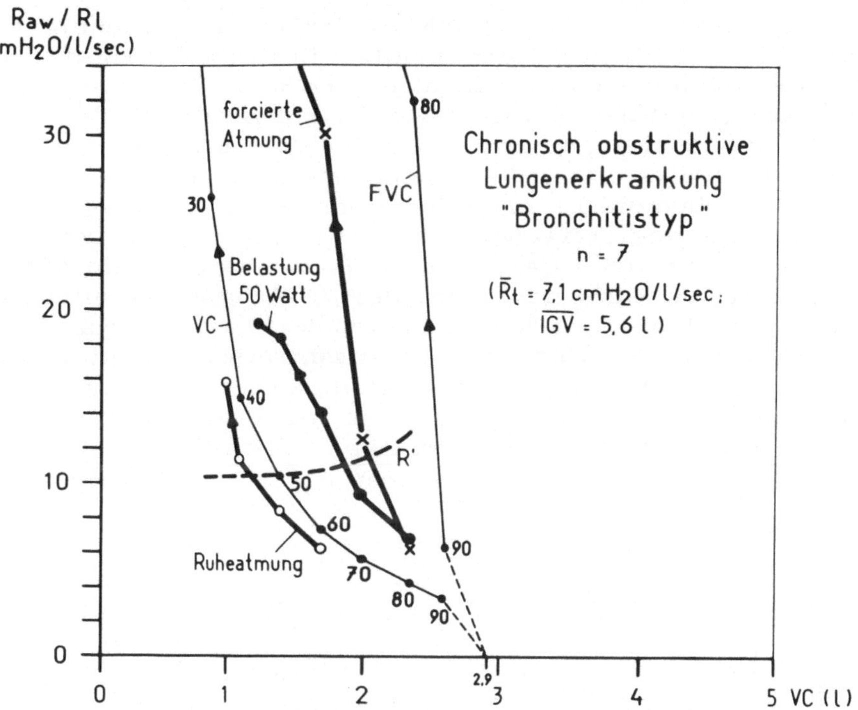

Abb. 7. Exspiratorischer Bronchialwiderstand (R_{aw} bzw. R_1) als Funktion des Lungenvolumens (VC, 1) bei langsamem Vitalkapazitätsmanöver (VC), bei maximal forciertem Vitalkapazitätsmanöver (FVC), bei Ruheatmung, bei forcierter Atmung und bei Belastung (50 Watt). Mittelwerte bei 7 Patienten vom "Bronchitistyp"; weitere Erklärungen siehe Abb. 3

Im Resistance-Volumen-Diagramm (Abb. 7) wird die Problematik der Anpassung des exspiratorischen Flows an den Ventilationsbedarf nochmals aus einer anderen Blickrichtung deutlich. Die VC-Kurve markiert den Verlauf der Resistance über die Vitalkapazität bei niedrigem Flow, die FVC-Kurve bei maximal forcierter Ausatmung. Die Volumenabhängigkeit der endobronchialen Resistance tritt deutlich in Erscheinung und spielt auch schon für den Ruheatmungsbereich eine große Rolle. Die R'-Linie markiert wiederum größenordnungsmäßig den Eintritt des Flow-Limitierungsmechanismus durch Atemwegskompression. Der im gesamten exspiratorischen Bereich deutlich erhöhte Bronchialwiderstand bei Ruheatmung wird bei der B-Gruppe bereits teilweise durch eine kompressionsbedingte Flow-Limitierung hervorgerufen. Das entspricht dem Bild der Kippkurve im zugehörigen Druck-Strömungsdiagramm bei 5 der 7 B-Patienten; dabei muß der Beginn des "Kippens" im Druck-Strömungsdiagramm nicht notwendig mit dem Beginn des Flow-Limitierungsmechanismus übereinstimmen (Nolte, 1967; Ulmer, 1970), da auch Effekte der gleichzeitigen Lungenvolumenänderung, des Bronchialmuskeltonus (Ulmer, 1970) und ausgeprägter ventilatorischer Inhomogenität (Nolte 1967) in das Kurvenbild eingehen können. Unter 50 Watt Belastung erfolgt eine Verschiebung des endexspiratorischen Volumenniveaus in Richtung der Inspiration, also in eine Richtung, in der einmal der endobronchiale Strömungswiderstand relativ geringer ist und gleichzeitig der kritische Transpulmonaldruck bzw. der kritische Flow höher liegt. Diese Verschiebungsmöglichkeit ist jedoch bei der Zunahme des Hubvolumens und bei der niedrigen VC durch die statischen Kräfte der Lunge und des Thorax begrenzt. Die trotz der Verschiebung des Volumenniveaus erkennbare Zunahme der Resistance bei gleichem Lungenvolumen gegenüber der Ruheatmung bzw. der VC-Atmung geht unterhalb von R' wahrscheinlich ausschließlich zu Lasten des höheren Flows. Trotzdem kann ein belastungsinduzierter Bronchospasmus nicht absolut ausgeschlossen werden. Oberhalb der R'-Linie, also im Bereich des limitierten Flows, erzeugt der überschießende, noch über dem Ruheniveau liegende, flowineffektive Druckaufbau den deutlichen Resistanceanstieg.

Bei der E-Gruppe (Abb. 8) ist der exspiratorische Bronchialwiderstand

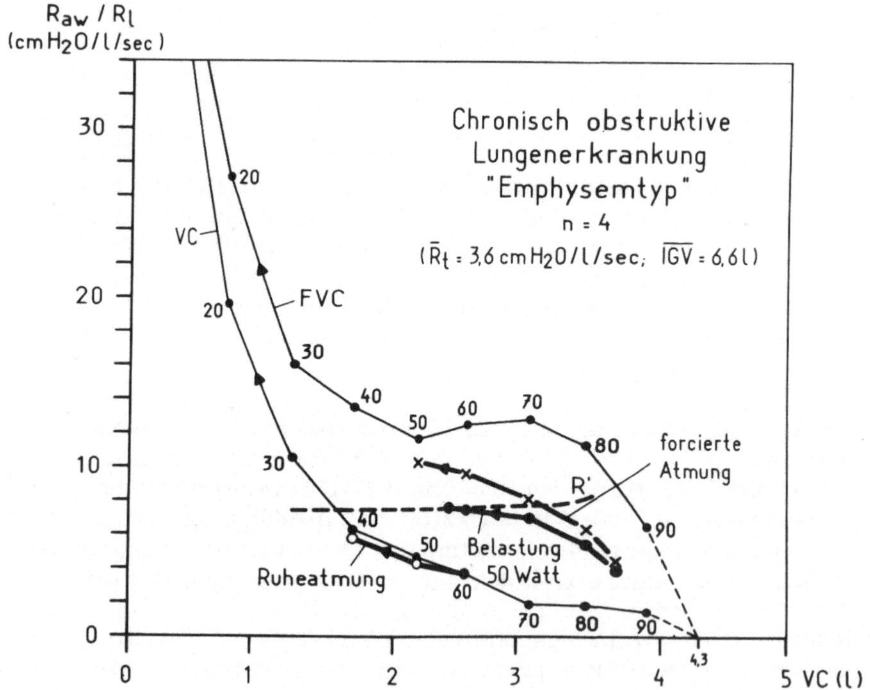

Abb. 8. Exspiratorischer Bronchialwiderstand (R_{aw} bzw. R_1) als Funktion des Lungenvolumens (VC, l) bei langsamem Vitalkapazitätsmanöver (VC), bei maximal forciertem Vitalkapazitätsmanöver (FVC), bei Ruheatmung, bei forcierter Atmung und bei Belastung (50 Watt). Mittelwerte bei 4 Patienten vom "Emphysemtyp"; weitere Erklärungen siehe Abb. 3

bei niedrigem Flow (VC-Kurve) weniger deutlich volumenabhängig als
bei der B-Gruppe. Es steht ein weiter Bereich mit normaler Resistance
zur Verfügung. Bei Ruheatmung nimmt zwar der Bronchialwiderstand
endexspiratorisch zu, jedoch wird die R'-Linie nicht erreicht. Eine Atemwegskompression findet also nicht statt. Unter der 50 Watt-Belastung erfolgt eine stärkere Verschiebung des endexspiratorischen Volumenniveaus
als bei der B-Gruppe. Diese stärkere Verschiebung bedeutet: erstens eine
Verschiebung in einen VC-Bereich mit noch niedrigerem endobronchialen
Strömungswiderstand und zweitens eine Verschiebung des kritischen maximalen Pleuradrucks bzw. kritischen Flows auf ein noch höheres Niveau
als bei den B-Patienten. Obwohl auch hier, wahrscheinlich wiederum durch
den höheren Flow, für ein bestimmtes Lungenvolumen die endobronchiale
Resistance ansteigt, wird die Zone der Flow-Limitierung durch Atemwegskompression im Mittel gerade erreicht.

Betrachten wir die zugehörigen statischen atemmechanischen Verhältnisse
im Zusammenhang. Aufgrund der bereits erwähnten unterschiedlichen Lun-
gendehnbarkeit, die vom Normalkollektiv über die B-Gruppe zur E-Gruppe
zunimmt, führt die deutliche, im Hinblick auf den Bronchialwiderstand und
den Flow-Limitierungsmechanismus günstige Verschiebung des endexspiratorischen Volumenniveaus bei den Patienten im Vergleich zu den Normalpersonen eher zu einer geringeren Zunahme der elastischen Atemarbeit
gegen die Lungenretraktion. Aus dem gleichen Grund führt die stärkere
Verschiebung der Atemmittellage bei der E-Gruppe zu keiner zusätzlichen
Steigerung der elastischen Atemarbeit gegenüber der B-Gruppe. Selbstverständlich darf die statische Druck-Volumen-Beziehung der Thoraxwand
nicht vernachlässigt werden. Vor allem bei erniedrigter Thoraxdehnbar-
keit, wie sie von Cherniak und Hodson (1963) sowie Krumholz und Albright
(1968) bei der chronisch obstruktiven Lungenerkrankung beschrieben wird,
ist eine Verschiebung des endexspiratorischen Volumenniveaus zur Inspirationsseite immer als energetisch ungünstig anzusehen. Das ist besonders auch deshalb bedeutungsvoll, weil, wie Grimby et al. (1973) nachgewiesen haben, die Ventilationssteigerung unter Belastung auch bei der
obstruktiven Ventilationsstörung fast ausschließlich durch Zunahme der
Thoraxatmung zustande kommt. Es ist in Fortsetzung dieser Überlegung
offensichtlich, daß die als Kompensationsmechanismus der Flow-Limitierung anzusehende Verschiebung der Atemmittellage bei weiterer Ventilationssteigerung mit Zunahme des Hubvolumens in Abhängigkeit von der
Größe der VC und des diese endgradig determinierenden Gleichgewichts
zwischen Inspirationsmuskelzug und Thorax-Lungen-Retraktion (Campbell
et al. , 1970) bei beiden Patientengruppen - bei der B-Gruppe rascher
als bei der E-Gruppe - erschöpfbar sein muß.

Zur Kompensation der begrenzten Anpassungsbreite des exspiratorischen
Flows an einen erhöhten Ventilationsbedarf stehen als weitere Mechanismen
zur Verfügung: Einmal die gegenüber der Änderung der Atemfrequenz relativ stärkere Zunahme des Atemhubvolumens und zweitens die Steigerung des inspiratorischen Flows unter Verschiebung des Atemzeitverhältnisses zugunsten einer langsameren Exspiration. Auch diese Kompensationsmöglichkeiten sind begrenzt. Die relativ starke Hubvolumenzunahme

konkurriert analog der Verschiebung der Atemmittellage mit den statischen
Gegenkräften der Lungen- und Thoraxretraktion. Die Steigerung des inspiratorischen Flows findet ihre Beschränkung in der Kraft-Geschwindigkeitsbe-
ziehung der Inspirationsmuskulatur, deren Spielraum im inspiratorischen
Teil der maximalen Flow-Volumen-Kurve zur Darstellung kommt; auch
hier stellt sich die B-Gruppe mit ihrer inspiratorisch wirksamen endobronchialen Obstruktion ungünstiger als die E-Gruppe.

Die Begrenzung der Ventilationssteigerung unter körperlicher Belastung
durch den Mechanismus der exspiratorischen Flow-Limitierung führt nach
Erschöpfung auch der Kompensationsmöglichkeiten in letzter Konsequenz
zur alveolären Hypoventilation. Der Abbruch einer Belastung ist jedoch
bei der chronisch obstruktiven Lungenerkrankung keineswegs notwendig an
eine grobe Störung des Gasaustausches gebunden, wie u.a. Grimby und
Stiksa (1970) gezeigt haben.

Aus unserer Untersuchung geht hervor, daß die Höhe des exspiratorischen
Pleuradruckpeaks bei 6 Patienten mit chronisch obstruktiver Lungenerkrankung (5 vom B- und 1 vom E-Typ) signifikant unter Belastung mit der
viskösen Atemarbeit des Druck-Volumendiagramms korreliert, auch wenn
hierbei Gaskompressionseffekte nicht quantitativ erfaßt werden. Die überschießende Druckentwicklung nach Eintritt der Flow-Limitierung, die
unter vergleichbarer Belastung bei B-Patienten deutlich stärker ausfällt
als bei E-Patienten, muß als zusätzliche frustrane Atemarbeit bewertet
werden. Der Grund für diesen unnötigen Druckaufbau ist wahrscheinlich
in dem grundsätzlich sinnvollen, mechanorezeptiv vermittelten Regelkreis
für den mechanischen Atemantrieb (Ulmer und Reichel, 1967; Ulmer et al.,
1975) zu suchen. Für diesen Regelkreis ist eine Erhöhung des Bronchialwiderstandes, wie sie bei B-Patienten dominiert, der adäquate Reiz. Es ist
vorstellbar, daß der zugehörige Mechanorezeptor eine Resistanceerhöhung
durch endobronchiale Obstruktion nicht von einer Resistanceerhöhung durch
dynamische Kompression unterscheiden kann.

Die frustrane Atemarbeit addiert sich zu jenen anderen Komponenten der
totalen Atemarbeit, die als Atemarbeit gegen endobronchiale Strömungswiderstände und gegen die elastischen Widerstände der Lunge und des Thorax
unter Belastung wiederum bei den B-Patienten stärker zunehmen als bei
den E-Patienten. Auf die ebenfalls für B-Patienten meistens relevantere
Komponente der totalen Atemtechnik, nämlich die kompressible Blindarbeit
bei Vorhandensein in- und exspiratorisch gefesselter Luft (Matthys und
Overrath, 1971; Hüttemann und Huckauf, 1971), soll hier nicht näher eingegangen werden.

Die totale Atemarbeit bzw. Atemleistung ist sicher ein gutes, wenn nicht
das beste Maß (Matthys, 1972) für den biologisch bedeutsamen Energieum-
satz des gesamten atemmechanischen Apparates unter Belastung. Aber abgesehen von der geringen Anschaulichkeit dieses Parameters für die klinische Praxis liefert auch eine stark erhöhte Atemleistung keine erschöpfende
Erklärung für den Abbruch einer Belastung. Jonson (1971) hat durchgerech-
net, daß die Atemleistung bei Obstruktion zum Zeitpunkt des Belastungsab-
bruchs geringer ist als die Atemleistung von Normalpersonen am Rande
ihrer Leistungskapazität. Die, wie wir gesehen haben, relativ günstige

atemmechanische Adaptation der E-Patienten an die Belastungsventilation
kontrastiert mit der Begrenzung ihrer Belastungstoleranz, lange vor
vollständiger Ausnutzung der Ventilationsreserven, so daß hier andere
Faktoren, wie Gasaustauschstörungen, im Vordergrund stehen müssen
(Marcus et al., 1970).

Es kann abschließend festgestellt werden, daß nur die Annahme eines
multifaktoriellen Systems dem Gesamtphänomen des "breaking point"
mit seinem Symptom Dyspnoe gerecht wird. Ein solches System muß auch
mögliche sensorische Mechanismen für die Perzeption und Übertragung
des Dyspnoeempfindung berücksichtigen, wie sie z. B. von Howell und
Campbell (1966), Guz et al. (1970) sowie Widdicombe (1971) mitgeteilt
wurden.

LITERATUR

Agostini, E., Fenn, W.O.: Velocity of muscle shorting as a limiting
    factor in respiratory air flow. J. appl. Physiol. 15, 349 (1960)
Asmussen, E.: Muscular exercise. In: Handbook of Physiology, Section 3,
    Respiration, Vol. II. 939 (1964)
Beil, M., Ulmer, W.T.: Funktionsanalytische Befundmuster bei chronisch
    obstruktiver Atemwegserkrankung und ihre Bedeutung für die klinische
    Kurzzeitprognose. Pneumonologie 153, 119 (1976)
Bouhuys, A., Jonson, B.: Alveolar pressure, air flow rate and lung infla-
    tion in man. J. appl. Physiol. 22, 1086 (1967)
Bouhuys, A.: Breathing. Physiology environment and lung disease, p. 156,
    160, 162. New York - London: Grune and Stratton 1974
Briscoe, W.A., DuBois, A.B.: The relationship between airway resist-
    ance, airway conductance and lung volume in subjects of different age
    and body size. J. clin. Invest. 37, 1279 (1958)
Burrows, B., Niden, A.H., Fletcher, C.M., Jones, N.L.: Clinical types
    of chronic obstructive lung disease in London and in Chicago. Amer. Rev
    resp. Dis. 90, 14 (1964)
Campbell, E.J.M., Agostini, E., Davis, J.N.: The respiratory muscles:
    Mechanism and neural control, p. 69 London: Lloyd-Luke 1970
Cherniak, R.M., Hodson, A.: Compliance of the chest wall in chronic
    bronchitis and emphysma. J. appl. Physiol. 18, 707 (1963)
Cotes, J.E.: Lung function, p. 276 Oxford: Blackwell Scientific Publ.
    1968
DuBois, A.B.: Significance of measurement of airway resistance. Int.
    Symposium on Body Plethysmograph, Nijmegen 1968
    Progr. Resp. Res. 4, 109 (1969)
Duffel, G.M., Marcus, J.H., Ingram, R.H.: Limitation of expiratory
    flow in chronic obstructive pulmonary disease. Relation of clinical
    characteristics, pathophysiological type, and mechanisms. Ann. Intern.
    Med. 72, 365 (1970)
Filley, G.F., Beckwitt, H.J., Reeves, J.T., Mitchell, R.S.: Chronic
    obstructive bronchopulmonary disease. II. Oxygen transport in two
    clinical types. Amer. J. Med. 44, 26 (1968)

Fry, D. L.: Theoretical considerations of the bronchial pressure-flow-volume relationships with particular reference to the maximum expiratory flow volume curve. Phys. Med. Biol. 3, 174 (1958)

Fry, D. L., Hyatt, R. E.: Pulmonary mechanics. A unified analysis of the relationship between pressure, volume, and gasflow in the lungs of normal and diseased human subjects. Amer. J. Med. 29, 672 (1960)

Grimby, G. E., Stiksa, J.: Flow-volume curves and breathing patterns during exercise in patients with obstructive lung disease. Scand. J. clin. Lab. Invest. 25, 303 (1970)

Grimby, G., Elgefors, B., Oxhöj, H.: Ventilatory levels and chest wall mechanics during exercise in obstructive lung disease. Scand. J. Resp. Dis. 54, 45 (1973)

Guz, A., Noble, M.I.M., Eisele, J.H., Trenchard, D.: Experimental results of vagal block in cardiopulmonary disease. In: Porter, R., Breathing, Hering-Breuer Centenary Symposium, Churchill, London: A.J. Churchill 1970

Howell, J.B.L., Campbell, E.J.M.: Breathlessness. Oxford: Blackwell Scientific Publ. 1966

Hüttemann, V., Schüren, K.P.: Chronisch obstruktive Lungenerkrankungen: Klinische Erscheinungsformen und ihre Korrelation zur gestörten Atmungsfunktion. Klin. Wschr. 50, 944 (1972)

Hüttemann, V., Huckauf, H.: Analyse elliptischer Druck/Fluß- und Druck/Volumen-Diagramme der Atemwege: Die kompressiv wirksame obstruktive Ventilationsstörung. Klin. Wschr. 49, 205 (1971)

Hyatt, R.E., Flath, R.E.: Relationship of air flow to pressure during maximal respiratory effort in man. J. appl. Physiol. 21, 477 (1966)

Islam, M.S., Ulmer, W. T.: Diagnostic value of "closing volume" in comparison to "airway resistance/lung volume plot". Respiration 31, 449 (1974)

Jones, I.G., Fraser, R.B., Nadel, J.A.: Prediction of maximum expiratory flow rate from area-transmural pressure curve of compressed airway. J. appl. Physiol. 38, 1002 (1975)

Jonson, B.: Pulmonary mechanics as a factor limiting the capacity for work in disease. Scand. J. resp. Dis. Suppl. 77, 94 (1971)

Krumholz, R.A., Albright, C.D.: The compliance of the chest wall and thorax in emphysema. Amer. Rev. resp. Dis. 97, 827 (1968)

Leaver, D.G., Pride, N.B.: Flow-volume curves and expiratory pressures during exercise in patients with chronic airway obstruction. Scand. J. resp. Dis. Suppl. 77, 23 (1971)

Macklem, P.T., Wilson, N.J.: Measurement of intrabronchial pressure in man. J. appl. Physiol. 20, 653 (1965)

Macklem, P.T., Mead, J.: Resistance of central and peripheral airways measured by a retrograde catheter. J. appl. Physiol. 22, 395 (1967)

Macklem, P.T., Fraser, R.G., Brown, W.G.: Bronchial pressure measurements in emphysema and bronchitis. J. clin. Invest. 44, 897 (1965)

Marcus, J.H., McLean, R.L., Duffell, G.M., Ingram, R.H.: Exercise performance in relation to the pathophysiologic type of chronic obstructive pulmonary disease. Amer. J. Med. 49, 14 (1970)

Matthys, H. , Orth, U. , Overrath, G. , Konietzko, N. : Verhalten von Druck,
Fluß, Volumen und verwandter Größen bei forcierter Atmung. Pneumono-
logie 147, 250 (1972)
Matthys, H. , Overrath, G. : Dynamics of gas and work breathing in ob-
structive lung disease. Bull. Physio-path. Resp. 7, 457 (1971)
Matthys, H. : Lungenfunktionsdiagnostik mittels Ganzkörperplethysmographie.
S. 93. Stuttgart - New York: F. K. Schattauer Verlag 1972
Mead, J. : Control of respiratory frequency. J. appl. Physiol. 15, 325
(1960)
Mead, J. , Whittenberger, J. L. : Physical properties of human lungs
measured during spontaneous respiration. J. appl. Physiol. 5, 779
(1953)
Mead, J. , Turner, J.M. , Macklem, P.T. , Little, J.B. : Significance of
the relationship between lung recoil and maximum expiratory flow.
J. appl. Physiol. 22, 95 (1967)
Nolte, D. : Mechanik der Trachea und Bronchien. In: Atemmechanik, Ver-
handlungen der Gesellschaft für Lungen- und Atmungsforschung, Bochum
1966, S. 197. Berlin - Heidelberg - New York: Springer-Verlag 1967
Olafsson, S. , Hyatt, R. E. : Ventilatory mechanics and expiratory flow
limitation during exercise in normal subjects. J. clin. Invest. 48, 564
(1969)
Otis, A. B. : The work of breathing. Physiol. Rev. 34, 449 (1954)
Otis, A. B. : The work of breathing. In: Handbook of Physiology, Section 3,
Respiration 1, 463 (1964)
Oullet, Y. , Poh, S. C. , Becklake, M.R. : Circulatory factors limiting
maximal aerobic exercise capacity. J. appl. Physiol. 27, 874 (1969)
Potter, W.A. , Oláfsson, S. , Hyatt, R.E. : Ventilatory mechanics and
expiratory flow limitation during exercise in patients with obstructive
lung disease. J. clin. Invest. 50, 910.(1971)
Pride, N. B. , Permutt, S. , Riley, R. L. , Bromberger-Barnea, B. :
Determinants of maximal expiratory flow from the lungs. J. appl.
Physiol. 23, 646 (1967)
Riley, R. L. : Pulmonary functions in relation to exercise. In: Science and
Medicine of Exercise and Sports. New York: Harper & Row 1960
Rohrer, F. : Der Strömungswiderstand in den menschlichen Atemwegen
und der Einfluß der unregelmäßigen Verzweigung des Bronchialsystems
auf den Atmungsablauf in verschiedenen Lungenbezirken. Pflüger' s
Arch. 162, 225 (1915)
Takishima, T. , Grimby, G. , Graham,W. , Knudson, R. , Macklem, P.T. ,
Mead, J. : Flow-volume curves during quiet breathing, maximum volun-
tary ventilation, and forced vital capacities in patients with obstructive
lung disease. Scand. J. resp. Dis. 48, 384 (1967)
Ulmer, W.T. , Reif, E. , Weller, W. : Die obstruktiven Atemwegserkrankun-
gen, S. 7. Stuttgart: G. Thieme 1966
Ulmer, W.T. , Reichel, G. : Die Atemregulation bei chronisch obstruktiven
Ventilationsstörungen. Med. thorac. 24, 338 (1967)
Ulmer, W.T. : Diskussionsbemerkung. In: Bronchitis III, Proceedings of
the third international symposium on bronchitis. Groningen 1969, S. 313.
Assen: Royal Vangorcum 1970

Ulmer, W.T., Islam, M.S., Chung, C.K.: Relation between the output of
the centers and the ventilation. In: Symposium "Acid-Base Homeostasis
of Brain Extracellular Fluid". Berlin-Heidelberg-New York: Springer
Verlag (im Druck) 1976
Vastag, E., Islam, M.S., Ulmer, W.T.: Der Zusammenhang zwischen
dem aktuellen Lungenvolumen und dem Strömungswiderstand in den
Atemwegen bei gesunden Versuchspersonen und bei Patienten mit chro-
nisch obstruktiver Atemwegserkrankung. Pneumonologie 147, 29 (1972)
Widdicombe, J.G., Nadel, J.A.: Airway volume, airway resistance, and
work and force of breathing: Theory. J. appl. Physiol. 18, 863 (1963)
Widdicombe, J.G.: Breathing and breathlessness in lung disease. Sci.
Basis Med. Ann. Revs., p. 148 (1971)
Yamashiro, S.M., Daubenspeck, J.A., Lauritzen, T.N., Grodins, F.S.:
Total work rate of breathing optimization in CO_2 inhalation and exercise
J. appl. Physiol. 38, 702 (1975)

Dr. Martin Beil
Silikoseforschungsinstitut
Hunscheidtstrasse 12
4630 Bochum

Pneumonologie Suppl. 1976, 61-74

Therapiemöglichkeiten bei Leistungsbegrenzung von seiten der Lunge: Rehabilitation chronischer Stadien

D. Nolte

Forschungsanstalt für Erkrankungen der Atmungsorgane und Innere Abteilung II des Städtischen Krankenhauses Bad Reichenhall

Possibilities for Treatment on Respiration as Limiting Factor for Working Capacity: Rehabilitation of Chronic Stages

---

Abstract. Physical therapy is an essential part in the rehabilitation of patients with stable chronic obstructive lung disease (COPD). Various physical measures to enhance the clearance and expectoration of sputum and breathing training or exercises to improve the marked dyspnoe are widely used. Most clinicians do not realize that up to now many methods of physical therapy are lacking a scientific background.

Using breathing exercise and intermittent positive pressure breathing (IPPB) as examples for two very different methods, the difficulty is demonstrated, to measure long-term effects of physical therapy. IPPB has some acute effects in patients with COPD, but it is uncertain, whether the course of the disease may be influenced in any way.

Breathing exercise as the oldest part of physical therapy now should be practised using modern conceptions of breathing mechanics. The different conditions of extrapulmonary factors on the one side (breathing muscles, thoraco-abdominal mechanics) and intrapulmonary factors on the other side (airway obstruction with check valve phenomenon, uneven distribution of ventilation) must be considered individually.

The necessity of controlled prospective studies in COPD patients is emphasized.

Zusammenfassung. Die Rehabilitation von chronisch kranken Lungenpatienten ist in hohem Maße auf physikalisch-therapeutische Maßnahmen angewiesen. Viele Methoden der physikalischen Therapie werden jedoch bis heute rein empirisch angewendet. Am Beispiel der Atemgymnastik und der IPPB-Therapie wird auf die Notwendigkeit hingewiesen, der physikalischen Therapie eine wissenschaftliche Grundlage zu geben.

Akute Effekte sind sowohl für die IPPB-Therapie als auch für die Atemgymnastik sicher nachgewiesen worden; problematisch ist aber die Frage des Langzeiteffekts. Hier kann bisher lediglich als gesichert gelten, daß eine IPPB-Heimbehandlung die Hospitalisierungsrate zu reduzieren vermag.

An Hand atemmechanischer Untersuchungen wird gezeigt, wie es möglich ist, die modernen Vorstellungen von der Pathophysiologie der Bronchialobstruktion auf die Atemgymnastik zu übertragen: Eine atemgymnastische Übung, bei welcher der obstruktive Patient seine Mittellage willkürlich erhöht, führt zu einer Verbesserung der intrapulmonalen Strömungsdynamik, des Ventilations-Perfusionsverhältnisses und der arteriellen Blutgase. Untersuchungen über die Längen-Spannungs-Beziehung der Inspirationsmuskulatur zeigen auf der anderen Seite, daß einer willkürlichen Erhöhung der Atemmittellage von der muskulären Seite her Grenzen gesetzt sind.

Die pathophysiologisch sinnvollste Atemgymnastik kann sich im Einzelfall nur an den Meßwerten einer eingehenden Lungenfunktionsanalyse orientieren.

Die Therapie bei chronischen Stadien, die Thema dieses Referates sein soll, unterscheidet sich von der Therapie akuter Stadien darin, daß ein stärkerer Akzent auf nicht-medikamentösen Maßnahmen liegt. Die folgenden Ausführungen konzentrieren sich daher bewußt auf Methoden der p h y - s i k a l i s c h e n   T h e r a p i e . Eine weitere Einengung des Themas ergibt sich dadurch, daß allein von Patienten die Rede sein soll, deren Leistungsbegrenzung durch eine c h r o n i s c h e   o b s t r u k t i v e   A t e m w e g s e r - k r a n k u n g bedingt ist und die sich in einem Terminalstadium befinden, das pharmakodynamisch nur noch wenig beeinflußbar ist. In der angelsächsischen Literatur wird dieser Zustand auch als "stable" chronic obstructive lung disease ("stable" COPD) bezeichnet.

R e h a b i l i t a t i o n bedeutet für die Pulmonologie etwas völlig anderes, als es von der Rehabilitation in der Kardiologie bekannt ist. Im Gegensatz zum Herzen ist die Lunge weder morphologisch noch funktionell zu Regenerationsvorgängen in der Lage; im Vergleich zum Infarktpatienten kann dem Emphysempatienten durch ein körperliches Training nur wenig geholfen werden. Es gibt umfangreiche Untersuchungen über den Effekt eines wochenlangen intensiven Trainings am Fahrradergometer oder am Laufband [12, 33]: Allein der Wirkungsgrad der Skelettmuskulatur wurde geringgradig verbessert; an der Lungenfunktion änderte sich nichts.

Eine entscheidende Rolle in der pulmonologischen Rehabilitation spielen heute Methoden der p h y s i k a l i s c h e n   T h e r a p i e . Tabelle 1 zeigt an einigen Beispielen, daß die Liste der b e h a u p t e t e n Effekte umfangreicher ist als die Liste der b e w i e s e n e n Effekte. Immerhin hat die in den letzten Jahren verfeinerte Lungenfunktionsdiagnostik dazu geführt, daß die im Vergleich zur Pharmako-Therapie viel schwerer objektivierbaren Effekte der physikalischen Therapie nach und nach mit Maß und Zahl belegt werden. Als Beispiel sei die B i n d e g e w e b s m a s s a g e genannt, die in einzelnen Fällen zu einer bodyplethysmographisch nachweisbaren Abnahme der Atemwegsresistance führt [32, 41]. Der Effekt ist jedoch nur nachweisbar, wenn die Atemwegsobstruktion partiell reversibel, also auch pharmakodynamisch beeinflußbar ist - eine Voraussetzung, die bei dem hier zu besprechenden Patientenkreis kaum noch gegeben ist.

Die Problematik der B e w e g u n g s t h e r a p i e bei Patienten mit chronischer Atemwegsobstruktion wurde bereits angedeutet; mehr als eine leich-

Tabelle 1. Effekte der physikalischen Therapie bei Patienten mit chronischer obstruktiver Lungenerkrankung

	Behaupteter Effekt	Bewiesener Effekt
LAGERUNGS - und VIBRATIONSTHERAPIE	Sekret-Drainage, Abnahme der R_{aw}, "Kaudalisation" der Ventilation, "Homogenisierung" des $\dot{V}/\dot{Q}$-Verhältnisses	Zunahme der Sputummenge, Abnahme der Sputumviskosität
BEWEGUNGSTHERAPIE	Trainingseffekte an der Atem- und Skelettmuskulatur	Leichte Besserung d. Belastbarkeit
BINDEGEWEBSMASSAGE	Bronchospasmolyse durch Reflexmechanismen	R_{aw}-Abnahme in einzelnen Fällen
ATEMGYMNASTIK	Verbesserung der diaphragmalen und costobasalen Atmung, "Kaudalisation" der Ventilation, Verhinderung des exspirator. Atemwegskollaps, Abnahme der Lungenüberblähung, "Ökonomisierung" der Atmung	Vertiefung und Verlangsamung der Atmung mit geringer Besserung der arteriellen Blutgase, Beeinflussung des Atemwegskollaps
O_2 - LANGZEITTHERAPIE	Beseitigung der art. Hypoxämie, Abnahme des pulmonalen Hochdrucks, Abnahme der R_{aw}, Verbesserung der körperlichen Belastbarkeit, Lebensverlängerung	Anstieg des pO_2 mit geringgradigem pCO_2-Anstieg, Abnahme des Pulmonalisdrucks, Besserung der Belastbarkeit
BEATMUNGSTHERAPIE mit IPPB	Bessere Applizierbarkeit von Aerosolen, Zunahme der alv. Vent., "Homogenisierung" von $\dot{V}/\dot{Q}$, Wiedereröffnung ("Reopening") peripherer Luftwege, Verringerung der Atemarbeit, Verbesserung der mukoziliären Clearance, Lebensverlängerung	Zunahme der alv. Vent. mit Besserung der art. Blutgase, Abnahme d. Atemarbeit, Abnahme der atemsynchronen Schlagvolumenschwankungen; Abnahme der Krankenhausaufenthalte

te Besserung der körperlichen Belastbarkeit läßt sich damit nicht erreichen.Für die Lagerungs - und Vibrations -Therapie ist bisher lediglich bewiesen, daß die Sputummenge zunimmt und die Sputumviskosität abnimmt. Der Beweis für eine behauptete "Homogenisierung" des $\dot{V}/\dot{Q}$-Verhältnisses oder für eine bessere Ventilation der kaudalen Lungenabschnitte ("Kaudalisation") steht jedoch bis heute noch aus. Dagegen sind für die Sauerstoff-Langzeit-Therapie zahlreiche der behaupteten Effekte inzwischen auch bewiesen worden. Ich bin darauf in einem hier vor zwei Jahren gehaltenen Übersichtsreferat ausführlich eingegangen [31]. Im folgenden möchte ich mich auf zwei Behandlungsmethoden der physikalischen Therapie konzentrieren, die sich scheinbar in jeder Beziehung voneinander unterscheiden: IPPB-Therapie und Atemgymnastik.

IPPB-THERAPIE

Die Beatmungs-Therapie mit intermittierendem Überdruck (IPPB) bei Patienten mit Atemwegsobstruktion geht ursprünglich auf die Arbeitsgruppe von Cournand [27] zurück. Sie ist innerhalb des letzten Jahrzehnts in den USA ungewöhnlich populär geworden [2, 7, 28, 36, 48]. Ein extremes Beispiel: Im Lomalinda University Hospital in Los Angeles, einer großen Universitätsklinik mit über 500 Betten, wurden 1973 allein 9% aller aufgenommenen Patienten irgendwann während ihres stationären Aufenthaltes mit IPPB behandelt [2].

In letzter Zeit werden im angelsächsischen Schrifttum jedoch Zweifel laut, ob der Kostenaufwand der IPPB-Therapie im rechten Verhältnis zum

Nutzen steht [7, 9, 11, 16, 19, 21]. In Europa ist dagegen die Einstellung zur IPPB-Therapie nach wie vor positiv: In Deutschland [13, 15, 39, 43, 44], Frankreich [10, 20], Schweden [8] oder in der Schweiz [34, 37] gehört das Beatmungsgerät zum Routineprogramm in der Behandlung chronischer Stadien der Atemwegsobstruktion.

Wie steht es um den objektiven Nutzen der IPPB-Therapie? Konkret gefragt: Ist der Respirator in der Lage, das Leben eines schwer obstruktiven Patienten zu verlängern?

Je nach Anwendungsweise, kann IPPB für den Patienten eine A e r o s o l - T h e r a p i e, eine S a u e r s t o f f - T h e r a p i e, vielleicht sogar eine Form der A t e m g y m n a s t i k bedeuten. Diese Differenzierung ist notwendig, um die zahlreichen IPPB-Studien der Literatur miteinander vergleichen zu können. Auf einem Symposion über IPPB, welches vor zwei Jahren in Amiens stattfand [10], zeigte sich, wie unterschiedlich die Beatmungs-Therapie von den einzelnen Arbeitsgruppen praktiziert wird. Teils wird mit Preßluft beatmet, teils mit einem Sauerstoffgemisch; oft wird gleichzeitig ein Broncholytikum oder ein Mukolytikum eingesetzt. Die Respiratoren unterscheiden sich in der Steuerung (Druck, Volumen, Flow) wie in der Energiequelle (Generator, Gasflasche). Die Frequenz der IPPB-Anwendung schwankt zwischen zwei- bis dreimal pro Woche und vier- bis sechsmal pro Tag. Teils kommen die Patienten ambulant ins Krankenhaus, teils behandeln sie sich selbst zu Hause.

Die meisten Autoren verbinden mit der IPPB-Therapie zwei Z i e l v o r - s t e l l u n g e n:

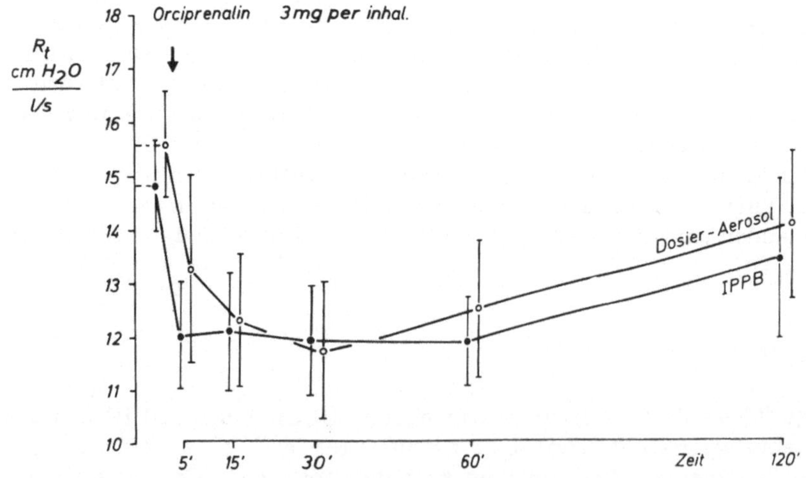

Abb. 1. Einfluß von O r c i p r e n a l i n auf die Atemwegs-Resistance (R_t) von 8 Patienten mit chronischer obstruktiver Lungenerkrankung bei Inhalation aus einem Dosier-Aerosol (4 Einzelhübe) und bei IPPB-Beatmung (Draeger-Assistor). Der Verlauf der beiden Zeit-Wirkungs-Kurven zeigt keine statistisch signifikanten Unterschiede

1. Ein pharmakologisch wirksames Aerosol soll besser in die Tiefe des Tracheobronchialbaums gebracht werden.

2. Das Gerät soll dem schwer dyspnoeischen Patienten einen Teil seiner Atemarbeit abnehmen.

ad 1:

Es ist unbestreitbar, daß man mit einem Respirator ein Aerosol erzeugen kann; aber das ist bekanntlich auch auf einfachere Weise möglich. In Abb. 1 sind Untersuchungsergebnisse von 8 Patienten mit schwerer chronisch obstruktiver Lungenerkrankung dargestellt, die an zwei verschiedenen Tagen morgens zwischen 8 und 10 Uhr eine einmalige Dosis von 3 mg Alupent® inhalierten, das eine Mal aus einem Dosier-Aerosol, das andere Mal während einer 5 Minuten langen IPPB-Beatmung mit einem Draeger-Assistor. Die Darstellung zeigt, daß der Effekt der IPPB-Beatmung nicht besser ist als der Effekt eines einfachen Taschen-Verneblers. Ergänzend muß allerdings bemerkt werden, daß die Patienten vor Beginn dieser Studie eine optimale Inhalationstechnik gelernt hatten - eine Voraussetzung, die in der täglichen Praxis nicht immer gegeben ist.

ad 2:

Es ist experimentell nachgewiesen worden, daß ein Beatmungsgerät dem obstruktiven Patienten einen Teil seiner Atemarbeit abnehmen kann [21]. Es muß aber bezweifelt werden, ob eine IPPB-Therapie, die einige Male am Tag für kurze Perioden durchgeführt wird, die gesamte Atemarbeit über 24 Stunden um einen wirklich relevanten Betrag zu senken vermag. Vielleicht dauern die akuten Wirkungen einer IPPB-Therapie auch in den Intervallen an: Es ist vorstellbar, daß durch Schleim verschlossene Atemwege, die durch den Respirator einmal geöffnet wurden, tatsächlich über Stunden hinweg offenbleiben. Bewiesen ist ein solches "Reopening" aber bis heute nicht [21].

Was bis heute einwandfrei experimentell belegt ist, das sind allein die akuten Effekte der IPPB-Beatmung [13, 15, 30, 39, 43, 44]:
Die alveoläre Ventilation nimmt zu, die arteriellen Blutgase bessern sich, die Atemarbeit nimmt ab. Eine Homogenisierung der Ventilation unter IPPB-Beatmung ließ sich dagegen bislang nicht objektivieren [46]. Nach unseren eigenen Messungen werden die starken atemsynchronen Druckschwankungen, die beim obstruktiven Patienten im Thorax, im Herzen und in den großen Gefäßen auftreten, unter der Beatmung erheblich reduziert. Dem steht aber der ungünstige Effekt entgegen, daß der intrathorakale Mitteldruck ansteigt, wodurch gelegentlich das Herz-Zeit-Volumen abnimmt [36]. Dies ist aber selten von klinischer Relevanz, ebensowenig wie die leichte Zunahme des funktionellen Totraums, die unter IPPB gemessen wurde (Übersicht bei [21]).
So sicher diese akuten Effekte nachgewiesen sind, so fraglich ist es, ob der Respirator dem Patienten auf längere Sicht zu einer besseren körperlichen Belastbarkeit verhilft oder sogar sein Leben zu verlängern vermag. Es gibt zu dieser Frage einige epidemiologische Untersuchun-

gen [13, 43, 44]; im gesamten Weltschrifttum ist mir aber keine prospektive Studie bekannt, in der man unter hieb- und stichfesten Versuchsbedingungen das Schicksal einer IPPB-Patientengruppe mit dem Schicksal einer klinisch und funktionsanalytisch wirklich identischen Kontrollgruppe verglichen hätte.

Eine umfangreiche Untersuchung an mehr als 100 Patienten läuft seit einigen Jahren in Winnipeg (Canada) im Rahmen eines Home Care Program. Cherniack hat vor kurzem ein vorläufiges Ergebnis mitgeteilt [9]: Er fand bisher weder im Verlauf der Lungenfunktionswerte noch in bezug auf die körperliche Belastbarkeit noch in den Überlebenszeiten einen Unterschied zwischen der IPPB-Gruppe einerseits und der Kontrollgruppe andererseits.

Unsere eigenen Patientenzahlen sind zu klein und die Beobachtungszeiten noch zu kurz, um zu der wichtigen Frage der Überlebenszeit Stellung nehmen zu können. Ein Teilergebnis steht bereits fest: Die Zahl der Hospitalisierungen pro Jahr nimmt unter einer Heimbehandlung mit IPPB ab. Diese Beobachtungen haben auch andere Autoren gemacht [8, 20, 44]. Damit entfällt das Argument des zu hohen Kostenaufwandes: Ein einziger eingesparter Krankenhausaufenthalt würde ausreichen, um die Anschaffung eines Respirators zu finanzieren.

ATEMGYMNASTIK

Unter dem Stichwort "Breathing Exercise" findet man im "Index Medicus" Jahr für Jahr eine Fülle von Publikationen, die sich mit dem Thema Atemgymnastik beschäftigen [3, 4, 5, 17, 18, 22, 23, 24, 25, 33, 38, 42, 45, 47]. Die meisten Arbeiten enthalten detaillierte Informationen über die Technik, mit welcher die Atemgymnastik durchgeführt wurde; nur selten finden sich Kommentare über den möglichen pathophysiologischen Hintergrund. Doppelblindstudien über den Effekt einer systematischen Atemgymnastik fehlen bis heute vollständig.

Während die in Tabelle 1 aufgeführten Soforteffekte der Atemgymnastik sicher belegt sind (Übersicht bei [18]), scheiterten bisher jegliche Versuche, Langzeiteffekte zu objektivieren [5, 19, 22, 35, 42].

Nach dem heutigen Stand unserer pathophysiologischen Vorstellungen könnte die Atemgymnastik bei einem Patienten mit fortgeschrittener Bronchialobstruktion folgende Effekte haben:

1. Durch ein Training der diaphragmalen Atmung und der costobasalen Atmung wird die Belüftung der kaudalen Lungenabschnitte verbessert ("Kaudalisation" der Ventilation). Grimby [14] hat mit Hilfe subtiler Radioisotopen-Untersuchungen jedoch feststellen müssen, daß eine wesentliche Änderung der Luftverteilung durch die Atemgymnastik nicht zu erreichen ist.

2. Der Wirkungsgrad der Atemmuskulatur wird durch Atemgymnastik erhöht; vielfach wird von "Ökonomisierung" der Atmung gesprochen. Dazu gehören u. a. Maßnahmen, die das Auftreten des exspiratorischen Bronchialkollaps verhindern sollen: "Lippenbremse", "Lippenpfeife",

"Pursed-lips-breathing" [26, 38, 40, 45]. Es gibt umfangreiche experimentelle Untersuchungen von Ingram und Schilder [17], welche belegen, daß der Patient auf diese Weise tatsächlich den exspiratorischen Bronchialkollaps verhindern kann.

3. Die Atemgymnastik führt zu einer Sekretmobilisierung (Übersicht bei [18]). Zweifellos hustet der Patient nach einer Atemgymnastik vermehrt Sputum ab. Wir wissen aber nicht, ob die erhöhte Sputummenge wirklich auf einer verbesserten Mobilisierung und nicht etwa auf einer Mehrproduktion von Bronchialsekret beruht.

Eine optimale Technik der Atemgymnastik ist nur zu erzielen, wenn die modernen pathophysiologischen Grundlagen der Atemmechanik berücksichtigt werden. Die Altmeister der Atemgymnastik wie Barach [3, 4] und Miller [24, 25] haben sich zu sehr auf die Atemmuskulatur , insbesondere auf das Zwerchfell, konzentriert; die Beeinflussung der gestörten intrapulmonalen Atemmechanik ist nach den gegenwärtigen pathophysiologischen Vorstellungen von mindestens ebenso großer Bedeutung.

Abb. 2 zeigt schematisch in einer dreidimensionalen Darstellung, wodurch die Ventilation und damit auch die Leistung bei einem Patienten mit fortgeschrittener Obstruktion begrenzt wird. Im Gegensatz zum Lungengesunden erreicht der schwer obstruktive Patient den "kritischen Fluß" schon unter Ruheatmung. Jede willkürliche Forcierung der Ausatmung über diese Grenze hinaus bedeutet zusätzliche Atemarbeit ("Blindarbeit"), eine Ventilationssteigerung wird dadurch nicht erreicht. Die in den 50-er Jahren noch vielfach vertretene Ansicht, Patienten mit Bronchialobstruktion müßten die Ausatmungsphase aktiv unterstützen [1, 24, 25, 47], kann heute nicht mehr aufrechterhalten werden.

Der Verlauf des Fluß-Volumen-Diagramms in Abb. 2 zeigt, daß der "kritische Fluß" vom aktuellen Lungenvolumen abhängt: Er wird um so eher erreicht, je tiefer die Atemlage des Patienten ist. Umgekehrt müßte eine Atemgymnastik, bei der der Patient seine Atemlage erhöht, die Strömungsdynamik der Exspirationsphase verbessern.

Wir haben mit dieser Fragestellung an 14 Patienten mit schwerer ob-

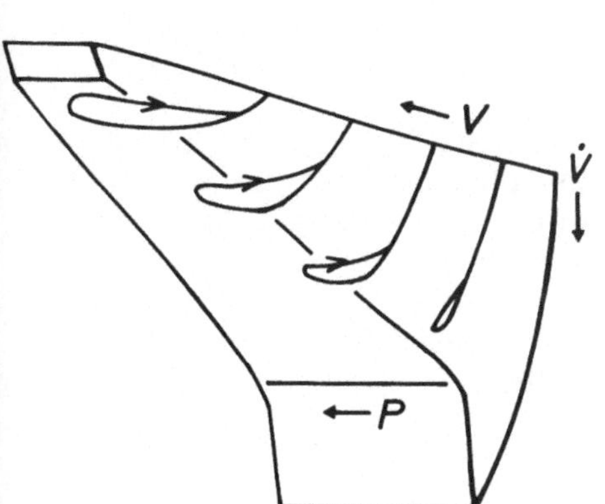

Abb. 2. Zusammenhänge zwischen Alveolardruck (P), exspiratorischer Atemstromstärke (V̇) und aktuellem Lungenvolumen (V) bei einem Patienten mit schwerer chronischer Bronchialobstruktion, dargestellt in einem 3-dimensionalen Diagramm. In das unter forcierter Exspiration gewonnene Fluß-Volumen-Diagramm (V̇/V) sind 4 Druck-Fluß-Diagramme (P/V̇) eingezeichnet, die sich in ihrer Form deutlich voneinander unterscheiden. Einzelheiten s. Text

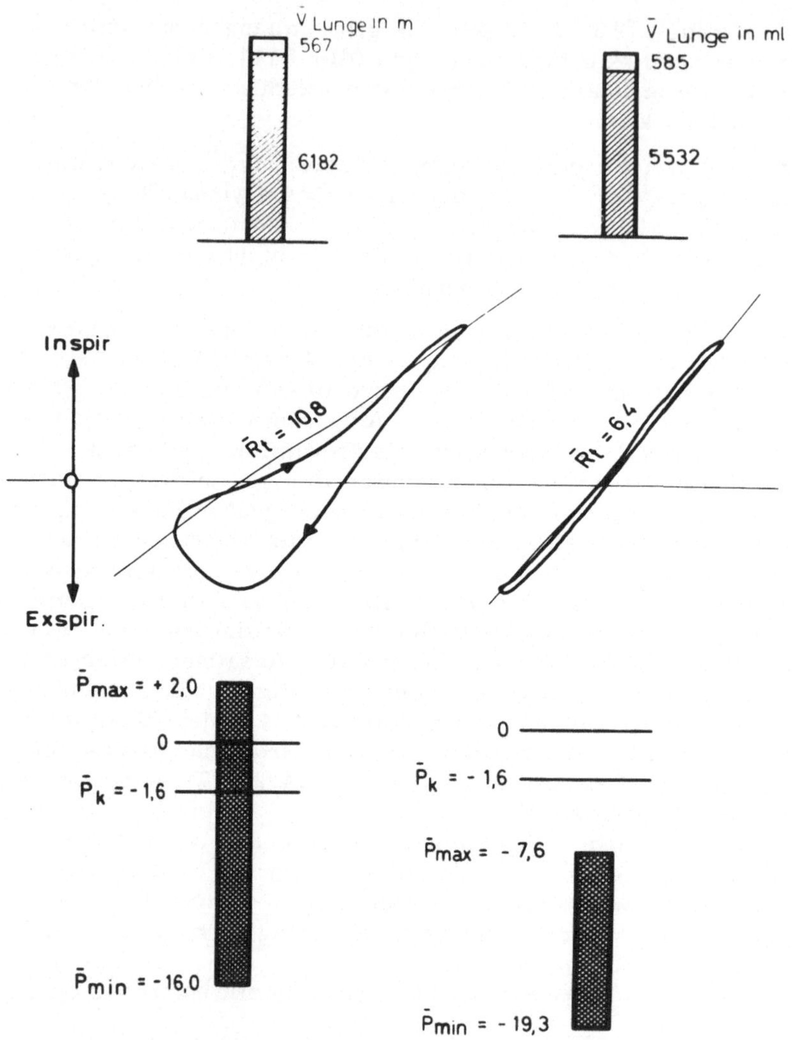

Abb. 3. Mittelwerte des aktuellen Lungenvolumens ($\bar{V}_{Lunge}$, oben), der Atemwegs-Resistance ($\bar{R}_t$, Mitte) und des Ösophagusdrucks (unten) von 14 Patienten mit chronischer obstruktiver Lungenerkrankung bei Spontanatmung (links) und bei Atmung mit willkürlich erhöhter Mittellage (rechts). $\bar{P}_{min}$ = niedrigster inspiratorischer Ösophagusdruck, $\bar{P}_{max}$ = höchster exspiratorischer Ösophagusdruck, $\bar{P}_k$ = Ösophagusdruck im Augenblick des exspiratorischen "Kippens" im Druck-Strömungs-Diagramm (Mitte)

struktiver Atemwegserkrankung atemmechanische Messungen durchgeführt.
Es erwies sich als außerordentlich schwierig, den Patienten einen willkürlichen Atemtyp beizubringen, der zwar die Atemmittellage verändert, nicht
jedoch Atemzugvolumen und Atemfrequenz.

In Abb. 3 sind die Mittelwerte des Gesamtkollektivs graphisch dargestellt. Man erkennt, daß die Atemlage im Mittel um 650 ml angehoben wurde (Anstieg der funktionellen Residualkapazität von 5532 ml auf 6182 ml);
Das Atemzugvolumen blieb dabei weitgehend konstant (567 ml gegenüber
vorher 585 ml). Aus dem unteren Teil der Abbildung geht hervor, daß unter dem künstlichen Atemmanöver der Ösophagusdruck erheblich in den
subatmosphärischen Bereich hinein verlagert wurde; das inspiratorische
Druckminimum verschob sich im Mittel um 3,3 cm H_2O. Die atemsynchronen Schwankungen des Ösophagusdrucks von vorher 18,0 cm H_2O fielen auf
11,7 cm H_2O ab. Der Verlauf des Druckströmungsdiagramms zeigt, wie
dieser Effekt zustande kommt: Durch das künstliche Atemmanöver gelingt
es dem Patienten, den exspiratorischen Bronchialkollaps zu verhindern
und damit unnötige Blindarbeit zu vermeiden: Das exspiratorische "Kip-
pen" des Druckströmungsdiagramms verschwindet, die Atemwegs-Resistance nimmt dadurch im Mittel von 10,8 auf 6,4 cm $H_2O/l/s$ ab.

Die willkürliche Erhöhung der Atemlage führt nicht allein zu einer Verbesserung der Atemmechanik; auch der Gasaustausch wird verbessert.
Abb. 4 zeigt, daß der arterielle Sauerstoffdruck bei einer Erhöhung der
Atemmittellage zunimmt und bei einer Erniedrigung der Atemmittellage
abnimmt. Dieser Effekt beruht auf Änderungen des Ventilations-Perfu-
sions-Verhältnisses.

Dazu paßt die Beobachtung, daß man bei Patienten mit Bronchialobstruktion unter leichter körperlicher Belastung eine Zunahme des arteriellen
pO_2 beobachten kann. Abb. 5 zeigt an einem Kollektiv von 14 Patienten mit
fortgeschrittener chronisch obstruktiver Lungenerkrankung, wie der arterielle Sauerstoffdruck beim Drehen einer ungebremsten Tretkurbel im Mittel von 52 Torr auf 58 Torr ansteigt. Es handelt sich um das gleiche Phänomen wie in Abb. 4: Grimby [14] hat nachgewiesen, daß der obstruktive
Patient unter Belastung spontan seine Atemlage erhöht.

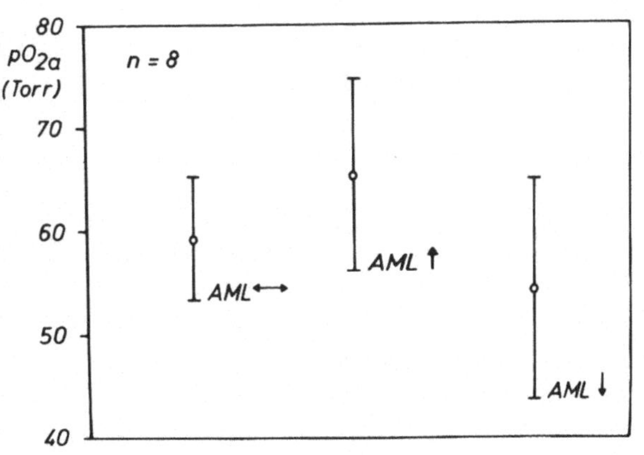

Abb. 4. Verhalten des ar-
teriellen Sauerstoffdrucks
(pO_2a) von 8 Patienten
mit chronischer obstruk-
tiver Lungenerkrankung
bei Spontanatmung, bei
willkürlich erhöhter und
bei willkürlich erniedrigter Atemmittellage (AML)

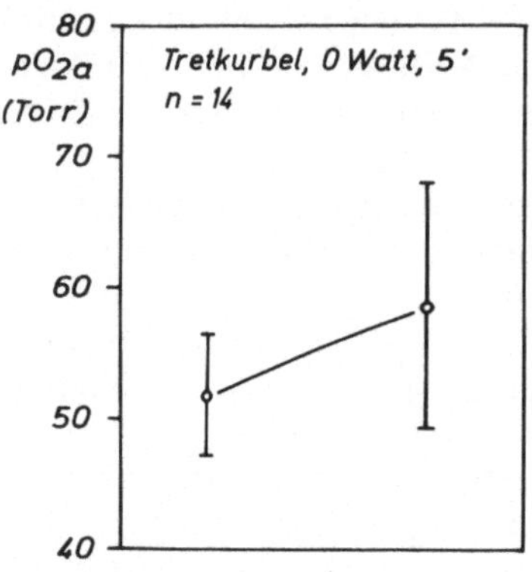

Abb. 5. Verhalten des arteriellen Sauerstoffdrucks (pO_{2a}) von 14 Patienten mit chronischer obstruktiver Lungenerkrankung unter leichter körperlicher Arbeit

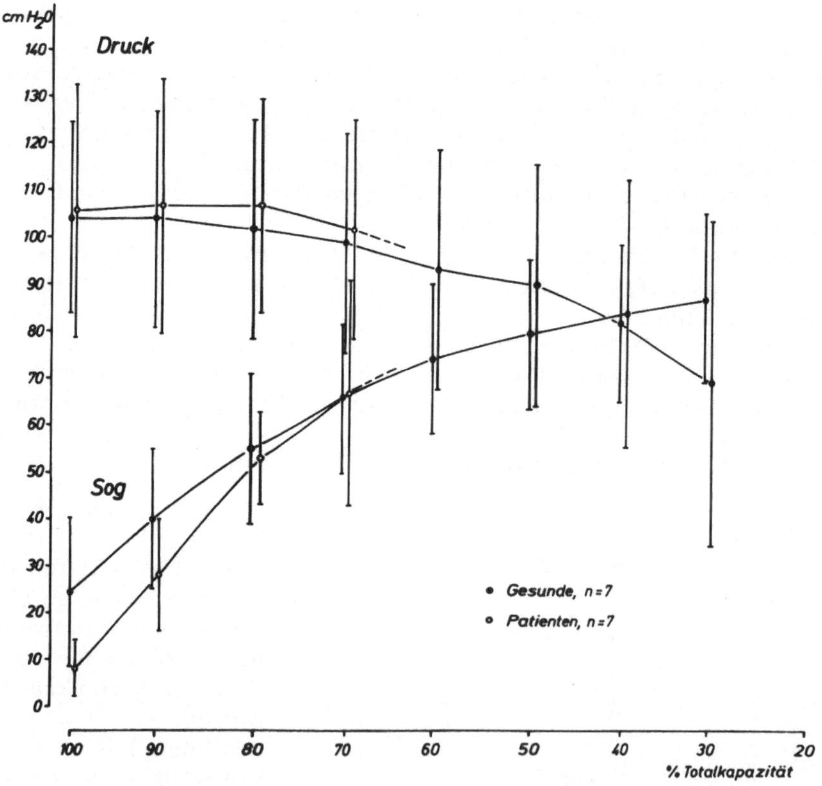

Abb. 6. Abhängigkeit des maximal möglichen Drucks bzw. Sogs gegen das verschlossene Mundstück (Ordinate) von der Atemlage (Abszisse). Einzelheiten s. Text

Leider stößt die Übertragung dieser Ergebnisse in die Praxis der Atemgymnastik auf zwei Schwierigkeiten:
1. Die Atemmittellage von Patienten mit chronischer Bronchialobstruktion ist meist ohnehin durch den Elastizitätsverlust der Lungen schon erhöht. Eine nochmalige willkürliche Erhöhung hätte zur Folge, daß Zwerchfell und inspiratorisch wirkende Interkostalmuskulatur immer mehr gegeneinander wirken: Zwerchfell-Thoraxwand-Antagonismus [46].
2. Die willkürliche Erhöhung der Atemlage führt dazu, daß der Nutzungsgrad der Inspirationsmuskulatur immer schlechter wird, bedingt durch die innere Längen-Spannungs-Beziehung der Muskelfasern [40].

Abb. 6 zeigt Meßergebnisse von 7 Lungengesunden und 7 Patienten mit schwerer chronischer Obstruktion. Ziel der Untersuchung war es, ein Äquivalent für die Kraftentfaltung der Inspirations- und der Exspirationsmuskulatur zu messen. Die einzelnen Probanden wurden aufgefordert, bei zahlreichen unterschiedlichen aktuellen Lungenvolumina gegen das verschlossene Mundstück einen maximalen Sog (= Inspirationsmuskulatur) oder einen maximalen Druck (= Exspirationsmuskulatur) auszuüben. Die Abbildung zeigt deutlich, daß die Kraft der inspiratorisch wirkenden Muskulatur bei niedrigemLungenvolumen größer ist als bei hohem Lungenvolumen. Die Patienten unterscheiden sich hierin prinzipiell nicht von den Gesunden. Abb. 6 zeigt, daß die Patientenkurve "verkürzt" ist; sie liegt in einem Bereich, in dem der Kranke nur noch 3/4 bis 1/4 seiner optimalen Inspirationskraft entwickeln kann. Einer künstlichen Erhöhung der Atemlage ist daher von der muskulären Seite her eine Grenze gesetzt. Dies macht deutlich, wie weit wir noch davon entfernt sind, diese oder jene Atemübung als die pathophysiologisch sinnvollste und für den Patienten nützlichste Form der Atemgymnastik empfehlen zu können.

LITERATUR

1. Allan, W. B. : The benefit of respiratory exercises in the emphysematous patient. Amer. J. Med. Sci. 224, 320 (1952)
2. Baker, J. P. : Magnitude of usage of intermittent positive pressure breathing. Amer. Rev. respir. Dis. 110, 170 (1974)
3. Barach, A. L. : Breathing exercises in pulmonary emphysema and allied chronic respiratory disease. Arch. Phys. Med. Rehabil. 36, 379 (1955)
4. Barach, A. L. : Diaphragmatic breathing in pulmonary emphysema. J. chronic Dis. 1, 211 (1955)
5. Becklake, M. R. , McGregor, M. , Goldman, H. I. , Braudo, J. L. : A study of the effects of physiotherapy in chronic hypertrophic emphysema using lung function tests. Dis. Chest 26, 180 (1954)
6. Berger, D. , Nolte, D. : Die Funktion der Atemmuskulatur bei Patienten mit chronisch obstruktiver Lungenerkrankung unter statischen Bedingungen. Verh. Dtsch. Ges. Inn. Med. im Druck (1976)
7. Birnbaum, M. L. , Cree, E. M. , Rasmussen, H. , Lewis, P. , Curtis, J. K. : Effects of intermittent positive pressure breathing on emphysematous patients. Amer. J. Med. 41, 552 (1966)

8. Brundin, A., Dahlstrom, G., Holmdahlson, M.H.: The indications for respirator treatment in chronic pulmonary disease and some practical views on its performance. Scand. J. resp. Dis., Suppl. 72, 27 (1970)

9. Cherniack, R.M.: Intermittent positive pressure breathing in management of chronic obstructive pulmonary disease: current state of the art. Amer. Rev. resp. Dis. 110, 188 (1974)

10. Colloque sur le traitement ambulatoire des insuffisants respiratoires chroniques graves par l'assistance ventilatoire et l'oxygénothérapie. Amien, France, 25.-26.5.1973

11. Curtis, J.K., Ashley, P.L., Rasmussen, H.K., Cree, E.M.: IPPB therapy in chronic obstructive pulmonary disease. J. Amer. med. Ass. 206, 1037 (1968)

12. Degre, S., Sergysels, R., Messin, R., Vandermoten, P., Salhadin, P., Denolin, H., Coster, A. de: Hemodynamic responses to physical training in patients with chronic lung disease. Amer. Rev. resp. Dis. 110, 395 (1974)

13. Ferlinz, R.: Der Effekt von Aerosolen mit und ohne intermittierende Überdruckbeatmung. Respiration 27 (Suppl.), 181 (1970)

14. Grimby, G.: Aspects of lung expansion in relation to pulmonary physiotherapy. Amer. Rev. resp. Dis. 110, 145 (1974)

15. Günthner, W., Greiner, L., Schmidt, O.P.: Zur Therapie des chronisch-obstruktiven Atemwegssyndroms: die intermittierend positive Druckbeatmung. Fortschr. Med. 92, 857 (1974)

16. Hyatt, R.E.: Intermittent positive breathing therapy. Introduction. Amer. Rev. resp. Dis. 110, 169 (1974)

17. Ingram, R.H., Schilder, D.P.: The effect of pursed lips expiration on the pulmonary pressure-flow relationship in obstructive lung disease. Amer. Rev. resp. Dis. 96, 381 (1967)

18. Jones, N.J.: Physical therapy - present state of the art. Amer. Rev. resp. Dis. 110, 132 (1974)

19. Lefcoe, N.M., Paterson, N.A.M.: Adjunct therapy in chronic obstructive pulmonary disease. Amer. J. Med. 54, 343 (1973)

20. Lévi-Valensi, P., Duwoos, H., Echter, E., Rousselin, L., Giroulle, H., Abric, J., Bernard, F., Lebris, P., Vonachen, P.: Les respirateurs à domicile dans le traitement des insuffisants respiratoires chroniques graves. Indications et conditions d'efficacité. Poumon 26, 1219 (1970)

21. Loke, J., Anthonisen, N.R.: Effect of intermittent positive pressure breathing on steady state chronic obstructive pulmonary disease. Amer. Rev. resp. Dis. 110, 178 (1974)

22. McNeil, R.S., McKenzie, J.M.: Assessment of the value of breathing exercises in chronic bronchitis and asthma. Thorax 10, 250 (1955)

23. Mellins, R.B.: Pulmonary physiotherapy in the pediatric group. Amer. Rev. resp. Dis. 110, 137 (1974)

24. Miller, W.F.: A physiologic evaluation of the effects of diaphragmatic breathing training in patients with chronic pulmonary emphysema. Amer. J. Med. 17, 471 (1954)

25. Miller, M. E. : Respiratory exercises for chronic pulmonary emphysema. Bull. John Hopkins Hosp. 92, 185 (1953)
26. Motley, H. L. : The effects of slow deep breathing on the blood gas exchange in emphysema. Amer. Rev. resp. Dis. 88, 485 (1963)
27. Motley, H. L., Werkö, L., Cournand, A., Richards, D. W. : Observations on the clinical use of intermittent positive pressure. J. Aviat. Med. 18, 417 (1947)
28. Murray, J. F. : Review of the state of the art in intermittent positive pressure breathing therapy. Amer. Rev. resp. Dis. 110, 193 (1974)
29. Nolte, D. : Die Strömungsmechanik der Atemwege bei der obstruktiven Ventilationsstörung. Habil.-Schrift, Gießen 1970
30. Nolte, D. : Endotracheale Respiratorbeatmung - Ultima ratio bei der chronischen respiratorischen Insuffizienz. Prax. Pneumol. 26, 22 (1972)
31. Nolte, D. : Hyperoxieatmung bei Patienten mit alveolärer Hypoventilation. Pneumonologie 149, 55 (1973)
32. Nolte, D. : Möglichkeiten der modernen Funktionsdiagnostik bei chronischen Lungenerkrankungen als Grundlage für die Anwendung physiotherapeutischer Maßnahmen. Physiother. 66, 663 (1975)
33. Paez, A., Eliot, P., Masangkay, M., Sproule, B. J. : The physiologic basis of training patients with emphysema. Amer. Rev. resp. Dis. 95, 944 (1967)
34. Perruchoud, A., Keller, R., Herzog, H. : Der Effekt kombinierter atemphysiotherapeutischer Maßnahmen auf den pulmonalen Gasaustausch und die Ventilation. 55. Wiss. Tag. Schweiz. Ges. Lungen- u. Tuberkuloseärzte, Genf, 25.-26. 4. 1975
35. Petty, Th. L. : Physical therapy. Introduction. Amer. Rev. resp. Dis. 110, 129 (1974)
36. Pierce, A. K. : Assisted respiration. Ann. Rev. Med. 20, 431 (1969)
37. Scherrer, M. : Hausbehandlung der chronischen Ateminsuffizienz. Schweiz. Rundschau Med. 59, 506 (1970)
38. Schmidt, R. W., Wasserman, K., Lillington, G. R. : The effect of air flow and oral pressure on the mechanics of breathing in patients with asthma and emphysema. Amer. Rev. resp. Dis. 90, 564 (1964)
39. Seith, U. : Inhalation mit intermittierendem Überdruck bei chronisch obstruktiven Lungenerkrankungen. Prax. Pneumol. 26, 353 (1972)
40. Sharp, J. T., Danon, J., Druz, W. S., Goldberg, N. B., Fishman, H., Machnach, W. : Respiratory muscle function in patients with chronic obstructive pulmonary disease: Its relationship to disability and to respiratory therapy. Amer. Rev. resp. Dis. 110, 154 (1974)
41. Siemon, G., Thoma, R., Ehrenberg, R. : Der Einfluß physikalischer Therapie auf den Bronchialwiderstand bei chronischen Atemwegserkrankungen. 6. Int. Kongr. Physikal. Med., Barcelona, 2.-6. 7. 1972
42. Sinclair, J. D. : The effects of breathing exercises in pulmonary emphysema. Thorax 10, 246 (1955)
43. Stadeler, H. J., Ferlinz, R., Püster, D. : Atemfunktionelle Untersuchungen über den Effekt einer Aerosoltherapie mittels ambulanter, assistierter Überdruckbeatmung beim chronisch-obstruktiven Syndrom. Verh. dtsch. Ges. inn. Med. 75, 944 (1969)

44. Steurich, F. : Hausbehandlung der chronischen obstruktiven Lungen-
    krankheiten durch intermittierende assistierte Überdruckbeatmung.
    Prax. Pneumol. 27, 730 (1973)
45. Thoman, R. L. , Stoker, G. L. , Ross, J. C. : The efficacy of pursed-
    lips breathing in patients with chronic obstructive pulmonary disease.
    Amer. Rev. resp. Dis. 93, 100 (1966)
46. Ulmer, W. T. , Reif, E. , Weller, W. : Die obstruktiven Atemwegser-
    krankungen. Stuttgart: Georg Thieme Verlag 1966
47. Weiser, H. I. : Respiratory disturbances treated by breathing exercise.
    Brit. J. Phys. Med. 13, 128 (1950)
48. Williams, M. H. : Ventilatory failure. Medicine (Baltimore) 45, 317
    (1966)

Prof. Dr. D. Nolte
Städtisches Krankenhaus
Riedelstraße 5
D-8230 Bad Reichenhall

E. Kehler, Bleckede: Ich möchte ganz konkret fragen, ob man sich einer
medizinischen Unterlassung schuldig macht, wenn man bei chronisch obstruktiven Lungenkrankheiten auf IPPB verzichtet.

D. Nolte, Bad Reichenhall: Die Polemik, die in dieser Frage steckt, geht
etwas über die Grenzen meines Referats hinaus. Ich habe darauf hinweisen
wollen, daß wir noch keine hieb- und stichfesten Befunde in der Hand haben,
die einen positiven Langzeiteffekt der IPPB-Behandlung beweisen könnten;
bei einem Patienten, an dem das gesamte konventionelle therapeutische
Repertoire schon versucht wurde, gibt es aber nicht nur streng-medizini-
sche Indikationen für eine Behandlungsmethode. Die Frage, ob man bei
der chronisch obstruktiven Lungenerkrankung mit IPPB behandeln soll
oder nicht, kann sich nur an den Besonderheiten jedes einzelnen Krank-
heitsfalles orientieren. Sie ist nach unserem heutigen Wissenstand noch
nicht allgemeinverbindlich zu beantworten und muß bis dahin dem Ermes-
sen, der Verantwortung und der persönlichen Erfahrung des jeweiligen be-
handelnden Arztes überlassen bleiben.

Pneumonologie Suppl. 1976, 75-96

Begutachtungsgrundlagen für die Leistungsbegrenzung von seiten der Lunge *

U. Smidt und G. Worth

Innere Abteilung des Krankenhaus Bethanien für die Grafschaft Moers, Moers

Principles for the assessment of working disability due to disorders of the lung

---

Abstract. In the frame of assessment of lung disorders we have to check not only, whether the lung is the limiting factor for the physical working capacity, but also the grade of a non-limiting functional disorder of the lung. Dyspnea is the most common complaint of such patients, but it is not specific for lung disorders.

It is shown by follow-up studies in 265 coal miners, which have been examined 2 to 6 times within 11 years, that neither vital capacity, nor arterial pO_2 nor airway resistance are stable enough to serve as a basis for our judgement, when we have only one of those parameters.

The evaluation of 1481 medical assessments of working disability in coal miners has shown, that the above mentioned functional parameters and FEV_1 do not play the main role for the physician, but more stable factors as age and the X-ray grade of pneumoconiosis have a higher importance.

From ergometric examinations in more than 3000 subjects we conclude that an increased specific ventilation besides an increase of airway resistance is an important measure for an increased work of breathing, which is sensitized as dyspnea. However, a pulmonary dyspnea may be caused also by pulmonary hypertension, so that in the single patient we have to apply all necessary methods to understand the causes of his dyspnea.

Key words: Assessment of functional pulmonary disturbances - Limiting factors for working capacity - Vital capacity - FEV_1 - Airway resistance - Arterial pO_2 - Specific ventilation - Pulmonary hypertension - Pneumoconiosis

---

* Mit Unterstützung durch die Hohe Kommission der Europäischen Gemeinschaften, Luxemburg, und die Deutsche Forschungsgemeinschaft.

Zusammenfassung: Im Rahmen der Begutachtung von Lungenerkrankungen ist nicht nur zu prüfen, ob die Lunge der limitierende Faktor für die Leistungsfähigkeit ist, sondern auch der Grad einer nicht leistungsbegrenzenden Funktionsstörung der Lunge zu ermitteln. Als Klage des Patienten steht die Dyspnoe ganz im Vordergrund, aber dies Symptom ist nicht spezifisch für eine Lungenerkrankung.

An Längsschnittuntersuchungen von 265 Kohlenbergarbeitern, die innerhalb von bis zu 11 Jahren bis zu 6mal untersucht wurden, wird gezeigt, daß weder die Vitalkapazität, noch der arterielle pO_2 noch die Resistance stabil genug sind, um allein auf eine dieser Größen ein gutachterliches Urteil zu stützen.

Die Auswertung von 1481 Gutachten an Kohlenbergarbeitern ergab, daß weder die drei genannten Funktionsgrößen, noch der Atemstoßwert die Hauptrolle für den Gutachter bei der Einschätzung der Minderung der Erwerbsfähigkeit spielen, sondern stabilere Faktoren wie das Lebensalter und der röntgenologische Pneumokoniosegrad.

Aus eingehenden ergometrischen Untersuchungen an über 3000 Probanden ergibt sich, daß eine im Verhältnis zur O_2-Aufnahme gesteigerte Ventilation, d. h. ein vergrößertes Atemäquivalent, neben erhöhten Strömungswiderständen ein wichtiges Maß für eine erhöhte Atemarbeit ist, die als Dyspnoe empfunden wird. Eine pulmonal bedingte Dyspnoe kann aber auch auf einer pulmonalen Hypertonie beruhen, so daß wir im Einzelfall mit allen verfügbaren Mitteln versuchen müssen, die Ursache einer Dyspnoe zu klären.

Schlüsselwörter: Beurteilung pulmonaler Funktionsstörungen - leistungsbegrenzende Faktoren - Vitalkapazität - Atemstoß - Atemwegsresistance - arterieller pO_2 - spezifische Ventilation - pulmonale Hypertonie - Pneumokoniose

---

Im Rahmen der Begutachtungsgrundlagen für die Leistungsbegrenzung vonseiten der Lunge geht es nicht um die Kausalitätsbeziehung zwischen verschiedenen Noxen und deren funktionellen Folgen, sondern um die Frage, ob bzw. inwieweit eine Begrenzung oder Einschränkung der körperlichen Leistungsfähigkeit ursächlich auf die Lunge, d. h. auf pulmonale Erkrankungen bezogen werden kann.

Beim Gesunden ist die Lunge sicher nicht der leistungsbegrenzende Faktor. Hier spielen vielmehr der Trainingszustand der Muskulatur, ihre Kapillarisierung und das kardiovaskuläre System die Hauptrolle.

Körperliches Training führt dagegen nicht zu einer wesentlichen Steigerung der Funktionsreserven einer gesunden Lunge (Hollmann, 1959). Weder für die Vitalkapazität, noch für den Einsekundenwert, das Residualvolumen, die Resistance oder die Blutgase in Ruhe oder während Belastung noch für den Atemgrenzwert gibt es wesentliche Unterschiede zwischen körperlich Trainierten und Untrainierten. Diese Tatsache sollte eigentlich die gutachterliche Beurteilung des Einzelfalles erleichtern, da eine Funktionsminderung eben nicht von dem vorherigen Trainingszustand abhängig ist. Andererseits ist aber die Streubreite der Norm - vor allem für die spirometrischen Werte - so groß, daß Unterschiede von 1 Liter oft noch keine sichere Zuordnung zum pathologischen Bereich erlauben.

Im Rahmen der Begutachtung von Lungenerkrankungen ist aber nicht nur zu prüfen, ob die Lunge der limitierende Faktor für die Leistungsfähigkeit ist (Becklake, 1975). Wäre das allein entscheidend, so wäre allen jenen Fällen keine Entschädigung für eine Lungenerkrankung zuzubilligen, bei denen ein anderes Organ, unabhängig von der Lungenerkrankung, die Leistungsfähigkeit begrenzt. Wenn z. B. ein Patient infolge eines angedehnten Herzinfarktes so stark leistungsgemindert ist, daß seine maximale O_2-Aufnahme weniger als 1 l/min beträgt, so müßte ihm eine Rente wegen einer davon unabhängigen pulmonalen Erkrankung verweigert werden, wenn seine Lunge noch eine O_2-Aufnahme von mehr als 1 l/min zuließe. Das hat der Gesetzgeber aber nicht vorgesehen, denn dann müßte auch eine wegen einer Lungenerkrankung gezahlte Rente wieder entzogen werden, wenn eines Tages eine andere Erkrankung, z. B. eine Koronarsklerose, hinzutritt und sich leistungsbegrenzend auswirkt. Lediglich in dem Fall, daß eine erstmalige Anerkennung einer berufsbedingten Lungenerkrankung erst dann erfolgt, wenn aus anderen Gründen schon eine Erwerbsunfähigkeit vorliegt, wird keine zusätzliche Entschädigung mehr gewährt.

In allen übrigen Fällen geht es bei der gutachterlichen Beurteilung von Lungenerkrankungen also nicht nur darum, ob die körperliche Leistungsfähigkeit durch die Lunge limitiert ist oder nicht, sondern auch um den Grad einer nicht leistungsbegrenzenden Funktionsstörung, d. h. darum, mit welchem Aufwand an Arbeit die jeweilige Ventilation und Perfusion und somit der Gasaustausch in der Lunge erzielt wird.

Dafür gibt es bis heute kein einzelnes Kriterium, das schon eine breitere Anerkennung gefunden hätte. Wassner (1961) empfahl den einseitigen CO_2-Rückatmungsversuch und definierte die untere Leistungsgrenze der Lunge als dann erreicht, wenn die andere Lungenseite in Ruhe nicht ausreicht, um soviel CO_2 abzuatmen, daß der arterielle pCO_2 nicht ansteigt. Das ist aber nur eine sehr grobe Definition, die allenfalls zur Beurteilung der Durchführbarkeit von Lungenresektionen geeignet ist. Hertz (1965, 1974) betont vor allem die Bedeutung des Abfalls des arteriellen pO_2 unter ansteigender Körperbelastung und weist darauf hin, daß dies durch einen ungenügenden Anstieg der Ventilation oder der Diffusionskapazität bedingt sein kann. Wenn infolge eines ungenügenden Herzminutenvolumens die Sauerstoffausschöpfung des Blutes größer wird, so daß der gemischt-venöse pO_2 absinkt, könnte es auch über einen - gleichbleibenden - Shuntanteil zu einem Abfall des arteriellen pO_2 kommen. Diese Hypothese ist aber noch nicht experimentell geprüft. Hertz empfiehlt, als "respiratorische Leistungsgrenze" diejenige Belastungsstufe - ausgedrückt durch die Sauerstoffaufnahme - zu definieren, bei der der arterielle pO_2 eben noch nicht abfällt. Man müsse jenseits dieses Punktes mindestens noch zwei Meßwerte mit erniedrigtem pO_2 haben, um einen Abfall mit genügender Sicherheit annehmen zu können. Hertz gibt aber zu, daß die Lungenfunktion auch ohne Beeinflussung der Blutgase gestört sein kann. Woitowitz (1971) und Reichel (1974) haben gezeigt, daß auch bei Gesunden z. T. ein recht erheblicher Abfall des arteriellen pO_2 unter Belastung vorkommt und messen deshalb ebenso wie Ulmer und Reichel (1963) dem Verhalten

der Blutgase bei Belastung keine große praktische Bedeutung für die Beurteilung der Leistungsfähigkeit zu.

Nach unseren Beobachtungen ist ein Anstieg des arteriellen pO_2 während Belastung selbst bei Lungenkranken weit häufiger als ein Abfall, ge-
schweige denn ein kontinuierlicher Abfall mit steigender Belastung. Es
wird also auch nicht wenige Kombinationsfälle geben, bei denen pathophysiologische Gründe für einen Anstieg und für einen Abfall so zusammenwirken,
daß die Belastungsstufe, bei der dieser Abfall eintritt, oder auch dessen
Ausmaß nicht dem Ausmaß der Lungenfunktionsstörung entspricht.

Wir erleben es bei ergometrischen Untersuchungen jedenfalls sehr häufig, daß die Kohlenbergarbeiter, die wir gutachterlich untersuchen, die
Belastung vorzeitig abbrechen, ohne daß der arterielle Sauerstoffdruck abfällt und auch ohne daß - als Ausdruck der kardialen Leistungsgrenze - eine
maximale Pulsfrequenz erreicht ist. Als Grund geben diese Patienten auch
keine allgemeine Erschöpfung an, wie man dies bei mangelhaft Trainierten
findet, sondern sie klagen über Atemnot.

Wenn ein Patient eine Begutachtung zum Zwecke der Entschädigung
wünscht, wird er in der Regel ebenfalls Atemnot als Hauptklage angeben
oder noch allgemeiner sagen, daß er körperlich nicht mehr so leistungs-
fähig oder schneller erschöpft sei als früher. Unsere Aufgabe im Rahmen
der Begutachtung ist es, diese Klage zu objektivieren, um so den versiche-
rungsrechtlichen Ansprüchen zu genügen und die Grundlage für eine gerech-
te Beurteilung zu schaffen. Die Begutachtung sollte auf Parametern basie-
ren, denen
- Spezifität für das Organ Lunge und
- Validität für die Beurteilung ihrer Funktionsstörung
zukommt.

Fletcher hat 1952 vier Grade der Dyspnoe unterschieden:
- Kurzatmigkeit beim Treppensteigen oder bei schnellem Gehen in der
  Ebene
- Kurzatmigkeit bei normalem Gehen in der Ebene
- Kurzatmigkeit bei langsamen Gehen in der Ebene
- Kurzatmigkeit in Ruhe

Wie läßt sich nun eine Dyspnoe objektivieren und feststellen, ob sie pulmonal verursacht ist?

Eine große Zahl von Begutachtungen - insbesondere auch bei der Pneumokoniose des Kohlenbergarbeiters - stützt sich heute noch auf das Verhalten von Pulsfrequenz, Blutdruck und Lippenzyanose nach 10 Kniebeugen,
obwohl diese Parameter nichts mit der Lunge zu tun haben, sondern allenfalls eine sehr grobes Maß für die Herz-Kreislauffunktion sind.

SPIROMETRIE

Ärzte, die nur ein einfaches Spirometer als technisches Hilfsmittel zur
Verfügung haben, stützen ihre Einschätzung der pulmonal bedingten Minderung der Erwerbsfähigkeit auf eine Verminderung der Vitalkapazität und
des Einsekundenwertes. Für eine Graduierung der MdE sind diese Größen
aber leider absolut ungeeignet, weil sie

1. zu stark von der Mitarbeit des Patienten und auch dem Engagement
   der MTA abhängen
2. bei wiederholten Messungen - auch bei gleichbleibender Mitarbeit -
   stark schwanken können
3. nur eine sehr lockere Beziehung zu einer pulmonal bedingten Leistungsbegrenzung haben.

Cotes (1975) hat Fletcher's Dyspnoe-Grade mit dem Atemstoßwert bei
125 Kohlenbergarbeitern, die im Rahmen einer ärztlichen Behandlung untersucht wurden, und bei 125 Kohlenbergarbeitern (mit vergleichbarem
Alter, Pneumokoniosegrad, Größe und Gewicht), die begutachtet wurden,
verglichen und gezeigt, daß letztere bei dem gleichen Atemstoßwert im
Schnitt einen signifikant höheren Dyspnoegrad angeben, also offenbar ihre
Dyspnoe stärker bewerten. Maas und Krause (1967) haben versucht, solche Diskrepanzen zwischen geklagten Beschwerden und objektivem Befund
durch zusätzliche psychologische Tests zu klären. Die Autoren weisen aber
auch mit Recht darauf hin, daß unsere klinischen Funktionsprüfungen bisher nur einzelne Sektoren des Spektrums erfassen, das insgesamt die
Leistungsfähigkeit im Alltag und am Arbeitsplatz bestimmt. Wir können
deshalb nicht unterstellen, daß unsere Funktionsprüfungen immer ein kor-
rekteres Bild als die Angaben des Patienten ergeben. Bei der Begutachtung stehen wir indessen grundsätzlich vor der Aufgabe, die Beschwerden
des Patienten zu objektivieren.

Statt von einem theoretischen Ansatz der zu erwartenden Pathomechanismen und ihrer Folgen auszugehen, seien hier zunächst einmal einige
Daten aus der gegenwärtigen Begutachtungspraxis vorangestellt.

Wir haben im letzten Jahr aus den Akten von 265 Kohlenbergarbeitern,
die zum zweiten bis sechsten Mal innerhalb der letzten 11 Jahre untersucht wurden, die funktionsanalytischen Daten dieser Untersuchungen her-
ausgezogen. Von den so ausgewerteten 978 Untersuchungen sind 685 bei
uns, 229 in Bochum, 40 in Aachen und 24 in verschiedenen anderen Kliniken durchgeführt worden.

Abb. 1 zeigt, wie groß die Schwankungen der Vitalkapazität von einer
Untersuchung bis zur nächsten, die im Mittel nach 2, 1 Jahren erfolgte, sind.
Es ist kaum anzunehmen, daß eine pulmonal bedingte Leistungsbegrenzung
oder auch nur Funktionsstörung ebenso große Schwankungen aufweist.
Sonst müßte jede gutachterliche Beurteilung mindestens nach Jahresfrist
überprüft werden. Das Ausmaß der Schwankungen der Vitalkapazität wird
auch nicht kleiner, wenn man nur die im gleichen Institut erhobenen Werte
vergleicht.

BLUTGASE

Wenn wir von den gleichen Fällen den arteriellen Sauerstoffdruck in Ruhe
betrachten, so ist die Schwankung nicht viel geringer (Abb. 2). Die Ursachen dieser Schwankungen sind bisher völlig ungeklärt. Wir sind aber
sicher, daß es sich nicht um Fehlmessungen handelt.

Einigkeit besteht wohl darüber, daß ein über 45 torr erhöhter arterieller pCO_2 Ausdruck einer fortgeschrittenen, meist obstruktiven Lungener-

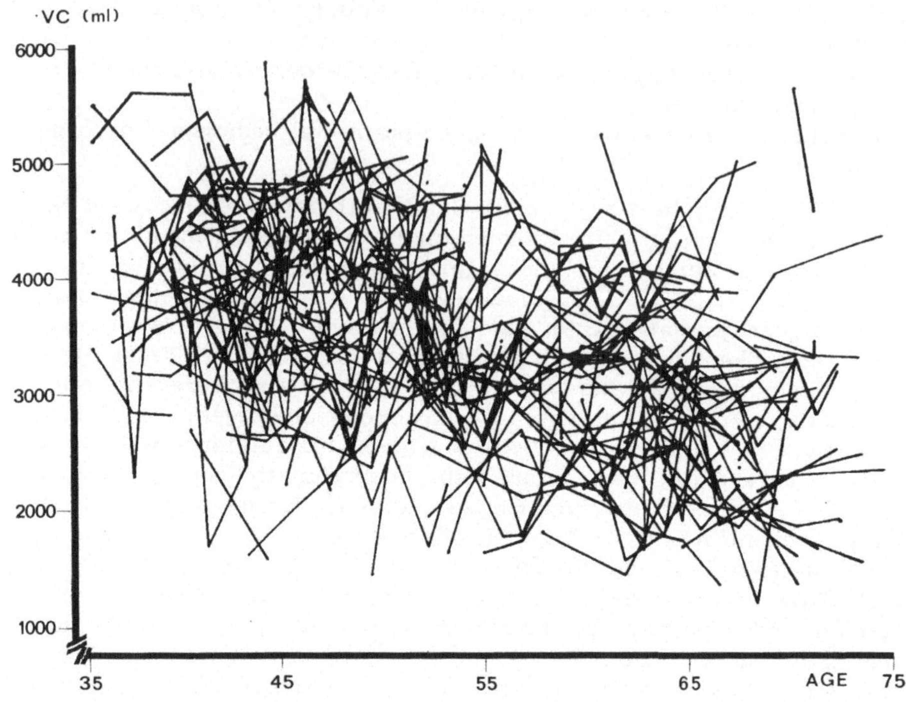

Abb. 1. Verlauf der Vitalkapazität in Abhängigkeit vom Lebensalter bei 265 Gutachtenpatienten, die im Verlauf von 2-11 Jahren 2-6mal untersucht wurden. Die Meßwerte des gleichen Patienten sind durch Striche verbunden

krankung ist, aber derartige Werte sind im Rahmen der Begutachtung eine Seltenheit. Mit prognostischen Aussagen sollte man auch bei stark pathologischen Blutgaswerten sehr vorsichtig sein. Wir haben bei einem Patienten, den wir innerhalb von 9 Jahren mehrmals gutachterlich untersucht haben, schon 1966 einen arteriellen pO_2 von 55 torr und einen pCO_2 von 44 torr gemessen.

STRÖMUNGSWIDERSTÄNDE IN DEN ATEMWEGEN

Daß die Bestimmung der Resistance nicht von der Mitarbeit des Probanden oder der MTA abhängt, sondern ein sehr objektives Maß einer endobronchialen Atemwegsobstruktion ist, wird allgemein anerkannt, ebenso daß eine deutliche Erhöhung eine Einschränkung der pulmonalen Leistungsbreite bedeutet. Wollten wir aber die Resistance zur Grundlage der Begutachtung machen, müßten wir ähnliche Schwankungen hinnehmen, wie bei der Vitalkapazität und dem arteriellen pO_2 (Abb. 3). Auch zum Grad der subjektiven Dyspnoe zeigt die Resistance nur eine relativ lockere Korrelation.

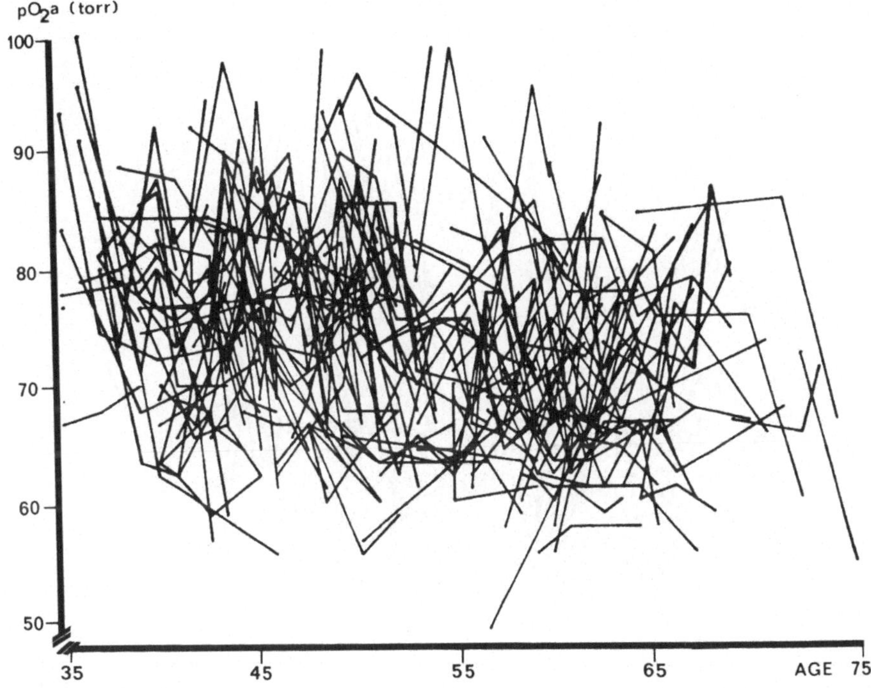

Abb. 2. Verlauf des arteriellen Sauerstoffdrucks bei den gleichen Patienten und in gleicher Darstellung wie in Abb. 1

Es wird zwar nur selten bei Patienten mit einer hohen Resistance eine Dyspnoe vermißt, aber auch viele Patienten mit normaler Resistance klagen über Dyspnoe, vor allem bei Belastung. Dies gilt vor allem für Patienten mit einem Lungenemphysem. Wir können also ähnlich wie beim starken Abfall des arteriellen pO_2 unter ansteigender Belastung sagen: eine erhöhte Resistance ist zwar ein spezifisches, aber kein sensibles Zeichen für eine pulmonale Funktionsstörung.

GEGENWÄRTIGE PRAXIS DER BEGUTACHTUNG

Wir haben weiterhin versucht, empirisch festzustellen, auf welche Befunde die Gutachter bei der Kohlenbergarbeiterpneumokoniose ihre Einschätzung der MdE stützen. Dazu haben wir von 1481 Bergarbeitern mit verschiedenen Graden der Pneumokoniose den Grad der MdE und die Häufigkeit pathologischer Werte für
- die Vitalkapazität
- den Atemstoßwert
- den arteriellen pO_2 in Ruhe und
- die Resistance
ermittelt (Abb. 4). Als Grenzen des Normalen nahmen wir für die Vital-

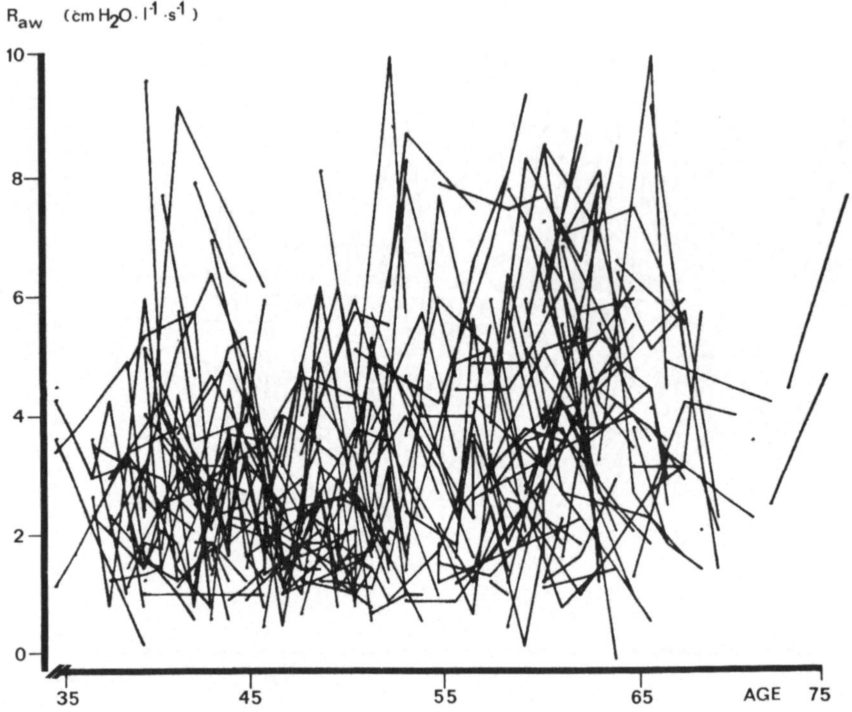

Abb. 3. Verlauf des Strömungswiderstandes in den Atemwegen bei den gleichen Patienten und in gleicher Darstellung wie in Abb. 1

kapazität und den Atemstoßwert jeweils 75% des Sollwertes, der anhand der Formeln

$$VK \ (1) = m^3 \cdot (1.03 - (\frac{a-25}{100})^2 \cdot 0.75) \qquad (1)$$

$$AST \ (1) = m^3 \cdot (0.82 - (\frac{a-22}{100})^2) \qquad (2)$$

m = Größe in Metern   a = Alter in Jahren

die Smidt et al. (1970) für die Sollwerttabellen der Europäischen Gemeinschaft aufgestellt haben, berechnet wurde.

Zur Sollwertbestimmung des arteriellen pO_2 benutzen wir die Beziehung

$$pO_2 a \ (torr) = 96.2 - 0.4 \cdot a \qquad (3)$$

und haben Werte unter 90% dieses Sollwertes als pathologisch angesehen.

Für die Resistance haben wir einen Grenzwert von 5 cmH_2O/l/s benutzt.

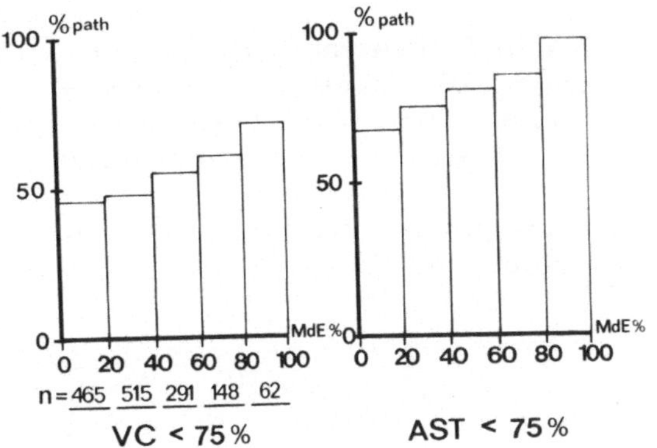

Abb. 4. Häufigkeit pathologischer Werte für die Vitalkapazität, den Atemstoßwert, den arteriellen pO_2 und die Resistance in Beziehung zu dem Prozentsatz der Minderung der Erwerbsfähigkeit bei 1481 Bergarbeitern mit verschiedenen Silikose-Graden

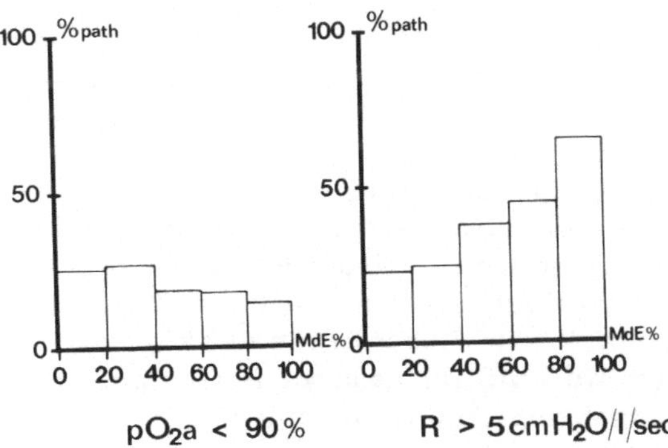

Die Vitalkapazität war schon in 46% derjenigen Fälle pathologisch, die weniger als 20% erwerbsgemindert waren, d. h. keine Entschädigung bekamen. Bei den Patienten mit einer MdE von 80-100% steigt die Häufigkeit einer erniedrigten VK auf 71% an. In der gleichen MdE-Spannweite steigt die Häufigkeit eines pathologischen Atemstoßwertes von 67% auf 96,8%.

Die Häufigkeit eines erniedrigten arteriellen pO_2 fällt mit steigender MdE sogar etwas ab, was aber nicht bedeutet, daß die Absolutwerte ansteigen.

Die Resistance zeigt mit 21% pathologischen Werten die geringste Häufigkeit in der Gruppe unter 20% MdE und den stärksten Häufigkeitsanstieg (63%) bis zur höchsten MdE-Gruppe.

Prüft man, wie oft gleichzeitig mehrere dieser Parameter in den verschiedenen Entschädigungsstufen pathologisch sind (Abb. 5), so ist der Unterschied zwischen der niedrigsten und der höchsten MdE-Gruppe erstaunlich gering. Schon in der niedrigsten MdE-Gruppe sind in 24% der Fälle 3 oder gar alle 4 dieser Parameter pathologisch, und selbst in der höchsten MdE-Gruppe steigt dieser Prozentsatz nur auf 55% an. In den Gruppen mit einer MdE unter 80% gibt es andererseits nicht wenige Patienten, bei denen alle 4 genannten Parameter im Normbereich liegen. Danach müssen noch andere Faktoren für den Gutachter bei der Einschätzung der MdE von Bedeutung sein. Vermutlich sind dies das Lebensalter und - beim Kohlenbergarbeiter - der Silikosegrad im Röntgenbild.

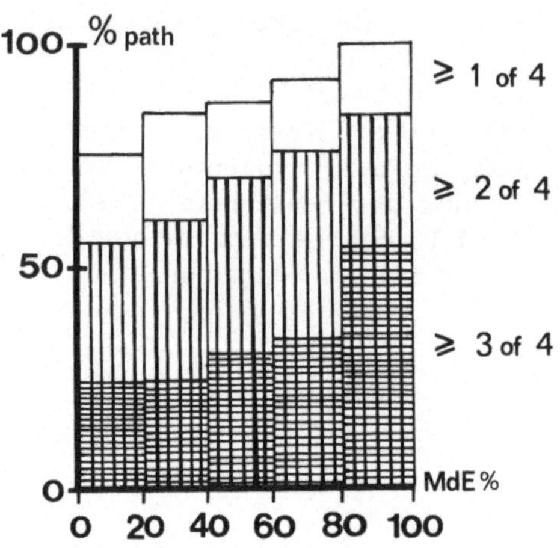

Abb. 5. Prozentuale Häufigkeit der Fälle, in denen mindestens einer, mindestens zwei bzw. mindestens drei der vier in Abb. 4 dargestellten Parameter bei den gleichen Probanden pathologisch sind

Wir haben deshalb die partiellen Korrelationskoeffizienten zwischen der MdE einerseits und den genannten Lungenfunktionsgrößen sowie dem Lebensalter und dem Silikosegrad (nach der Johannesburger Klassifikation) andererseits ausgerechnet. Mit dieser Berechnung wird die übrige gegenseitige Abhängigkeit der Parameter eliminiert. Da die Vitalkapazität, der Atemstoßwert und der arterielle pO_2 stark vom Lebensalter abhängen, verschwand dabei ihre Korrelation zur MdE völlig, denn auch die MdE hängt stark vom Lebensalter ab. So ergab sich die Gleichung

$$\%MdE = 0.2 \text{ x Alter} + 16.5 \text{ x Si-Grad} + 0.6 \text{ x R} + Const \quad (4)$$

und bei Einsetzen der Mittelwerte

$$39 = \quad 11 \quad + \quad 38,5 \quad + \quad 3,1 - 13,5$$

Wie man sieht, spielen der röntgenologische Silikosegrad und das Lebensalter in der Praxis der Begutachtung die Hauptrolle, und man mag sich fragen, ob diese Kriterien für die Einschätzung der MdE relevant sind oder nicht. Zumindest haben sie gegenüber den genannten Lungenfunktionsgrößen den Vorteil der Stabilität. Daß die Leistungsfähigkeit, auch die der Lunge, mit zunehmendem Lebensalter abnimmt, wird niemand bestreiten, aber das ist kein pathologischer, sondern zunächst ein normaler Alterungs prozeß, der in der Begutachtung von den pathologischen Veränderungen abzutrennen ist. Daß der röntgenologische Silikosegrad bei der Silikosebegutachtung eine Rolle spielt, steht hier am Rande der Thematik, erklärt aber die enge Korrelation zur MdE, weil hier ja nur solche Funktionsstörungen entschädigt werden, die ursächlich auf die Silikose, deren Klassifizierung röntgenologisch erfolgt, zu beziehen sind.

DIE DIFFERENZIERUNG DER URSACHEN EINER DYSPNOE

Nicht nur bei den Kohlenbergarbeitern mit einer Pneumokoniose, sondern praktisch bei allen Begutachtungsfällen chronischer Lungenerkrankungen steht subjektiv die Dyspnoe im Vordergrund. Das sollte eigentlich die

Begutachtung vereinfachen, aber neben der Subjektivität bereitet vor allem
die Unspezifität dieses Symptoms Schwierigkeiten. In der Begutachtung stehen wir vor der Aufgabe, pulmonale Dyspnoeformen von kardialen und anderen abzugrenzen.

Die bisher genannten Parameter - VK, AST, pO_2a und R_{aw} - können
zwar mit genügender Spezifität auf die Lunge bezogen werden, aber sie
sind, wie wir gesehen haben, nicht sensibel genug, um damit jede pulmonal bedingte Dyspnoe zu entdecken.

Da die Dyspnoe in der Regel zunächst bei körperlicher Belastung auf-
tritt, liegt es nahe, nach dem Auftreten pathologischer Veränderungen im
Rahmen einer Belastungsprüfung zu suchen.

Wir haben nun, um Parameter zur Differenzierung der Ursachen einer
Belastungsdyspnoe zu gewinnen, bei 2.415 Hüttenarbeitern, die wir im Rahmen der DFG-Studie über die Ursachen der chronischen Bronchitis untersuchten, und bei 602 aktiven Steinkohlenbergarbeitern eine sehr eingehende
lungenfunktionsanalytische Untersuchung in Ruhe und während ansteigender
Körperbelastung (6 Minuten, mit 60 Watt beginnend und um 10 Watt/min ansteigend) durchgeführt.

Um die verschiedenen Ursachenfaktoren für eine Belastungsdyspnoe zu
differenzieren, galt es, Probandengruppen zu bilden, die entweder primär
kardial oder primär pulmonal geschädigt waren oder aber eine Belastungsdyspnoe unbekannter Ursache hatten. Bei fortgeschritteneren Krankheits-
stadien würden sicher wesentlich geringere Probandenzahlen ausreichen,
um zu signifikanten Unterschieden zu kommen.

Wir haben diejenigen Probanden als pulmonal erkrankt angesehen, die
angaben, wegen einer chronischen Bronchitis in hausärztlicher Behandlung
zu stehen oder gestanden zu haben. Analog wurden diejenigen Probanden
als kardial geschädigt angesehen, die angaben, wegen einer Herzerkrankung in hausärztlicher Behandlung zu stehen oder gestanden zu haben. Die
dritte Gruppe umfaßt diejenigen Probanden, die über eine Kurzatmigkeit -
mindestens beim schnellen Gehen in der Ebene oder bei leichtem Bergan-
gehen - klagten, jedoch weder von einer Bronchitis noch von einer Herzerkrankung zu berichten wußten. Probanden mit einer Bronchitis und einer
Herzerkrankung wurden aus der Gegenüberstellung ausgeschlossen. Alle
übrigen Probanden dienten als gesunde Vergleichsgruppe.

Man könnte einwenden, daß diese Kriterien nur anamnestisch begründet
sind, so daß sie nicht ausreichend gesichert sind. Dennoch halten wir diese Kriterien für geeignet, weil meistens anamnestische Angaben Anlaß zu
eingehenden Funktionsanalysen geben und zum anderen, weil hier nicht
Einzelfälle beurteilt, sondern die Mittelwerte größerer Untersuchungsgruppen verglichen werden sollen.

Die kontinuierlich anfallenden Meßsignale des Pneumotachogramms, der
massenspektrometrischen O_2 - und CO_2-Messung der Atemluft und die Pulsfrequenz sowie der minütlich gemessene Blutdruck wurden on-line von einem Prozeßrechner (PDP-12) verarbeitet (Smidt und Finkenzeller, 1972),
die arteriellen Blutgase wurden in Ruhe und während der 6. Belastungsminute bestimmt.

In Tabelle 1 sind die anthropometrischen Daten der Gruppen zusammengestellt. Sie zeigen eine gute Vergleichbarkeit. Aus der Fülle der Meß-

Tabelle 1. Mittelwerte und deren Standardabweichungen von anthropometrischen Daten der Untersuchten

| Parameter | Gesunde | | Herzkranke | | Pat. mit Bronchitis | | Pat. mit Dyspnoe unbekannter Ursache | |
| | n = 1810 | | n = 162 | | n = 318 | | n = 348 | |
	$\bar{x}$	$s_{\bar{x}}$	$\bar{x}$	$s_{\bar{x}}$	$\bar{x}$	$s_{\bar{x}}$	$\bar{x}$	$s_{\bar{x}}$
Alter	43,2	0,22	44,1	0,1	44,0	0,08	43,8	0,1
Größe	173,5	0,2	172,6	0,5	172,2	0,4	172,7	0,5
Gewicht	79,5	0,2	79,5	0,8	77,1	0,6	78,4	0,8

größen, die in Tabelle 2 zusammengestellt sind, sollen hier nur diejenigen herausgegriffen werden, die signifikante Unterschiede zwischen wenigstens zwei der vier verglichenen Gruppen aufweisen (Tabelle 3 und 4). Folgende Größen haben weder in Ruhe noch bei der Belastungsstufe von 110 Watt signifikante Mittelwertsunterschiede zwischen wenigstens 2 der 4 verglichenen Gruppen gezeigt:
- Sauerstoffaufnahme pro Minute
- alveolare Ventilation
- Sauerstoffpuls
- Sauerstoffaufnahme pro Atemzug
- Kohlensäureabgabe pro Atemzug
- Zeit zwischen 25% und 75% der O_2-Amplitude einer Exspiration
- Zeit zwischen 25% und 75% der CO_2-Amplitude einer Exspiration
- Atemzugvolumen
- Zunahme des pCO_2 in den letzten 300 ml Exspirationsluft
Lediglich in Ruhe zeigten außerdem
- der arterielle pCO_2
- der arterielle pH-Wert
- die Gesamtpufferbasen
- die Atemfrequenz
- die Kohlensäureabgabe
keinerlei signifikante Unterschiede.

Vergleichen wir die Größe der gefundenen Gruppendifferenzen zwischen der Ruhe- (Tabelle 3) und der Belastungsuntersuchung (Tabelle 4), so nehmen die Differenzen fast durchweg bei Belastung deutlich zu. Daraus läßt sich auf die Überlegenheit der ergometrischen gegenüber der Ruheuntersuchung zur Differenzierung zwischen Gesunden und den hier betrachteten Krankheitsgruppen schließen. In Abb. 6 sind noch einmal diejenigen Parameter namentlich aufgeführt, deren Mittelwerte sich signifikant zwischen den Gesunden und wenigstens einer der Patientengruppen unterscheiden. Vergleichen wir die Anzahl der Differenzen zwischen den einzelnen

Tabelle 2. Meßgrößen, die während der Ruhe- und Belastungsphase bestimmt wurden.

V_{O_2}	ml/min	Sauerstoffaufnahme
V_{CO_2}	ml/min	Kohlensäureabgabe
pO_2A	torr	endexspiratorischer Sauerstoffdruck gemittelt aus allen Atemzügen dieser Minute
pCO_2A	torr	endexspiratorischer Kohlensäuredruck
AMV	l/min	Atemminutenvolumen
AF	/min	Atemfrequenz
P	/min	Pulsfrequenz
RRsy	torr	systolischer Blutdruck
$AeqO_2$	ml/ml	ml Atemvolumen/ml Sauerstoffaufnahme
V_{alv}	%	alveolare Ventilation
RQ	ml/ml	respiratorischer Quotient
O_2P	ml/Schlag	Sauerstoffaufnahme pro Pulsschlag
pH		Wasserstoffionenkonzentration
BB	mval/l	Pufferbasen

Außerdem werden aus jedem Atemzug folgende Werte berechnet:

V_{dtO_2}	ml	geatmetes Volumen zwischen 25% und 75% der exspiratorischen pO_2-Amplitude
V_{O_2}	ml	Sauerstoffaufnahme
dtO_2	sec	Zeitraum zwischen 25% und 75% der exspiratorischen pO_2-Amplitude
V_{dtCO_2}	ml	geatmetes Volumen zwischen 25% und 75% der exspiratorischen pCO_2-Amplitude
V_{CO_2}	ml	Kohlensäureabgabe
$dtCO_2$	sec	Zeitraum zwischen 25% und 75% der exspiratorischen pCO_2-Amplitude
AV	ml	Atemzugvolumen
dpO_2	torr	Abnahme des pO_2 während der letzten 300 ml einer Exspiration
$dpCO_2$	torr	Zunahme des pCO_2 während der letzten 300 ml einer Exspiration

Tabelle 3. Mittelwerte und deren Standardabweichungen von Funktionsparametern, die während der Ruhephase gemessen wurden. Abkürzungen und Dimensionen siehe Tabelle 1

Parameter	Gesunde		Herzkranke		Pat. mit Bronchitis		Pat. mit Dyspnoe	
	$\bar{x}$	$s_{\bar{x}}$	$\bar{x}$	$s_{\bar{x}}$	$\bar{x}$	$s_{\bar{x}}$	$\bar{x}$	$s_{\bar{x}}$
pO_2a	76,7	0,25	73,7	0,8	73,8	0,5	81,8	0,6
pO_2A	107,2	0,14	108,7	0,6	108,7	0,5	108,0	0,14
pCO_2A	34,0	0,1			32,5	0,4	33,0	0,3
AMV	9,6	0,06			10,5	0,1		
AF	15,8	0,1			17,0	0,2		
P	75,3	0,1	77,2	0,7	81,7	0,9	78,4	0,8
RRsy	132,0	0,3	136,5	1,1				
$AeqO_2$	33,9	0,1			40,8	0,3		
RQ	0,975	0,003					1,005	0,01
V_{dtO_2}	210,8	0,8			267,2	0,6		
V_{dtCO_2}	168,6	0,7			219,2	0,5	145,8	1,9
dP_{O_2}	3,4	0,03			4,7	0,1		

Krankheitsgruppen, so zeigen die Patienten mit einer Bronchitis die meisten Unterschiede zu den Gesunden. An zweiter Stelle folgen die Patienten mit einer Dyspnoe ohne anamnestische Hinweise auf eine Herz- oder Lungenerkrankung, und am Schluß stehen die Herzkranken.

Die gleiche Rangordnung erhalten wir für das Ausmaß der Differenzen zwischen den verschiedenen Gruppen. Vergleichen wir das Muster der Funktionsstörungen bei den verschiedenen Gruppen, so ergeben sich deutliche Unterschiede:

Die Patienten mit einer Herzerkrankung zeigen als einzige in Ruhe einen erhöhten Blutdruck. Der arterielle pO_2 liegt in Ruhe und wäh-

Tabelle 4. Mittelwerte und deren Standardabweichungen von Funktionsparametern, die während der 5. Belastungsminute gemessen wurden. Abkürzungen und Dimensionen siehe Tabelle 1

Parameter	Gesunde		Herzkranke		Pat. mit Bronchitis		Pat. mit Dyspnoe	
	$\bar{x}$	$s_{\bar{x}}$	$\bar{x}$	$s_{\bar{x}}$	$\bar{x}$	$s_{\bar{x}}$	$\bar{x}$	$s_{\bar{x}}$
$\dot{V}_{CO_2}$	975,0	2,4					987,0	7,2
AMV	25,4	0,11			26,0	0,2	26.0	0,4
AF	23,2	0,12			24,4	0,16	30,1	0,4
P	121,6	0,3	148,7	1,3			125,1	1,1
RRsy	144,7	0,3					161,7	0,9
$AeqO_2$	27,6	0,1			29,1	0,4		
RQ	1,06	0,005			1,09	0,01	1,09	0,006
V_{dtO_2}	297,0	1,3			334,1	3,7		
V_{dtCO_2}	237,2	1,2			256,3	3,4		
pO_2A	100,8	0,16	104,0	0,7	104,2	0,5	103,5	0,5
pCO_2A	40,4	0,14			37,0	0,4	38,5	0,3
dpO_2	3,5	0,04			4,7	0,1		
pO_2a	81,1	0,27	79,6	0,8	79,2	0,6		
pCO_2a	42,3	0,06					40,8	0,12
Puffer-basen	47,0	0,5					44,5	1,5
pH	7,443	0,001					7,411	0,003

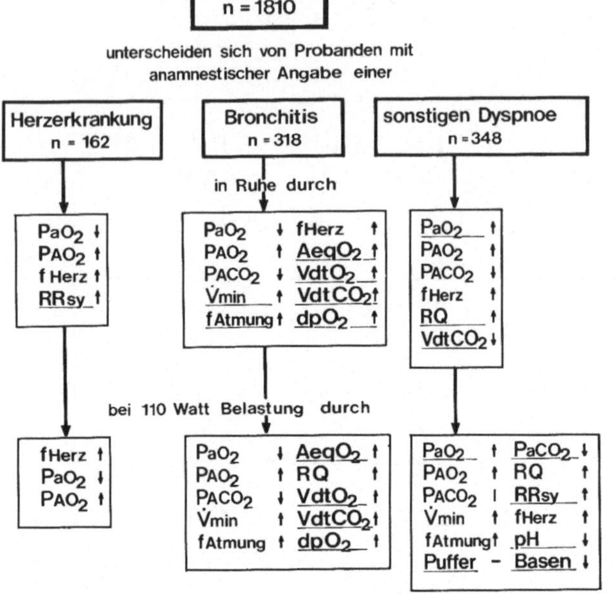

Abb. 6. Zusammenfassung derjenigen kardiopulmonalen Funktionsgrößen aus Tabelle 1, deren Mittelwert sich signifikant zwischen den Gesunden und mindestens einer der anderen Gruppen unterscheidet. Diejenigen Parameter, deren Unterschied für eine Patientengruppen spezifisch ist, sind unterstrichen. Aufwärts gerichtete Pfeile bedeuten eine Vergrößerung, abwärts gerichtete eine Verminderung. Symbole siehe Tabelle 1

rend der Ergometerbelastung niedriger, der alveolare pO_2 höher als bei den Gesunden. Das ist aber gleichermaßen bei den Bronchitikern der Fall. Ebenso liegt die Pulsfrequenz in Ruhe bei beiden Gruppen höher. Den größten Unterschied zeigen die Herzkranken in der Pulsfrequenz bei Belastung, die 27 Schl/min höher liegt als bei den Gesunden.

Da die meisten übrigen Parameter die Effektivität der Ventilation und des intrapulmonalen Gasaustausches charakterisieren, ist es nicht überraschend, daß sie für die Herzkranken keine anderen Werte als für die Gesunden aufweisen. Aber auch der respiratorische Quotient, der ebenso von der Zirkulation oder von einer extrapulmonal bedingten Hyperventilation beeinflußt wird, zeigt keine Besonderheiten. Selbst der systolische Blutdruck ist unter Belastung nicht mehr erhöht.

Bei den Patienten mit einer Bronchitis weichen alle diejenigen Parameter von denen der Gesunden ab, die sich auf eine verschlechterte Ökonomie der Atmung beziehen. Die Bronchitiker haben eine erhöhte Atemfrequenz, ein erhöhtes Atemminutenvolumen, ein erhöhtes O_2-Atemäquivalent, erniedrigte arterielle pO_2- und pCO_2-Werte (letztere vermutlich infolge der für die Aufrechterhaltung eines genügenden pO_2 notwendigen stärkeren Ventilation), sowie niedrigere alveolare CO_2-Drucke und höhere alveolare O_2-Drucke. Infolge der Inhomogenitäten in der Lunge sind auch die im Mischluftanteil der exspiratorischen O_2- und CO_2-Kurven exspirierten Volumina (V_{dtO_2} und V_{dtCO_2}) vergrößert, ebenso erklärt sich der stärkere Abfall des exspiratorischen pO_2 während der letzten 300 ml einer Exspiration. Unter Körperbelastung ist auch der respiratorische Quotient erhöht, da der Gasaustausch für CO_2 durch die Inhomogenitäten weniger behindert wird als derjenige für O_2.

Die Patienten mit einer Dyspnoe unklarer Genese zeigen bei Belastung einen erniedrigten pH-Wert bei ebenfalls niedrigem pCO_2, so daß sich ein verminderter Gesamtpufferwert errechnet, ohne daß jedoch eine Anämie vorliegt oder bereits in Ruhe ein Basendefizit bestand. Die alveolaren O_2- und CO_2-Drucke zeigen die gleiche Verschiebung wie bei den Patienten mit einer Bronchitis, jedoch ohne erniedrigten arteriellen pO_2, so daß man keine Inhomogenitäten, sondern eine Hyperventilation annehmen muß. Ausdruck eines respiratorischen Kompensationsversuches der metabolischen Azidose sind auch die gesteigerte CO_2-Abgabe, der RQ und der erniedrigte arterielle pCO_2. Als weitere auffällige Befunde sind eine erhöhte Pulsfrequenz in Ruhe und vor allem ein stark erhöhter systolischer Blutdruck bei Belastung festzustellen. Man möchte nach dieser Befundkonstellation am ehesten eine ungenügende periphere Zirkulation und eine konsekutive Zunahme des anaeroben Stoffwechsels infolge Trainingsmangels annehmen.

Kommen wir zurück auf die Patienten mit einer Bronchitis, so war ihre auffälligste Besonderheit das erhöhte Atemäquivalent für Sauerstoff, auch "spezifische Ventilation" genannt, also die Vergrößerung des Atemminutenvolumens im Verhältnis zur Sauerstoffaufnahme. Diese Vergrößerung wird mehr über die Atemfrequenz als über das Atemzugvolumen erreicht. Bei Gesunden fällt das Atemäquivalent während einer mittelschweren Belastung typischerweise ab, da die normalen Inhomogenitäten geringer werden. Bei den Bronchitikern bleibt es dagegen unverändert hoch. Beim Gesunden steigt das Atemäquivalent erst mit Erreichen der Leistungsgrenze an.

Das erhöhte Atemminutenvolumen des Bronchitikers bedeutet eine erhöhte Atemarbeit, die als Dyspnoe empfunden wird. Bei entsprechend erhöhter Atemarbeit hindert die Dyspnoe den Patienten, seine körperliche Leistung weiter zu steigern, obgleich er in Ruhe bei einer willkürlichen Hyperventilation - wie im Rahmen der Atemgrenzwertbestimmung - oft noch wesentlich höhere Werte erreichen kann. Aber bekanntlich wird weder vom Gesunden noch vom Lungenkranken bei maximaler körperlicher Anstrengung der Atemgrenzwert erreicht, wahrscheinlich weil er nicht genügend lange aufrechterhalten werden kann.

Aufgrund dieser Überlegungen möchten wir als ein Kriterium für eine pulmonal bedingte Leistungsbegrenzung ein Atemäquivalent, das in Ruhe sowie während einer ansteigenden Belastung konstant über 38 ml Ventilation pro ml O_2-Aufnahme liegt, vorschlagen, vorausgesetzt daß nicht gleichzeitig ein erniedrigter arterieller pCO_2, ein erhöhter pO_2 oder ein erhöhter pH-Wert vorliegen, die auf eine Hyperventilation ohne metabolische Notwendigkeit hindeuten. Anstelle der relativ aufwendigen Messung des O_2-Atemäquivalents dürfte aber auch die Bestimmung des Atemminutenvolumens genügen, wenn gleichzeitig aus der Ergometerbelastung die O_2-Aufnahme geschätzt werden kann und durch Blutgasanalyse eine Hyperventilation ausgeschlossen werden kann.

In dem Faktor Atemarbeit ist aber nicht nur das bewegte Volumen, sondern auch der für die Bewegung notwendige Kraftaufwand, d. h. der transpulmonale und transpleurale Druck enthalten. Müssen diese Drucke wegen erhöhter intrabronchialer Strömungswiderstände, wegen einer verminderten Compliance oder wegen einer Phasenverschiebung zwischen Druck und Strömung infolge mechanischer Inhomogenitäten erhöht werden, so tritt über diese Erhöhung der Atemarbeit ebenfalls eine leistungsbegrenzende Dyspnoe auf.

Die Korrelation zwischen Dyspnoe und Resistance ist von Ulmer et al. (1970) und vielen anderen überzeugend nachgewiesen worden. Das Gleiche gilt für eine erniedrigte Compliance. Solange wir die Resistance und die Compliance während einer Körperbelastung nicht zuverlässig und zumutbar messen können, müssen wir uns mit einer Extrapolation der in Ruhe gemessenen Werte begnügen.

So entscheidend die Strömungswiderstände in den Atemwegen in vielen Fällen sind, so dürfen sie doch nicht als alleinbestimmende für die gutachterliche Entscheidung über eine pulmonale Leistungsminderung gelten. Auch die zusätzliche Bestimmung des Atemminutenvolumens reicht nicht immer aus, denn bei der körperlichen Belastung nimmt nicht nur die Atemarbeit, sondern auch die Herzarbeit als Produkt von mittlerem systolischem Druck und ausgeworfenem Volumen zu. Erhöht sich durch eine Lungenerkrankung - am häufigsten durch ein Emphysem - der Druck im kleinen Kreislauf, so führt diese Erhöhung der Herzarbeit ebenfalls zu einer Dyspnoe und Leistungsbegrenzung, wenn das Blut in den rechten Vorhof und die großen Venen zurückgestaut wird und dort die Dehnungsrezeptoren reizt, die eine Steigerung der Atmung und die Dyspnoe verursachen.

Bei Patienten mit einer Belastungsdyspnoe, die wir nicht durch eine erhöhte Atemarbeit oder eine extrapulmonale Ursache erklären können, müssen wir deshalb auch den Pulmonalisdruck und den zentralen Venendruck nicht nur in Ruhe, sondern auch während einer Körperbelastung messen, um eine pulmonale Ursache nachzuweisen oder unwahrscheinlich zu machen (Rosenkranz et al., 1965; Konetzke und Schlegel, 1972).

So vereinfacht sich einerseits das Problem der Begutachtung von Patienten mit einer Funktionsstörung der Lunge dadurch, daß praktisch alle diese Patienten eine Dyspnoe bei Belastung angeben, wie unterschiedlich die pathophysiologische Ursache auch sein mag. Andererseits kann es aber sehr schwer sein und einen hohen Aufwand erfordern, im Einzelfall pulmonale von extrapulmonalen Ursachen abzugrenzen.

Die entscheidenden Parameter für den Nachweis einer pulmonal bedingten Dyspnoe sind
- die Blutgase
- das Atemäquivalent für Sauerstoff während Belastung
- die Resistance und Compliance
- der Pulmonalisdruck und der zentrale Venendruck.
Häufig werden wir nicht mit einem dieser Parameter auskommen, sondern erst aus der Synopsis eines breiten Befundspektrums zu einem gerechten Urteil kommen (Claasen und Kaufmann, 1973). Es steht auch noch dahin, inwieweit wir durch einen 6- oder auch 20-minütigen Belastungsversuch unter Laborbedingungen der Situation gerecht werden, wie sie für den Patienten im Alltag oder während einer 8-stündigen Arbeitsschicht gegeben ist.

LITERATUR

Becklake, M.: Summary of the Conference "Respiratory Impairment Including Assessment of Disability". Bull. Physiopathol. Respir. (Nancy) 11, 203-209 (1975)

Claasen, W., Kaufmann, F. W.: Zur Beurteilung der Leistungsfähigkeit bei Atembeschwerden. Lebensversicherungsmedizin 25, 139-142 (1973)

Cotes, J. E.: Assessment of Disability due to Impaired Respiratory Function. Bull. Physiopathol. Respir. (Nancy) 11, 210-217 (1975)

Deutsche Forschungsgemeinschaft: Chronische Bronchitis. Bericht über das Schwerpunktprogramm. Boppard: Boldt 1975

Fletcher, C. M.: The Clinical Diagnosis of Pulmonary Emphysema - an experimental study. Proc. roy. Soc. med. 45, 577-578 (1952)

Hertz, C. W.: Zur Begutachtung von Lungenfunktionsstörungen durch den Arbeitsversuch. Dtsch. Med. Wschr. 90, 461-468 (1965)

Hertz, C. W.: Blutgase. Diagnostik 7, 118-122 (1974)

Hollmann, W.: Der Arbeits- und Trainingseinfluß auf Kreislauf und Atmung. Darmstadt: Dr. Dietrich Steinkopff 1959

Konetzke, G. W., Schlegel, M.: Zur gutachterlichen Beurteilung von Silikosen unter besonderer Berücksichtigung ihrer Auswirkungen auf Atmung, Herz und Kreislauf. Dtsch. Ges. wesen 27, 135-145 (1972)

Maas, G., Krause, St.: Erweiterte Silikosebegutachtung mit psychodiagnostischen Verfahren. Mschr. Tbk.-Bekpfg. 10, 240-245 (1967)

Reichel, G.: Die Bedeutung der arteriellen Blutgasanalyse für die Lungenfunktionsdiagnostik und Begutachtung. Wien. Med. Wschr. Suppl. 28, 4-10 (1975)

Rosenkranz, K. A., Drews, A., Holling, J., Buschmann, G.: Zur Hämodynamik des kleinen Kreislaufs bei leicht- und mittelgradiger Silikose. In: Grundfragen der Silikoseforschung VI, 557-560 (1964)

Smidt, U., Muysers, K., Nieding, G. v.: Nicht-lineare Formeln zur Berechnung spirometrischer Sollwerte. Pneumonologie 144, 52-58 (1971)

Smidt, U., Finkenzeller, P.: Ein Computerprogramm für die Ergometrie. Pneumonologie 147, 245-250 (1972)

Ulmer, W. T., Reichel, G., Nolte, D.: Die Lungenfunktion. Stuttgart: Georg Thieme 1970

Ulmer, W. T., Reichel, G.: Untersuchungen über die Altersabhängigkeit der alveolären und arteriellen O_2- und CO_2-Drucke. Klin. Wschr. 41, 1-6 (1963)

Wassner, U. J.: Die untere Leistungsgrenze der Lunge. Die Tbc und ihre Grenzgebiete in Einzeldarstellungen, Band 12. Berlin-Göttingen-Heidelberg: Springer Verlag 1961

Woitowitz, H. J.: Die Blutgasanalyse in der Beurteilung der Arbeitsinsuffizienz aus pulmonaler Ursache. Dtsch. Med. Wschr. 96, 862-871 (1971)

Dr. U. Smidt
Innere Abteilung des
Krankenhaus Bethanien
4130 Moers

DISKUSSION

G. Fruhmann, München: Herr Smidt, bevor Ihre Diagramme von den erheblichen Schwankungen der Lungenfunktions-Parameter zwischen den Kontroll-Zeiträumen für lange Zeit in das Bewußtsein zahlreicher mit Begutachtungsfragen befaßter Personen eingehen, bitte ich noch einmal, die Art Ihres Ausgangskollektivs zu präzisieren. Haben Sie in vergleichbaren Untersuchungen von Patienten, bei denen n i c h t die Frage einer Rentengewährung dahintersteckt, auch so große Variationen von Vitalkapazität, Atemstoßtest usw. gefunden?

Schließlich fällt auf, daß in der von Ihnen angegebenen empirischen Gleichung der Prozentsatz der MdE sehr stark von dem Röntgenbefund der Lunge abhängt. Nach den gültigen Bestimmungen sollte sich aber die Entschädigung ganz überwiegend an der Einschränkung der Funktion orientieren. Wurde nach Ihrer Meinung im Mittel unzulässig begutachtet? Haben Sie auch einen ähnlichen Korrelations-Versuch bei pulmonalen Erkrankungen ohne stärkere Veränderungen im Thorax-Röntgenbild, beispielsweise bei obstruktiver Bronchitis und Lungenemphysem unternommen?

C. W. Hertz, Malente: In meiner von Herrn Smidt zitierten Arbeit in der Deutschen Medizinischen Wochenschrift 1965 wird ausdrücklich darauf hingewiesen, daß mit dem genannten Verfahren nur Störungen der Arterialisierung unter Belastung erfaßt werden. Es wird betont, daß selbstverständlich auch atemmechanische Funktionsstörungen ohne Störung des Gasaustausches zu einer Erwerbsminderung führen können. In der genannten Arbeit ging es mir darum, den Versuch zu machen, eine quantitative Grundlage für die Beurteilung der Erwerbsminderung zu finden, um von der arbiträren Abschätzung von Prozentsätzen abzukommen. Es wird ausdrücklich darauf hingewiesen, daß hiermit nur Gasaustauschstörungen erfaßt werden. Inzwischen haben wir in Zusammenarbeit mit Herrn Hub gleichzeitige blutgasanalytische und atemmechanische Untersuchungen unter körperlicher Belastung angestellt. Hierbei zeigte sich, daß bei den Patienten mit Absinken des arteriellen Sauerstoffdruckes unter körperlicher Arbeit der Anstieg der Atemleistung unter Arbeit im Mittel höher lag, als bei chronischen Bronchitikern mit behinderter Atemmechanik ohne Gasaustauschstörung. Diese Ergebnisse wurden kürzlich auf der Tagung der Europäischen Gesellschaft für Pathophysiologie der Atmung in Budapest vorgetragen. Das kontinuierliche Absinken der arteriellen Sauerstoffspannung bei stufenweiser Belastung beweist eine Gasaustauschstörung; die Lunge kann unter Belastungsbedingungen ihre Aufgabe, das Blut regelrecht zu arterialisieren, nicht erfüllen.

J. Meier-Sydow, Frankfurt/Main: Bei der Besprechung der Gutachtertabellen von Hertz geht die Diskussion immer um Berechtigung oder Nicht-Berechtigung des Kriteriums Sauerstoffabfall. Zu dieser Frage hat soeben der Autor selbst noch einmal Stellung genommen.

M. E. liegt aber der besondere Wert der Tabellen von Hertz in dem Vorschlag einer verbindlichen Festlegung von drei Dingen, die der Vergleichbarkeit von Gutachten verschiedener Provenienz, d. h. aber der Vereinheitlichung der Begutachtung dienen sollen:

1. Ersatz der Angabe in Watt durch solche der Sauerstoffaufnahme: Jeder Untersucher wird zur Eichung seines Ergometers durch ein Probekollektiv aufgefordert; falls die Eichung sich als konstant erweist, braucht im Einzelfall bei Gutachten die Sauerstoffaufnahme nicht gemessen zu werden.

2. Tabellarische Angaben der MdE/Prozente, alters- und geschlechtsabhängig, errechnet unter Zugrundelegung des Verhältnisses von zumutbarer Dauerbelastung zu zumutbarer Kurzbelastung von 40 : 100 ("respiratorische Leistungsgrenze").

3. "Respiratorische Mindest-Leistungsgrenze" für die verschiedensten Berufe, zur Festlegung einer Berufsunfähigkeit.

Natürlich wird mit (übrigens genau erläuterten) Approximationen gearbeitet; Diese Tabellen sind m. E. aber dennoch die übersichtlichste Form einer solchen Zusammenstellung, die bisher erschienen ist, basierend auf exakten Messungen der Funktionsanalyse und der Arbeitsphysiologie.

Wir selbst benutzen diese Tabellen seit ihrem Erscheinen, wobei wir kardio-vaskuläre und auch klinische neben Lungenfunktions-Kriterien anwenden, die die Erschöpfung des Probanden feststellen lassen. Aber je nach Arbeitsrichtung könnten auch andere Kriterien erarbeitet werden, etwa atemmechanische (s. z. B. Beiträge Grimby, Beil, Wylicil dieser Tagung).

Sowie man festgelegt hat, welche Kriterien der Erschöpfung man anerkennt, kann man diese Tabellen benutzen, ganz unabhängig von einem evtl. auftretenden Sauerstoffabfall unter Belastung.

LITERATUR

Hertz, C.Q.: Dtsch. med. Wschr. 90, 461-647 (1965)
Meier-Sydow, J.: Fortschr. Med. 92, 1451-1456 (1974)

U. Smidt, Moers: Zunächst zu Herrn Fruhmann: Unser Ausgangskollektiv waren, wie gesagt, Bergleute mit einer Pneumokoniose, bei denen immer die Frage der Rentenhöhe besteht. Ein anderes Kollektiv haben wir nicht ausgewertet. Wenn die Langzeitschwankungen nur bei denjenigen Parametern, die - wie VK und AST - von der Mitarbeit abhängig sind, zu beobachten wären, müßte man in der Tat wohl am ehesten an Unregelmäßigkeiten in der Mitarbeit als Ursache der Schwankungen denken. Aber Sie haben ja gesehen, daß die Schwankungen bei der Resistance und bei dem arteriellen Sauerstoffdruck nicht geringer sind.

Da sich unser Referat mit den Begutachtungsgrundlagen zu beschäftigen hatte und da die Begutachtung in vielen Fällen zu Vorschlägen einer Rentenhöhe führt, erschien es uns legitim, das Langzeitverhalten der Lungenfunktionsparameter an einem solchen Kollektiv zu prüfen.

Selbst wenn die Schwankungen in einem Kollektiv, wo nicht die Frage der Rente dahintersteht, geringer wären, so könnte man daraus noch nicht auf eine Eignung dieser Parameter für die Begutachtung schließen.

Wenn man sich in die Abbildungen die altersbezogene Grenzlinie zwischen normalen und pathologischen Werten eingezeichnet denkt, zeigt sich auch, daß sich die Schwankungen nicht nur innerhalb des Normalbereichs abspielen, sondern diese Linie in beiden Richtungen kreuzen.

Sie sagen richtig, daß in der angegebenen empirischen Gleichung der Prozentsatz der MdE viel stärker vom Röntgenbefund der Silikose als von den Lungenfunktionsgrößen abhängt. Ich meine aber nicht, daß man daraus auf eine im Mittel unzulässige Begutachtung schließen kann, denn der Gesetzgeber fordert nur für die prinzipielle Anerkennung eine Einschränkung der kardiopulmonalen Funktion. Er verlangt nicht, daß der Grad der MdE-Einschätzung von einem bestimmten Grad einer kardio-pulmonalen Funktionsstörung abhängig gemacht wird. Wäre dies der Fall, so können Sie sich anhand unserer Ergebnisse leicht vorstellen, welches Hin und Her dabei herauskäme.

Analoge Korrelationen bei Patienten ohne stärkere Veränderungen im Thorax-Röntgenbild haben wir nicht berechnet, da uns ein solches Kollektiv nicht zur Verfügung stand.

Zu Herrn Meier-Sydow: Ihren Vorschlag, anstelle des Hertz' schen Kriteriums des arteriellen Sauerstoffdruckabfalls andere lungenfunktionsanalytische, klinische oder kardio-vaskuläre Kriterien zur Objektivierung der Erschöpfung heranzuziehen, finde ich sehr gut, wenn unsere Aufgabe darin besteht, zur globalen Leistungsfähigkeit eines Patienten Stellung zu nehmen. Wir müssen aber immer die Fragestellung im Auge behalten, d. h. hier die Feststellung der r e s p i r a t o r i s c h e n Leistungsgrenze oder auch nur der respiratorischen Funktionsstörung. Und da bezweifle ich eben den Wert des arteriellen Sauerstoffdruckabfalls, weil der durch andere Faktoren verschoben oder verhindert werden kann, so daß wir lediglich dann, wenn er eintritt, sagen können, daß s p ä t e s t e n s bei dieser Belastungsstufe die respiratorische Leistungsgrenze erreicht ist. Dies Kriterium hat also zwar eine sehr gute Spezifität, aber nach unseren Erfahrungen eine sehr geringe Sensibilität.

Das bestätigt eigentlich auch Prof. Hertz in seiner Diskussionsbemerkung, wenn er sagt, daß die Atemleistung bei den Patienten, die einen Abfall des arteriellen Sauerstoffdrucks zeigen, stärker ansteigt als bei chronischen Bronchitikern mit behinderter Atemmechanik, aber ohne Gasaustauschstörung.

Damit erweist sich der Abfall des arteriellen Sauerstoffdrucks als Spätsymptom, bei dessen Fehlen wir aber nicht schließen dürfen, daß keine Gasaustauschstörung vorliegt, sondern - im Falle eines erhöhten Ventilations- oder Druckaufwandes - besser von einer kompensierten Gasaustauschstörung sprechen sollten.

Pneumonologie Suppl. 1976, 97-104

Zur Objektivierung der pulmonalen Leistungsgrenze

H. H. Marx und H. Erwes

Medizinische Klinik im Diakonissenkrankenhaus Stuttgart

Abstract. An objective assessment of the pulmonary function limit is only secured where an exact clinical and radiological examination including spirographic and gas analytical pulmonary function test is possible. The examination should be completed by a tolerance test with control of capillary blood gases and pH value, unless indications of an overall insufficiency during the resting period were found, since only in this way the "continuous function limit" can be determined. Special attention should be paid to the proportions of the acid base balance and their relation to the blood gas reaction.

In case of particular questions further important indications as to the condition of the cardiopulmonary system are obtained by intracardiac pressure measuring. Pulmonary pressure and oxygen pressure are in statistical correlation during resting periods, might work however in opposite directions under strain. This occurs especially in cases where the oxygen pressure under strain improves, whereas because of mainly restrictive dysfunction, the right ventricular pression increases. Therefore, on principal the measuring of blood gases does not substitute the recording of the intracardiac pressure reaction under strain.

Zusammenfassung. Eine objektive Beurteilung der pulmonalen Leistungsgrenze ist nur dort sichergestellt, wo eine exakte klinische und röntgenologische Untersuchung einschließlich spirographischer und gasanalytischer Lungenfunktionsprüfung möglich ist. Sofern nicht Hinweise auf eine globale Ruheinsuffizienz bestehen, sollte die Untersuchung durch eine Belastung mit Kontrolle der kapillaren Blutgase und des pH-Wertes ergänzt werden, weil nur so die "Dauerleistungsgrenze" definiert werden kann. Die Verhältnisse des Säure-Basengleichgewichtes und ihre Beziehung zum Verhalten der Blutgase verdienen besondere Beachtung.

In speziellen Fragestellungen gibt die intrakardiale Druckmessung weitere wichtige Hinweise auf die Situation des kardio-pulmonalen Systems. Pulmonalisdruck und Sauerstoffdruck stehen in Ruhe in statistischer Korrelation, können sich aber unter Belastung gegensinnig verändern. Dies trifft insbesondere für solche Fälle zu, in denen sich der Sauerstoffdruck unter Belastung verbessert, während wegen überwiegend restriktiver Funktionsstörung der rechtsventrikuläre Druck ansteigt. Deshalb ersetzt die Messung der Blutgase grundsätzlich nicht die Registrierung des intrakardialen Druckverhaltens unter Belastung.

Jedem Gutachter ist die ebenso häufige wie unangenehme Erfahrung bekannt, daß die Objektivierung einer Leistungseinschränkung der Atmung mittels Lungenfunktionsprüfung bei den verschiedensten Fragestellungen im Verlauf eines Rentenverfahrens noch immer zu den Ausnahmen zählt. Wenn dann Nachuntersuchungen angeordnet oder Verschlimmerungsanträge vorgelegt werden, sieht sich der Gutachter mangels vergleichbarer Meßdaten häufig außerstande, eine Änderung der pulmonalen Leistungsfähigkeit festzustellen. Damit die zuständigen Behörden in Zukunft objektiv brauchbare Befundunterlagen verwenden können, ist es erforderlich, daß die mit solchen Untersuchungen beauftragten Fachleute auch einheitliche Kriterien anbieten. Nur dann werden in möglichst jedem Fall vergleichbare Untersuchungsergebnisse zur Verfügung stehen. Obwohl immer wieder einmal Versuche zur Vereinheitlichung der Untersuchungsmethoden unternommen wurden [4], ist die Bewertung der Einzelkriterien in den verschiedenen Kliniken und Instituten noch recht unterschiedlich, weshalb hier anhand eigener Erfahrungen Vorschläge zu einer einheitlichen Leistungsbewertung des kardiopulmonalen Systems vorgelegt werden sollen.

Mit diesem Ziel haben wir die bei 25 Gutachten-Patienten während des letzten Jahres erhobenen Untersuchungsbefunde zusammengestellt und unter Einschluß früherer Erfahrungen und Untersuchungen aus den Jahren 1965-1968 ausgewertet. Es handelt sich bei den jetzt in der Stuttgarter Klinik untersuchten Patienten um 19 Männer und 6 Frauen, mit dem Durchschnittsalter von 59 Jahren, überwiegend mit gemischt obstruktiv-restriktiver Ventilationsstörung, die allerdings recht unterschiedlich verursacht war, z. B. durch Thoraxverletzungen, inaktive Tuberkulose der Lungen oder der Pleura, chronische Bronchitis oder obstruktives Lungenemphysem. In allen Fällen bestand nach den klinischen und elektrokardiographischen Befunden Verdacht auf eine pulmonale Hypertonie, die es zu objektivieren galt. Deshalb wurde bei allen Fällen eine intrakardiale Druckmessung im rechten Ventrikel mittels Einschwemmkatheter nach Grandjean in Ruhe durchgeführt [2].

Außerdem wurden die üblichen spirographischen Ventilationsgrößen registriert und die kapillar entnommenen Blutgase mittels "Gascheck" bestimmt. Exakte klinische Untersuchung, Röntgenuntersuchung des Thorax in 2 Ebenen, Elektrokardiogramm, Kreislaufverhalten einschließlich Blutdruck und Pulsfrequenz ergänzten die Untersuchungen. In 15 von 25 Fällen konnte liegend am Fahrradergometer eine Belastung durchgeführt werden, die prinzipiell 1 Watt/kg Körpergewicht betrug und die möglichst 6 Minuten im relativen steady state, in einigen Fällen allerdings auch weniger lang, durchgeführt wurde. Am Ende der Belastung wurden erneut kapillare Blutgase entnommen sowie das Elektrokardiogramm und das Pulsverhalten festgehalten.

Schwierigkeiten einer Auswertung und allgemeinen Aussage über die Objektivität der einzelnen Kriterien entstanden durch das recht unterschiedlich zusammengesetzte Krankengut sowie durch die nicht immer gleichmäßig durchgehaltene Belastungsintensität. Auch die Katheterisierung des rechten Herzens ist nicht problemlos, zumal die Pulmonalarterie nicht immer mit dieser Methode erreicht wurde. Wir haben uns deshalb - in Kenntnis gewisser Auswertungsschwierigkeiten - mit der Registrierung des systolischen rechtsventrikulären Druckes begnügt. Dabei ist uns weiterhin bekannt, wie viele unterschiedliche Faktoren auf diesen Ventrikeldruck Einfluß nehmen, vor allem Schlagvolumen, Herzfrequenz, Rezirkulation, Klappenstatus, Zustand der Koronarien und auch die Blutviskosität.

Nach vergleichender Betrachtung der an unserem Krankengut gewonnenen Untersuchungsergebnisse halten wir folgende Kriterien zur Bewertung der individuellen pulmonalen Leistungsfähigkeit für unentbehrlich:

1. KLINISCHER UNTERSUCHUNGSBEFUND

Hierzu gehört nicht nur eine exakte Auskultation und Perkussion, sondern auch die Berücksichtigung der wichtigen Symptome Zyanose und Dyspnoe, die Beschreibung der Thoraxelastizität und Dehnbarkeit, Prüfung des Atemstoßes und der Zwerchfellverschieblichkeit. Ergänzt werden diese Befunde durch das Thoraxröntgenbild in 2 Ebenen, den Ruheblutdruck, das Pulsverhalten und ein Elektrokardiogramm sowie die Bestimmung des Hämoblobins und des Hämatokrits, da diese zur Beurteilung der Zyanose bedeutsam sind.

Der klinische Befund basiert selbstredend auf einer vollständigen Anamnese, bei der nicht nur frühere Beschädigungen und Erkrankungen des kardio-pulmonalen Systems, sondern vor allem auch die früheren und jetzigen Lebensgewohnheiten (Nikotinkonsum!) und die derzeitige Medikation festgehalten werden müssen. Ein Gutachter handelt fahrlässig, wenn er eine chronische Bronchitis oder ähnliches als Kriegsschadensfolge ansieht, ohne frühere und derzeitige Rauchgewohnheiten mit in seine Beurteilung einzubeziehen.

2. SPIROGRAPHISCHE RUHEUNTERSUCHUNG

Dieses Untersuchungsverfahren ist mancherorts - zu Unrecht, meinen wir - in Mißkredit geraten. Meßwerte wie maximales Atemvolume, Atemgrenzwert und Atemstoß unterliegen gewiß stets einer großen Schwankungsbreite; trotzdem kann auf sie nicht verzichtet werden, insbesondere dann, wenn nicht nur das zahlenmäßige Ergebnis, sondern auch das figürliche Verhalten in bezug auf Schwankungen der Atemmittellage beim Atemgrenzwert in die Beurteilung eingehen. Die Bestimmung des Residualvolumens kann eine sinnvolle Ergänzung sein, jedoch sollte deren Ergebnis nur qualitativ, nicht quantitativ berücksichtigt werden. Die funktionelle Bedeutung eines obstruktiven Emphysems läßt sich genauer an den Blutgasen und am Atemgrenzwert als an der Höhe des Residualvolumens ablesen.

3. UNTERSUCHUNGEN DER ATEMMECHANIK

Die Bestimmung der Resistance, vor allem bei obstruktiven Ventilationsstörungen, eventuell auch der Compliance, dies vor allem bei restriktiven Störungen, sind nicht allerorts praktikabel, sie können auch nicht als un-

abdingbar angesehen werden. Auch diese Verfahren unterliegen einer erheblichen Schwankungsbreite, sie sind jedoch für die Beurteilung der Ventilationsleistung von Bedeutung.

4. ARTERIELL BZW. KAPILLAR ENTNOMMENE BLUTGASE [3]

Von entscheidender Bedeutung ist die Aussage über die in Ruhe vorhande-
nen Gasdrucke, den pH-Wert und das Basendefizit, zumal die heute verfügbaren Methoden objektiv gut brauchbar sind. In Zweifelsfällen, insbesondere bei erheblicher Polyglobulie, sollte die Blutentnahme allerdings
arteriell erfolgen. Ergibt die Blutgasanalyse Hinweise auf eine nicht nur
vorübergehende alveolare Minderbelüftung mit Hypoxämie und Hyperkapnie, so engt sich die Anwendung weiterer belastender Untersuchungsverfahren erheblich ein, insbesondere wenn diese Befunde mit einer starken
Einschränkung der Ventilationsleistung im Atemgrenzwert und Anzeichen
eines bereits klinisch manifesten Cor pulmonale korrespondieren [10].

5. INTRAKARDIALE DRUCKMESSUNG [9, 10]

Wo nicht bereits das klinische Bild eine Rechtsherzinsuffizienz erkennen
läßt oder das Ergebnis der Blutgase (PO_2 unter 60 mm Hg, PCO_2 über 50
mm Hg), des Elektrokardiogramms und des Röntgenbildes eine pulmonale
Hypertonie wahrscheinlich machen, ist die Registrierung des rechtsventrikulären und Pulmonalarterien-Druckes anzustreben. Es sollte in solchen Fällen allerdings die Möglichkeit einer ergometrischen Belastung
vorhanden sein, da das Ruheergebnis allein in vielen Fällen nicht genügend
aussagefähig ist. Bei in Ruhe bereits erhöhten Ventrikeldrucken wird
man im allgemeinen auf eine ergometrische Belastung am Fahrradergometer verzichten können.

6. ERGOMETRIE [7, 11]

In möglichst vielen Fällen sollte die pulmonale Leistungsgrenze unter Belastung exakt definiert werden, sofern nicht bereits in Ruhe Anzeichen
einer globalen Minderbelüftung nachgewiesen werden. Wie früher im einzelnen begründet, muß eine ergometrische Untersuchung

adäquat und unschädlich,
objektiv und reproduzierbar sein
und im steady state erfolgen.

Die Belastung erfolgt stufenweise ansteigend, jeweils 5-6 Minuten, zunächst 1 Watt, später eventuell 2 Watt/kg Körpergewicht. Sogenannte
"Maximalleistungen" sind für Patienten nicht reproduzierbar. Ziel einer
solchen Untersuchung ist vielmehr die Austestung der sogenannten Dauer
leistungsgrenze. Darunter verstehen wir jene Belastungsstufe, die
wenigstens 6 Minuten im relativen Stoffwechselgleichgewicht geleistet

werden kann, bei der der Sauerstoffdruck nicht unter den Ausgangswert
und der pH-Wert nicht unter 7, 35 abfällt [7].

Je nach apparativen Voraussetzungen werden unter Belastung die Ventilationsgrößen sowie der Sauerstoffverbrauch und das Pulsverhalten und die daraus errechneten Quotienten gewertet, wobei ein Atemäquivalent über 3, 5 und eine fehlende Sauerstoffmehraufnahme Kriterien der Leistungsgrenze sind. Diese Verfahren sind jedoch von verschiedenen technischen Voraussetzungen, insbesondere von einer exakten Volumen- und Gasdruckstabilisierung und von den mechanischen Gerätewiderständen stark abhängig. Vor allem ist die synchrone Registrierung der Atemvolumina und der Gasdrucke problematisch.

Wir haben deshalb in unserer Klinik inzwischen auf die Bestimmung der Ventilationsgrößen unter Belastung vollständig verzichtet und registrieren nur noch die kapillaren Blutgase vor, während und nach Belastung sowie das Elektrokardiogramm und die Pulsfrequenz, in Einzelfällen dazu die intrakardialen Drucke.

1965 habe ich nachgewiesen, daß bei Patienten mit Atmungsinsuffizienz arterieller Sauerstoffdruck, Kohlensäuredruck und auch der pH-Wert in enger statistisch gesicherter Korrelation stehen. Vielfache Untersuchungen seit Cournand haben gezeigt, daß die Korrelation auch den rechtsventrikulären Druck einbeziehen kann [1]. Unter ergometrischer Belastung sind die Beziehungen weniger einheitlich [11].

Bei dem Bemühen, die bei unseren Gutachten-Patienten unter Belastung erhaltenen Druckwerte zueinander in Beziehung zu setzen, konnten wir feststellen, daß trotz unterschiedlich zusammengesetzten Patientenguts statistisch signifikante Beziehungen zwischen der Erniedrigung des arteriellen Sauerstoffdrucks und dem Anstieg des rechtsventrikulären Ruhedrucks festzustellen waren. Der Korrelationskoeffizient lag bei $r = -0,44$; $x/y = 40,9/68,8$ Regressionsgrade; $a = -0,39$ (Abb. 1).

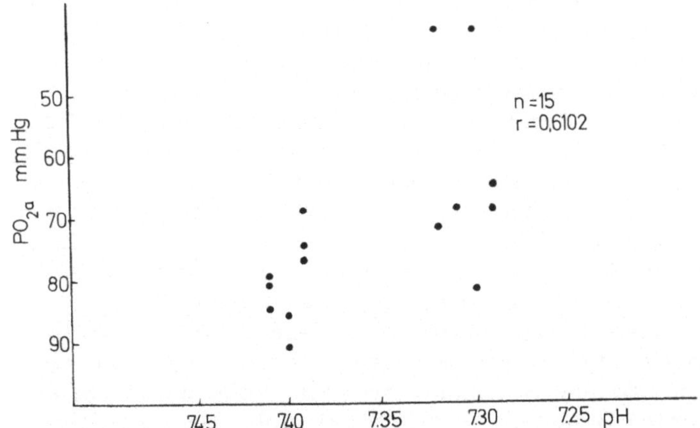

Abb. 1. Kapillarer Sauerstoffdruck in Beziehung zum rechtsventrikulären Druck bei 25 Patienten mit Atmungsinsuffizienz in Ruhe

Da bei unseren routinemäßigen Untersuchungen die Ausgangswerte, das Maß der Funktionsstörung und auch die Belastungsintensität nicht einheitlich waren, war zu erwarten, daß ein einheitliches Verhalten der Intrakardialdrucke und der Sauerstoffdrucke unter der Belastung nicht bestätigt werden konnte. Auffällig war jedoch, daß in fast allen Fällen unter der Belastung der rechtsventrikuläre Druck deutlich anstieg, wobei die Steigerung 7-34 mm Hg ausmachte. Dagegen fanden wir das Pulsverhalten weniger aufschlußreich, da die in Ruhe bereits häufig vorhandene Sinustachykardie des Cor pulmonale differenzierte Schlüsse über die Belastungsreserven nicht zuläßt. Hier liegen die Verhältnisse offensichtlich grundsätzlich anders als bei den vielfach untersuchten Jugendlichen und Sportlern. Überdies verbietet sich bei diesen Patienten eine sogenannte "Ausbelastung" bis in höchste Wattstufen.

Der Sauerstoffdruck unter Belastung verhielt sich ganz unterschiedlich, was früher bereits Hertz [3], zuletzt wieder Vogel und Mitarb. [11] gezeigt haben. In 4 Fällen unserer Patienten stieg der Sauerstoffdruck nach 4-6 Minuten Belastung an, in 10 Fällen sank er ab. Einen Anstieg des Sauerstoffdrucks sahen wir vereinzelt aber auch in solchen Fällen, in denen bereits in Ruhe oder dann unter Belastung eine pulmonale Hypertonie nachzuweisen war.

Würde man also in solchen Fällen den Sauerstoffdruck unter Belastung als entscheidendes oder einziges Kriterium anwenden, so könnte dies zu einem Fehlschluß führen. Derartige Diskrepanzen im Verhalten des Sauerstoffdrucks und des Ventrikeldrucks sind offensichtlich vor allem dann zu erwarten, wenn es sich um restriktive Ventilationsstörungen mit starker mechanischer Einschränkung der Ventilationsfläche und Beeinträchtigung des Pulmonalkreislaufs handelt.

Andererseits sahen wir auch immer wieder Patienten, die sich zu einer höheren Leistung zu einem Zeitpunkt bereits außerstande erklärten, bei denen weder intrakardiale noch arterielle Sauerstoffdrucke eindeutig pathologisch geworden waren.

Auf diese Krankheitsfälle, die frühzeitig bereits unter ansteigender Belastung ihren echten Atemgrenzwert erreichen, hatten wir bereits früher hingewiesen [8]. Offensichtlich erreichen in diesen Fällen die Atemwegswiderstände und die dadurch verursachte Dyspnoe unter ansteigender Belastung ein derart hohes Maß, daß dem Patienten die Fortführung der Belastung nicht mehr möglich ist. Man muß sich in solchen Fällen hüten, die Probanden als nicht genügend kooperativ zu beurteilen.

Die Verhältnisse im Säure-Basenhaushalt sind als Kriterien der muskulären und metabolischen Leistung ebenfalls von Interesse, in erster Linie der pH-Wert, der die Möglichkeit gibt, eine periphere Übersäuerung als Hinweis auf eine muskuläre Leistungsbegrenzung zu erkennen [6]. Kubicek hat dann die Wertung des Basendefizits unter ansteigender Belastung als Kriterium vorgeschlagen [5]. In unseren jetzigen Untersuchungen wurde dies aber weniger deutlich als eine Beziehung zwischen abfallendem Sauerstoffdruck und pH-Wert unter Belastung (r = 0,6102) (Abb. 2). Zwischen Säure-Basengehalt und Ventrikeldruck fanden wir keine Korrelation.

Außerdem läßt sich folgern, daß die Lungenfunktion in Ruhe und unter Belastung um so stärker eingeschränkt ist, je ausgeprägter die Hypoxämie,

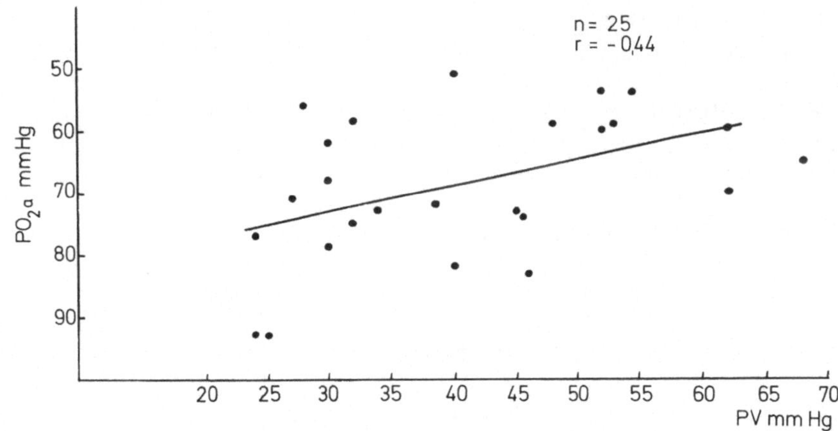

Abb. 2. Kapillarer Sauerstoffdruck im Verhältnis zum pH-Wert bei 15 Patienten mit Atmungsinsuffizienz unter Belastung (1 Watt/kg Körpergewicht)

je früher eine metabolisch oder respiratorisch bedingte Azidose erkennbar werden. Die Messungen des Ventrikeldrucks oder des Pulmonalarterien-Mitteldrucks bilden hierzu eine wichtige Ergänzung, zumal sie in manchen Fällen hinsichtlich der Aussage in unterschiedliche Richtung weisen.

LITERATUR

1. Cournand, A. : Some aspects of the pulmonary circulation in normal man and in chronic cardiopulmonary diseases. Circulation 2, 641 (1950)
2. Gaissmaier, U. , Klaus, D. , Sadowski, P. , Gauss, D. , Trübestein, G. : Erfahrungen mit der Mikrokathetertechnik nach Grandjean zur Rechtsherzsondierung. Med. Klin. 66, 1558-1564 (1971)
3. Hertz, C.W. : Zur Begutachtung von Lungenfunktionsstörungen durch den Arbeitsversuch. Dtsch. Med. Wschr. 90, 461 (1965)
4. Hertz, C.W. : Begutachtung von Lungenfunktionsstörungen. Stuttgart: Georg Thieme 1968
5. Kubicek, F. : Über das Verhalten des Basendefizits beim spiroergometrischen Arbeitsversuch. Wien. Klin. Wschr. 78, 590-595 (1966)
6. Marx, H.H. : Die Verschiebung des Säure-Basengleichgewichts bei chron. pulmonaler Insuffizienz. Verh. Dtsch. Ges. inn. Med. 71, 314 (1965)
7. Marx, H.H. , Zühlke, E. , Schütze, H. : Möglichkeiten und Grenzen der Ergometrie für klinische Fragestellungen. Z. Kreislaufforschg. 54, 1054 (1965)
8. Marx, H.H. : Die Beurteilung der Lungenfunktion und der Belastungsfähigkeit in der Klinischen Praxis. Münch. Med. Wschr. 110, 2952-2958 (1968)

9.   Meister, R. , Klempt, H. W. , Heine, J. : Pulmonalarterienmitteldruck und Lungenfunktion bei Skoliosepatienten. Med. Welt (N. F.) 26, 1397-1399 (1975)

10. Schüren, K. P. , Hüttemann, U. : Chron. obstruktive Lungenerkrankungen: Lungenkreislauf, Herzfunktion und Sauerstofftransport bei unterschiedlichen klin. Erscheinungsformen. Klin. Wschr. 51, 605-614 (1973)

11. Vogel, F. , Rost, H. D. , Geisler, L. S. : Der Arbeitsversuch in der Diagnostik von Lungenfunktionsstörungen. Therapiewoche 1975, 7079-7093

Prof. Dr. H. H. Marx
Medizinische Klinik im
Diakonissenkrankenhaus
Rosenbergstraße 38
D-7000 Stuttgart

Pneumonologie Suppl. 1976, 105-113
by Springer-Verlag 1976

Kardiopulmonale Funktionsstörungen in Ruhe und unter körperlicher Belastung bei Patienten mit einseitiger Pleuraschwarte *

N. Konietzko, H. Schlehe, K.H. Rühle, J. Brandstetter und H. Matthys

Sektion Pulmonologie des Departments Innere Medizin der Universität Ulm

---

Abstract. Patients with unilateral fibrothorax are limited in their working capacity to an extent, which can be estimated from the amount of restriction at spirometry. The limiting factor is the inability to increase the tidal volume during muscular work to an adequate degree. In addition, there is evidence of permanently increased dead space ventilation, which is thought to be due to an abnormally high $\dot{V}_A/\dot{Q}$ - ratio in the normal lung. During exertion, there is an increased work as well for the respiratory muscle as for the heart muscle: the latter is due to an increase in precapillary pulmonary vascular resistance and a hyperkinetic state of the circulation.

Key words: Pleural disease - Exercise - Ventilation/perfusion-imbalance - Dead space ventilation - Pulmonary hypertension

Zusammenfassung: Die körperliche Leistungsfähigkeit von Patienten mit einseitiger Pleuraschwarte ist reduziert in einem Ausmaß, das sich aus dem Grad der restriktiven Ventilationsstörung abschätzen läßt. Limitierend für die körperliche Belastbarkeit ist das Unvermögen, das Atemzugvolumen adäquat zu steigern. Hinzu kommt eine permanente Totraumhyperventilation, bedingt durch ein abnorm hohes Ventilations-/Perfusionsverhältnis in der gesunden Lunge. Die körperliche Arbeit wird erbracht mit einer erhöhten Atemarbeit, elastisch und teilweise viskös, und einer erhöhten Herzarbeit. Diese wiederum ist bedingt durch eine präkapillare pulmonale Widerstandserhöhung,die gut mit dem Ausmaß der Restriktion korreliert, und eine hyperkinetische Kreislaufregulationsstörung.

---

* Mit Unterstützung der Deutschen Forschungsgemeinschaft Ma. 466/6

I. EINLEITUNG

Patienten mit Pleuraschwarte sind in ihrer körperlichen Leistungsfähigkeit
eingeschränkt (Sommerwerck, 1974). In der prä- und postoperativen Funktionsdiagnostik und für gutachterliche Fragestellungen kann es bedeutsam
sein, daß Außmaß der Störung quantitativ zu erfassen. Unter nachfolgender
Fragestellung wurde deshalb ein Kollektiv von 49 Patienten mit einseitiger
oder vorwiegend einseitiger Pleuraverschwartung unterschiedlicher Ausdehnung und unterschiedlicher Ätiologie untersucht:

1. In welchem Ausmaß ist die körperliche Belastbarkeit von Patienten mit
   Pleuraschwarte gegenüber einem Normalkollektiv herabgesetzt?
2. Welche Störung limitiert die körperliche Leistungsfähigkeit?
3. Unter welchen Bedingungen wird die körperliche Leistung erbracht?
4. Läßt sich aus den in Ruhe durchgeführten spirometrischen Untersuchungen
   auf das Verhalten bei körperlicher Belastung rückschließen?

II. METHODIK

Lungenvolumina und Atemwegswiderstand wurden ganzkörperplethysmographisch bestimmt (Matthys, 1972), die Diffusionskapazität der Lunge für
CO im Einatemzugverfahren in der Modifikation nach Ogilvie et al. (1957).
Regionale Ventilation und Perfusion wurden bei Atemmittellage unter Verwendung von 133 Xenon und einer Szintilationskamera gemessen und mit
einem Rechner off-line bestimmt (Konietzko et al., 1974). Die bisher auf-
gezählten Untersuchungen wurden am sitzenden Patienten durchgeführt,
die folgenden hämodynamischen und respiratorischen Meßwerte am liegenden Patienten und ohne vorangegangene Prämedikation erhoben:
Der Einschwemmkatheter wurde nach der Grandjean-Technik in die
Pulmonalarterie eingeführt, die Drucke über ein Statham-Element gemessen. Blutproben wurden arteriell und zentralvenös entnommen und auf
folgende Werte analysiert: Hämatokrit, PO_2, PCO_2 und pH. Die Ventilation wurde im offenen System exspiratorisch gemessen, wie von Schlehe
et al. (1973) beschrieben. Dabei wurden folgende Parameter gemessen oder
errechnet: Sauerstoffaufnahme ($\dot{V}O_2$), CO_2-Abgase ($\dot{V}CO_2$), respiratorischer Quotient, arterio-venöse Sauerstoffdifferenz (C $(a-\bar{v})$ O_2), Herzzeitvolumen nach dem Fick-Prinzip ($\dot{Q}$), Drucke in der Pulmonalarterie
(Pap) einschließlich Mitteldruck ($\overline{P}ap$), Gesamtlungengefäßwiderstand
($R_L = \overline{P}ap/\dot{Q}$), alveo-arterieller O_2-Gradient nach der Alveolarluftformel
(P $(A-a)$ O_2) und prozentuelle Totraumventilation mit Hilfe von $PaCO_2$
(V_D/V_T). Nachdem die Ruhewerte erfaßt waren, wurden die Patienten im
allgemeinen in drei stufenförmig ansteigenden Belastungsstufen submaximal
belastet und die Messungen jeweils in kardiopulmonalen steady state in der
6. Minute durchgeführt.

III. PATIENTEN

Die Patienten waren im Durchschnitt 49 ± 6 Jahre alt, der jüngste 30,
der älteste 65 Jahre. Es wurden nur 3 Frauen untersucht. Bei 22 Patienten
handelte es sich um eine posttraumatische Pleuraschwarte, bei 27 Patienten
um eine postinfektiöse, zumeist posttuberkulöse. 20 Patienten hatten eine
einseitige "Mantelschwarte", der Rest wies umschriebene Schwielen auf,
die nicht den gesamten Hemithorax einnahmen, jedoch bis auf 2 Ausnahmen
das Zwerchfell miterfaßten.

IV. ERGEBNISSE

Tabelle 1 faßt die Ergebnisse der Messung von Lungenvolumina, Atemwegswiderstand und Diffusionskapazität für CO zusammen. Im Einzelfall
lagen bei 3 Patienten alle aufgeführten Werte im Normbereich, 10 Patienten zeigten eine gemischt restriktiv-obstruktive Ventilationsstörung, der
Rest war in unterschiedlichem Ausmaß restriktiv. Die bereits beim Gesamtkollektiv gegenüber der Norm nicht signifikant verschiedene funktionelle
Residualkapazität (FRK) blieb auch nach Unterteilung des Kollektivs in
obstruktive und nicht obstruktive Patienten gegenüber dem Sollwert nicht
verschieden.
    In Tabelle 2 sind die wichtigsten für die Ventilation, den Gasaustausch
und die Hämodynamik repräsentativen Meßwerte als Mittelwerte in Ruhe
und bei der letzten Belastungsstufe zusammengestellt. Eine statistisch
zu sichernde Korrelation zwischen Sauerstoffaufnahme oder Watt als Funktion der Leistung und den arteriellen Blutgasen wurde nicht gefunden, dagegen nahm die relative Totraumventilation von einem Ruhewert von 53%
exponentiell ab (V_D/V_T = 0, 346 - 0, 1137 $\dot{V}O_2$ (in Litern pro Minute)).
Das Herzzeitvolumen als Funktion der Sauerstoffaufnahme lag deutlich
über dem Sollwert (lg $\dot{Q}$ = 1, 103 + 0, 503 x lg $\dot{V}O_2$), bedingt durch einen
unproportionierten Pulsanstieg. Der Pulmonalarteriendruck stieg diastolisch
nur geringfügig, systolisch deutlich an, bedingt sowohl durch eine Erhöhung
des Flußes ($\dot{Q}$) als auch des Widerstandes (R_L).
    Abb. 1 zeigt die Steigerung des Atemvolumens als Funktion der Sauer-
stoffaufnahme bei dem Gesamtkollektiv, verglichen mit einem Normalkollektiv. In Abb. 2 ist der Gesamt-Lungengefäßwiderstand in Ruhe als
Funktion des Quotienten Vitalkapazität-Ist gegen Vitalkapazität-Soll aufgetragen.
    Tabelle 3 zeigt die regionale Lungenfunktion, am sitzenden Probanden
mit konstantem mittlerem Lungenvolumen gemessen und für den gesamten
gesunden bzw. kranken Lungenflügel ausgewertet.

Tabelle 1. Lungenvolumina, Atemwiderstand und Diffusionskapazität für CO beim Gesamtkollektiv, angegeben als Mittelwert mit einfacher Standardabweichung ($x \pm s$).

Parameter	Sollwert	Meßwert	Statistik	
	$\bar{x} \pm S$	$\bar{x} \pm S$	t	p
IVC (1)	4,95 $\pm$ 0,71	3,36 $\pm$ 0,88	14,134	< 0,001
RV (1)	1,93 $\pm$ 0,23	2,27 $\pm$ 0,94	2,857	< 0,005
FRC (1)	3,58 $\pm$ 0,46	3,49 $\pm$ 1,04	n.s.	
TLC (1)	6,86 $\pm$ 0,77	5,64 $\pm$ 1,33	6,611	< 0,001
FEV_1/IVC (%)	73,10 $\pm$ 2,62	69,16 $\pm$ 13,24	2,098	< 0,025
Raw* (cmH_2O/1 $\cdot$ sec^{-1})	1,85 $\pm$ 0,13	3,12 $\pm$ 1,90	4,546	< 0,001
$D_{L_{CO}}$-SB** (ml/min/mm Hg)	33,65 $\pm$ 4,41	28,05 $\pm$ 8,11	4,664	< 0,001
D_L/TLC_{He}^{**} (ml/min/mm Hg/1)	4,96 $\pm$ 0,24	4,91 $\pm$ 1,02	n.s.	
TLC_{He}/TLC_{BP}	1,02	0,99	n.s.	

n = 49 *n = 47 **n = 30

Tabelle 2. Mittelwert der wichtigsten Parameter für die Ventilation, den Gasaustausch und die Hämodynamik in Ruhe und in der letzten Belastungsstufe beim Gesamtkollektiv

Meßwert	Ruhe			Letzte Belastungsstufe		
$\dot{V}_{O_2}$ (1/min)	0,274	$\pm$	0,093	1,202	$\pm$	0,387
BE (mval/l)	- 0,28	$\pm$	2,01	- 3,01	$\pm$	2,10
Pa_{CO_2} (mm Hg)	37,6	$\pm$	5,1	37,6	$\pm$	5,0
Pa_{O_2} (mm Hg)	77,5	$\pm$	8,5	77,6	$\pm$	12,7
P (A-a) O_2 (mm Hg)	21,4	$\pm$	9,3	25,8	$\pm$	12,3
V_D/V_T	0,49	$\pm$	0,08	0,34	$\pm$	0,10
$\bar{P}ap$ (mm Hg)	16,8	$\pm$	4,6	32,5	$\pm$	9,1
$\dot{Q}$ (1/min)	7,28	$\pm$	3,27	13,66	$\pm$	4,11
R_1 (dyn $\cdot$ sec $\cdot$ cm^{-5})	209	$\pm$	93	202	$\pm$	95

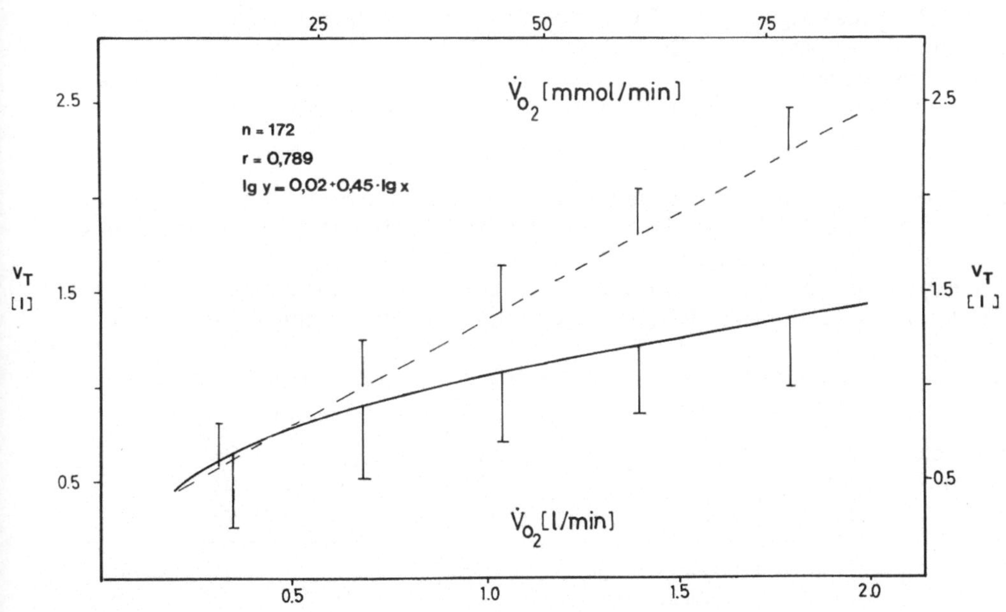

Abb. 1. Atemzugvolumen (V_T) in Litern (l) als Funktion der Sauerstoffaufnahme (V_{O_2}) in Litern pro Minute (l/min) beim Gesamtkollektiv der Patienten mit Pleuraschwarte (durchgezogene Linie) verglichen mit einem Normalkollektiv (gestrichelte Linie).

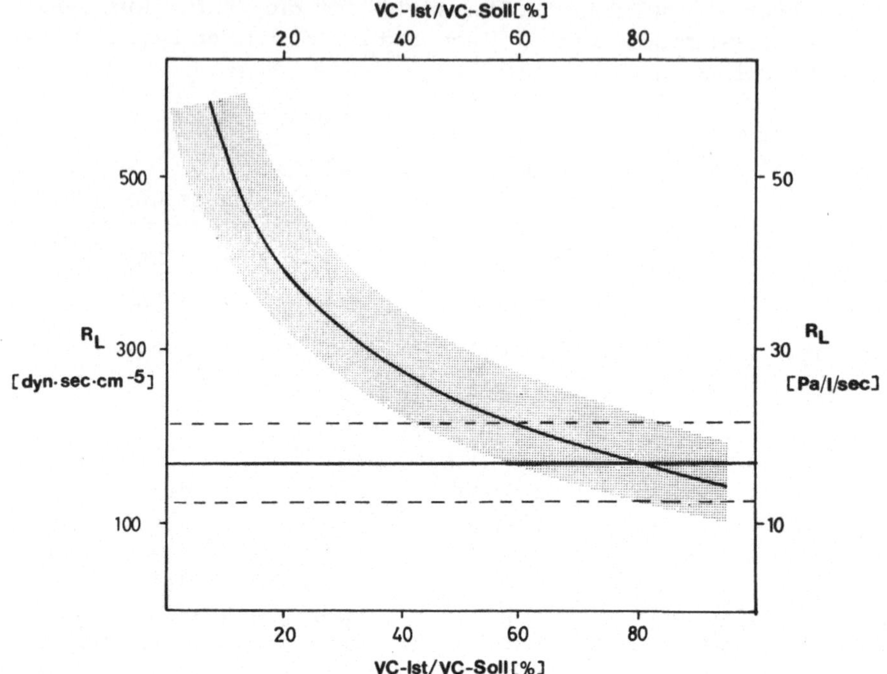

Abb. 2. Abhängigkeit des Lungengefäßgesamtwiderstandes ($R_L = \dfrac{\overline{P}_{ap}}{\dot{Q}}$) in Ruhe als Funktion der Ist-Vitalkapazität in Prozent des Sollwertes bei dem Gesamtkollektiv der Patienten mit einseitiger Pleuraschwarte. Die Horizontallinien repräsentieren den Normwert $\pm$ 2 s.

Tabelle 3. Ergebnisse der regionalen Lungenfunktionsdiagnostik, radiospirometrich mit 133 Xenon an 9 sitzenden Patienten bei Atemmittellage gemessen. Ventilation und Perfusion pro Einheit Lungenvolumen ($\dot{V}$-Index bzw. $\dot{Q}$-Index) und das Verhältnis beider zueinander sind jeweils für den gesamten gesunden, bzw. kranken Lungenflügel ausgewertet

Meßwert	gesunde Seite	kranke Seite	Statistik	
			t	p
$\dot{V}$-Index	120 $\pm$ 24	81 $\pm$ 14	3,44	< 0,005
$\dot{Q}$-Index	105 $\pm$ 7	90 $\pm$ 15	2,01	< 0,05
$\dot{V}/\dot{Q}$	1,13 $\pm$ 0,20	0,90 $\pm$ 0,11	2,84	< 0,01

n=9

V. DISKUSSION

Leistungslimitierend ist bei Patienten mit Pleuraschwarte die restriktive Ventilationsstörung. Die Verminderung der Brustwandcompliance erhöht die Atemarbeit direkt (Colp et al.; 1975; Sommerwerck, 1974) und indirekt: Die Atemmittellage steigt an und bei Erhöhung des Atemzugvolumens muß die Lunge im mechanisch ungünstigen, flacheren Teil der Compliancekurve bewegt werden (Caro et al., 1960). Das Atemzugvolumen wird während körperlicher Belastung weit weniger gesteigert als bei Normalpersonen (Abb. 1), die Möglichkeit über eine Steigerung der Atemfrequenz - vom energetischen Standpunkt aus gesehen günstiger - zu kompensieren, ist begrenzt, Eine zugleich bestehende Obstruktion schmälert diese Möglichkeit weiter. Zudem bewegen die Patienten sowohl in Ruhe als auch unter körperlicher Belastung einen deutlich größeren Totraumanteil pro Atemzugvolumen. Der Grund ist in einer Imbalance im Verhältnis von Ventilation zu Perfusion mit erhöhtem Ventilations-/Perfusions-Quotienten ("Luftshunt" in der gesunden Lunge zu sehen (Tabelle 3). Diese Befunde stehen im Gegensatz zu Schlußfolgerungen, die aus bronchospirometrischen Untersuchungen von Patienten mit einseitiger Pleuraschwarte gezogen werden (Patton et al. 1952, Siebens et al., 1956; Auteo, 1959). Die Erklärung ist darin zu suchen, daß die Perfusion über die Sauerstoffaufnahme berechnet wird und Areale der Lunge, die durchblutet, aber schlecht belüftet sind, wenig Sauerstoff aufnehmen werden. Die Perfusion wird also quantitativ mit dieser Methode unterschätzt. Kompartimente mit erniedrigtem Ventilations-/Perfusionsquotient ("Blutshunt") erscheinen im statistischen Mittel kein charakteristisches Merkmal der Pathophysiologie der Pleuraschwarte zu sein, wenn auch im Einzelfall, insbesondere bei zusätzlich bestehender Obstruktion mit inhomogener Ventilation, Hypoxämien mit Besserung unter Belastung beobachtet wurden (Hertz, 1954). Diffusionsstörungen sind ohne Bedeutung. Hämodynamisch ist die leichte, präkapillare pulmonale Hypertonie über eine disproportionierte Steigerung des Herzzeitvolumens und eine mäßige Erhöhung des Gefäßwiderstandes im präkapillären Schenkel der Lungenstrombahn erklärt. Diese Befunde decken sich mit kasuistischen Beiträgen über pulmonale Hypertonie bei Pleuraschwarten und ihre Besserung nach Decortication (Hughes et al., 1975; Robin et al., 1966; Petty et al., 1961). Ob die herzfrequenz-bedingte Steigerung des Herzeitvolumens die primäre Störung ist, wie etwa bei der Lungenfibrose, oder eine unzureichende venöse Ausschöpfung mit Erniedrigung der arteriovenösen Sauerstoffdifferenz, wie beim Untrainierten, die dann sekundär zu einer kompensatorischen Steigerung des Herzzeitvolumens führt, ist nicht zu entscheiden. Die Widerstandserhöhung ist korreliert mit dem Ausmaß der Restriktion und muß ins Kalkül gezogen werden, wenn die Vitalkapazität auf die Hälfte der Norm reduziert ist (Abb. 2).

LITERATUR

1. Autio, V.: The reduction of respiratory function by parenchymal and pleural lesions. A bronchospirometric study of patients with unilateral involvement. Acta Tuberc. Scand. 37, 112 (1959)

2. Caro, C. G., Butler, J., DuBois, A. B.: Some effects of pleural effusion on pulmonary function. Amer. Rev. Resp. Dis. 89, 55 (1964)

3. Colp, Ch., Reichel, J., Suh Park, S.: Severe pleural restriction: the maximum static pulmonary recoil pressure as an aid in diagnosis. Chest 67, 658 (1975)

4. Hertz, C. W.: Pleuraschwarte und Lungenfunktion II. Beitr. Klin. Tuberk. 112, 503 (1954)

5. Hughes, R. L., Jensik, R. J., Faber, L. P., Bliss, K.: Evaluation of unilateral decortication. Ann. Thorac. Surg. 19, 704 (1975)

6. Konietzko, N., Adam, W. E., Matthys, H.: Radioisotope in der modernen Lungenfunktionsdiagnostik. Münch. med. Wschr. 116, 159 (1974)

7. Matthys, H.: Lungenfunktionsdiagnostik mittels Ganzkörperplethys.-mographie. Stuttgart: F. K. Schattauer 1972

8. Ogilvie, C. M., Forster, R. E., Blakemore, W. S., Morton, J. W.: A standardized breath holding technique for clinical measurement of diffusing capacity of the lung for carbon monoxide. J. clin. Jnvest. 36, 1 (1957)

9. Patton, W. E., Waton, T. R., Gaensler, E. A.: Pulmonary function before and at intervals after surgical decortication of the lungs. Surg. Gynecol. Obstet. 32, 53 (1952)

10. Petty, T. L., Filley, G. F., Metchel, R. S.: Objective functional improvement by decortication after twenty years of artificial pneumothorax for pulmonary tuberculosis. Amer. Rev. Resp. Dis. 84, 572 (1961)

11. Robin, E. C.: Pulmonary hypertension and unilateral pleura constriction with speculation on pulmonary vasoconstrictive substances. Arch. Int. Med. 118, 391 (1966)

12. Rühle, K. H., Konietzko, N., Orth, U., Matthys, H.: Nominal values for a computer program to calculate ventilatory and hemodynamic parameters at rest and during exercise. General meeting on respiratory impairment including assessment of disablement (SEPCR), Budapest (1975)

13. Schlehe, H., Matthys, H., Härich, B., Nissen, H., Konietzko, N.: Vergleichende Herzminutenvolumenbestimmungen in Ruhe und bei körperlicher Belastung mittels Thermodilution und Fickschem Prinzip. Schweiz. med. Wschr. 103, 1773 (1973)

14. Siebens, A.: The physiologic effects of fibrothorax and the functional results of surgical treatment. J. Thorac. Surg. 32, 53 (1956)

15. Sommerwerck, D. : Funktionelle Ergebnisse nach Dekortikation
Thoraxchirurgie 22, 430 (1974)

Priv. -Doz. Dr. N. Konietzko
Ruhrlandklinik
4300 Essen 16

DISKUSSION

G. Fruhmann, München: Aus früheren Untersuchungen ist bekannt, daß
durch Pleuraschwarten die Entwicklung eines Lungenemphysems und
einer chronischen Bronchitis begünstigt wird. Ich möchte annehmen, daß
ein Teil der von Ihnen gefundenen Funktionsstörungen durch diese Sekundär-
erkrankungen hervorgerufen wird.

N. Konietzko, Essen: Dies trifft zu. Bei fast jedem 4. Patienten der vorliegenden Studie wurde eine Atemwegsobstruktion unterschiedlichen Ausmaßes diagnostiziert, bei allen bestand klinisch die Symptomatik einer
chronischen Bronchitis. Als pathogenetische Faktoren können Verziehung,
Abknickung und Torquierung des Bronchialsystems der befallenen Seite,
häufig mit Bronchiektasenbildung sowie eine Störung des Hustenmechanismus angenommen werden (die zum Erreichen hoher Strömungsgeschwindigkeit beim Hustenstoß wesentliche Kompression der Bronchien ist imkom-
plett). Hinweise auf das Bestehen eines perifokalen Lungenemphysems
im Bereich der Schwarte fanden sich in Form eines erhöhten Residualvolumens und eines erhöhten RV/TLC-Verhältnisses im Bereich der
kranken Lunge, verglichen zur gesunden Lunge, bei der regionalen Funktionsdiagnostik mit 133 Xenon.

Pneumonologie Suppl. 1976, 115-124

Atemfunktion und Lungenkreislauf bei thorakaler „Fesselung" der Lunge

R. Meister und H.-W. Klempt

Medizinische Klinik und Poliklinik der Westfälischen Wilhelms-Universität Münster

Kardiologische Abteilung der Medizinischen Klinik der Westfälischen Wilhelms-Universität Münster

Lung Function and Pulmonary Circulation in Patients with "Captive Lung" due to Chest Deformity

Abstract. The pulmonary dysfunction in patients with thoracic scoliosis is due to captivation of the lungs in a rib cage that is not only deformed but also restricted in its movements. A characteristic feature of the "captive lung" is the restricted ventilatory defect, the degree of impairment being determined by the degree of the deformity. Inspite of a reduction in ventilatory and circulatory reserves the arterial blood gases and the pulmonary artery pressure are normal during the early stages. Only if the lung volume has been reduced to a higher degree arterial hypoxaemia and pulmonary hypertension during exercise occur. There is a close negative correlation between arterial oxygen tension and pulmonary artery mean pressure. In addition correlations exist between vital capacity (% of predicted value) and some haemodynamic parameters (pressure gradient $\bar{P}_{PA} - \bar{P}_{PCV}$ at rest, PVR at rest and during exercise, $\Delta\bar{P}_{PA}$ from rest to exercise). - The presented results are based on investigations of cardiopulmonary function in 52 patients with moderate to severe thoracic scoliosis.

Key words: "Captive lung" - Chest deformity - Scoliosis - Lung function and haemodynamic

Zusammenfassung: Am Beispiel der skoliotischen Thoraxdeformität wurde untersucht, welchen Effekt die thorakale "Fesselung" der Lunge auf die Atemfunktion und Hämodynamik im kleinen Kreislauf hat. Als Probanden dienten 52 Skoliosepatienten (25 Jugendliche, 27 Erwachsene). In allen Fällen erfolgten Lungenfunktionsprüfungen sowie Druckmessungen im kleinen Kreislauf bei Körperruhe und unter Belastung. Bei 19 Erwachsenen wurde zusätzlich das Herzzeitvolumen bestimmt.

Lungenfunktionsanalytisch fand sich eine restriktive Ventilationsstörung, deren Ausmaß vom Schweregrad der Thoraxdeformität bestimmt wurde. Auch bei schwerer Einschränkung des Lungenvolumens blieb der Pulmonalarterienmitteldruck in Ruhe noch im Normalbereich. Es zeigte sich aber, daß der pulmonale Gefäßwiderstand mit abnehmendem Lungenvolumen leicht anstieg. Im Arbeitsversuch war sogar ein weiterer Anstieg über den Ruhewert zu beobachten. Zwischen dem Gefäßwiderstand und der Vitalkapazität (% des Sollwertes) ließ sich in Ruhe und unter Belastung eine negative Korrelation nachweisen. Auch das Verhalten des Pulmonalarterienmitteldruckes unter Belastung wies eine Abhängigkeit vom Grad der Restriktion auf. Der Druck stieg umso höher an, je stärker die Vitalkapazität eingeschränkt war. Weiterhin fanden sich eine negative Korrelation zwischen dem arteriellen Sauerstoffpartialdruck und dem Pulmonalarterienmitteldruck sowie eine Abhängigkeit des Gradienten zwischen Pulmonalarterienmitteldruck und mittlerem Pulmonalkapillardruck von der gemischtvenösen Sauerstoffsättigung.

Die Hinwendung verschiedener Parameter zum Pathologischen bei körperlicher Belastung machte deutlich, daß das Funktionsmuster der "gefesselten Lunge" im wesentlichen von dem Mangel an ventilatorischen und zirkulatorischen Reserven bestimmt wird.

Die Lunge ist als ein mechanisch tätiges Organ allein nicht funktionstüchtig, sondern in hohem Maße abhängig von der Intaktheit der sie umgebenden Strukturen wie Pleura, Thoraxwand und Zwerchfell, mit denen sie eine funktionelle Einheit bildet. Verlieren diese Strukturen ihre Beweglichkeit oder Dehnbarkeit, so resultiert daraus eine Behinderung der Pumpfunktion sowie eine Einschränkung des Luftfassungsvermögens der Lunge. Pleuraschwarten und Thoraxdeformitäten sind die häufigsten Ursachen für diese Form der extrapulmonalen Atemfunktionsstörung, deren Merkmal die "Fesselung" der Lunge ist.

Der Effekt der "Fesselung" läßt sich modellhaft am Beispiel der skoliotischen Thoraxdeformität studieren, da das Lungenparenchym beim Skoliotiker primär nicht krankhaft geschädigt ist, was vor allem für den jugendlichen Patienten gilt. Allfällige Atemfunktionsstörungen können darum als unmittelbare Folge der Fesselung gedeutet werden. Anders bei Pleuraschwarten. Sie sind häufig mit intrapulmonalen Läsionen kombiniert, so daß die Interpretation von Funktionsstörungen mehrerer Ursachen zu berücksichtigen hat.

Die vorliegende Untersuchung geht der Frage nach, welche Beziehungen zwischen Atemfunktion und Hämodynamik in der gefesselten Lunge bestehen.

UNTERSUCHUNGSGUT

Als Probanden dienten 52 Skoliosepatienten mit mittelgradigen bis schweren
Thoraxdeformitäten, bei denen ein primäres Lungenleiden ausgeschlossen
werden konnte. Das Kollektiv setzte sich aus 25 Jugendlichen und 27 Erwachsenen zusammen. Ätiologisch handelte es sich überwiegend um idio-
pathische Skoliosen. Hinsichtlich des Schweregrades der Thoraxdeformität
waren die Patienten beider Altersgruppen vergleichbar. Über den mittleren
Skoliosewinkel, das durchschnittliche Alter und die wichtigsten anthropometrischen Daten gibt Tabelle 1 Auskunft.

METHODIK

Bei allen Probanden wurden zunächst die Lungenvolumina und der bronchiale
Strömungswiderstand in einem volumenkonstanten Ganzkörperplethysmographen (Fa. Siemens) gemessen. Anschließend wurden am liegenden Patienten mit Hilfe eines mehrlumigen Ballon-Einschwemmkatheters die
Drucke im kleinen Kreislauf in Ruhe und unter Belastung gemessen. Die
Belastung am Fahrradergometer betrug bei den Jugendlichen 1 Watt/kg, bei
den Erwachsenen, deren Relativgewicht höher lag, 0,75 Watt/kg Körpergewicht. Der Arbeitsversuch erstreckte sich im Mittel über 7 Minuten. Bei
19 Erwachsenen wurde neben den Druckmessungen auch das Herzzeitvolumen
mit Hilfe der Thermodilutionsmethode [9] bestimmt. In allen Fällen wurde
gleichzeitig mit den Druckmessungen Kapillarblut aus dem hyperämisierten
Ohrläppchen zur Blutgasanalyse entnommen. Bei 17 Patienten konnte zusätzlich die gemischtvenöse Sauerstoffsättigung in Ruhe und unter Belastung
bestimmt werden. Als Analysegeräte dienten der Combi-Analysator der
Fa. Eschweiler sowie das IL-182-CO-Oximeter.
    Zur Festsetzung der Sollwerte für die Lungenvolumina wurde die Ist-
Körpergröße der Skoliotiker in der von Bjure et al. [2] beschriebenen Weise
auf die "wahre" Größe korrigiert. Die Referenzwerte für die Jugendlichen
wurden der Zusammenstellung von Polgar und Promadhat [18] entnommen.
Für die Erwachsenen wurden die Basler Sollwerte [1] zugrunde gelegt.

ERGEBNISSE UND DISKUSSION

Die wichtigsten lungenfunktionsanalytischen und hämodynamischen Daten
sind in Tabelle 1 und 2 zusammengefaßt.
    Die Messung der Lungenvolumina ergab - übereinstimmend mit den
Angaben in der Literatur [10, 12-14, 20-22] - eine Einschränkung der
Vital- und Totalkapazität in Abhängigkeit vom Schweregrad der Deformität.
Die Vitalkapazität war stets stärker von der Fesselung betroffen als die
Totalkapazität. Sie erwies sich damit als der empfindlichere Gradmesser
für die thorakogene Restriktion. Zwischen der Vitalkapazität (% Soll) und

Tabelle 1. Zusammenstellung der wichtigsten anthropometrischen und lungenfunktionsanalytischen Daten mit Angabe der Mittelwerte und Standardabweichungen. VC = Vitalkapazität; TLC = Totalkapazität; RV = Residualvolumen; IGV = intrathorakales Gasvolumen; R_t = totale Resistance

		Winkel ^{o} Cobb	Alter Jahre	Größe cm	Gewicht kg	VC % Soll	TLC % Soll	RV % TLC	IGV l	R_t cmH$_2$O/l
Jugendliche	$\bar{x}$	91,08	15,68	163,84	44,96	52,52	66,40	39,68	2,00	2,75
(n = 25)	± s	26,63	1,81	7,65	9,23	13,86	15,06	8,93	0,63	1,38
Erwachsene	$\bar{x}$	99,74	36,81	170,57	59,94	56,28	67,78	39,85	2,26	2,30
(n = 27)	± s	22,88	10,01	10,04	13,24	18,65	16,13	8,91	0,63	1,46

dem thorakalen Skoliosewinkel (^{o}Cobb) bestand eine negative Korrelation, die sich für die Patienten beider Altersgruppen nachweisen ließ (Jugendliche: r = -0,571; p < 0,01. Erwachsene: r = -0,683; p < 0,001). Eine ähnliche Abhängigkeit galt auch für die Totalkapazität (% Soll). Im Gegensatz dazu war das Residualvolumen zumeist normal oder nur wenig eingeschränkt. Folglich war sein Anteil innerhalb der reduzierten Totalkapazität erhöht und lag bei den Jugendlichen und Erwachsenen im Mittel zwischen 39 und 40%. Der bronchiale Strömungswiderstand verhielt sich in der Regel normal. Nur bei stark reduziertem Lungenvolumen (IGV) wurden leicht erhöhte Werte gemessen, was jedoch aufgrund der Volumen-abhängigkeit des bronchialen Strömungswiderstandes als physiologisch zu bewerten ist [4, 14, 17].

Der Lungenfunktionsbefund macht deutlich, daß durch die thorakale Fesselung vor allem die ventilatorischen Reserven, die sich gut in der Größe der Vitalkapazität wiederspiegeln, beschnitten werden. Da die Lunge

Tabelle 2. Zusammenstellung der wichtigsten blutgasanalytischen und hämodynamischen Daten mit Angabe der Mittelwerte und Standardabweichungen. PaO_2 = arterieller Sauerstoffpartialdruck; $PaCO_2$ = arterieller Kohlendioxydpartialdruck; $\bar{P}_{PA}$ = Pulmonalarterienmitteldruck; $\bar{P}_{PCV}$ = mittlerer Pulmonalkapillardruck; HF = Herzfrequenz; $\dot{Q}$ = Lungendurchfluß (= Herzzeitvolumen); PVR = pulmonal-vaskuläre Resistance

		PaO_2 mm Hg	$PaCO_2$ mm Hg	$\bar{P}_{PA}$ mm Hg	$\bar{P}_{PCV}$ mm Hg	HF min^{-1}	$\dot{Q}$ 1/min	PVR mm Hg/1/min
Ruhe								
Jugendliche	$\bar{x}$	80,80	38,79	16,20	9,29	87,66		
(n = 25)	$\pm$ s	5,82	2,42	3,73	3,24	15,50		
Erwachsene	$\bar{x}$	78,06	37,48	17,94	9,52	78,87	5,75[*]	1,61[*]
(n = 27)	$\pm$ s	11,50	4,07	4,89	2,51	12,11	1,01	1,19
Belastung								
Jugendliche	$\bar{x}$	77,16	38,83	23,47	10,11	158,25		
(n = 25)	$\pm$ s	12,38	3,10	5,23	4,45	15,54		
Erwachsene	$\bar{x}$	72,95	37,96	31,37	12,23	132,71	10,29[*]	1,93[*]
(n = 27)	$\pm$ s	14,94	5,08	12,29	4,24	23,18	1,87	1,97

[*] n = 19

jedoch von der Anlage her über große Reserven verfügt, kann sie bei Körperruhe oder leichter Belastung den Anforderungen im Gasaustausch häufig noch gerecht werden.

Ähnlich verhält es sich mit der Hämodynamik im Lungenkreislauf. Der Mangel an Perfusionsreserven macht sich bei Körperruhe und normalem Lungendurchfluß von 4-6 1/min nicht oder nur wenig bemerkbar. Der Pulmonalarterienmitteldruck bleibt auch bei schwerer Restriktion - solange noch nicht das Stadium der Globalinsuffizienz erreicht ist - zumeist im altersentsprechenden Normalbereich. Eine Abhängigkeit vom Skoliosewinkel ließ sich im eigenen Untersuchungsgut nicht nachweisen (r = 0,0033).

Obwohl der Pulmonalarterienmitteldruck bei Körperruhe den oberen Normalbereich gewöhnlich nicht überschreitet, finden sich doch bei

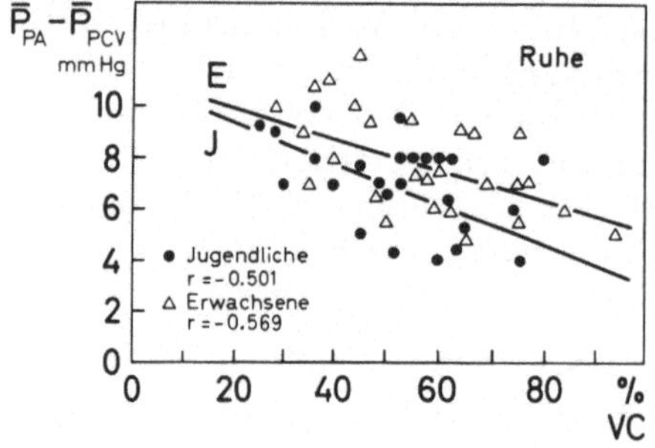

Abb. 1 a. Abhängigkeit des Gradienten zwischen Pulmonalarterienmitteldruck und mittlerem Pulmonalkapillardruck ($\bar{P}_{PA} - \bar{P}_{PCV}$) vom Grad der Restriktion, gemessen an der Größe der Vitalkapazität (VC in % des Sollwertes). J = Jugendliche (n = 25); E = Erwachsene (n = 27)

genauerer Betrachtung Anzeichen für eine veränderte Druck-Fluß-Beziehung im Lungenkreislauf. Wie aus Abb. 1 a hervorgeht, vergrößert sich mit abnehmendem Lugenvolumen der Gradient zwischen Pulmonalarterienmitteldruck und mittlerem Pulmonalkapillardruck. Zwischen dem Druckgradienten und der Vitalkapazität (% Soll) besteht eine negative lineare Korrelation, die für die Patienten beider Altersgruppen nachweisbar ist. Es ist danach zu vermuten, daß der pulmonale Gefäßwiderstand eine Abhängigkeit vom Grad der Restriktion aufweist. Diese Vermutung konnte durch die Untersuchungen an 19 Erwachsenen bestätigt werden, bei denen neben den Druckmessungen auch das Herzzeitvolumen bestimmt wurde. Es zeigte sich, daß der pulmonale Gefäßwiderstand mit abnehmender Vitalkapazität (% Soll) leicht ansteigt (r = -0,534; p <0,025). Die sich in Ruhe bereits ankündigende Störung der Druck-Fluß-Beziehung tritt unter Belastung bei vergrößertem Herzzeitvolumen stärker in Erscheinung. Während bei leichter Restriktion der Gefäßwiderstand unter Belastung noch gesenkt werden kann, steigt er bei stärkerer Einschränkung des Lungenvolumens sogar über den Ruhewert an und zeigt damit ein pathologisches Verhalten [5]. Zwischen dem Gefäßwiderstand und der Vitalkapazität (% Soll) besteht eine negative Korrelation (r = -0,692; p < 0,01).

Der sich in dem erhöhten Gefäßwiderstand wiederspiegelnde Mangel an Perfusionsreserven in der gefesselten Lunge macht verständlich, daß der Pulmonalarteriendruck unter Belastung stärker ansteigt als bei

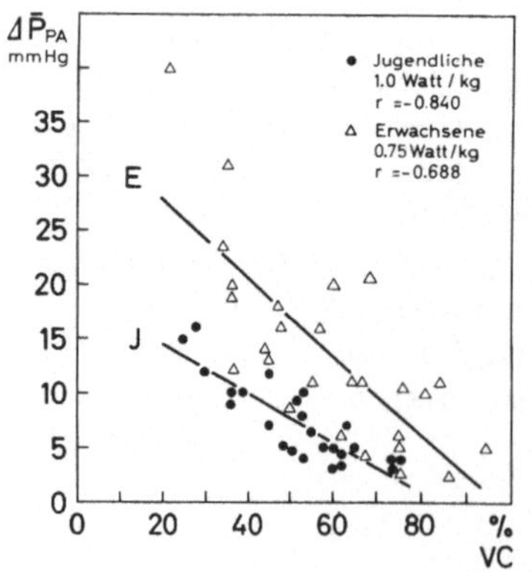

Abb. 1 b. Anstieg des Pulmonalarterienmitteldruckes unter Belastung in Abhängigkeit vom Grad der Restriktion, gemessen an der Größe der Vitalkapazität (VC in % des Sollwertes). $\Delta \bar{P}_{PA}$ = Differenz zwischen Pulmonalarterienmitteldruck in Ruhe und unter Belastung. J = Jugendliche (n = 25); E = Erwachsene (n = 27)

Normalpersonen. Auch hier zeigt sich die Abhängigkeit des Druckverhaltens vom Grad der Restriktion. Je tiefer die Vitalkapazität unter dem Sollwert liegt, umso höher steigt bei einer definierten Belastung der Pulmonalarteriendruck an (Abb. 1 b). Jugendliche und Erwachsene unterscheiden sich nur quantitativ in der Höhe des Druckanstiegs, was aus dem getrennten Verlauf der Regressionsgeraden hervorgeht. Das unterschiedliche Druckverhalten in beiden Altersgruppen findet wahrscheinlich seine Erklärung in sekundären Gefäßwandveränderungen beim Erwachsenen [16].

Der Pulmonalarterienmitteldruck korreliert nicht nur mit der Vitalkapazität, sondern weist auch eine enge Beziehung zum arteriellen Sauerstoffpartialdruck auf. Im eigenen Untersuchungsgut ließ sich eine negative lineare Korrelation zwischen beiden Größen herstellen (Abb. 2 a). Die Abhängigkeit war für die Werte in Ruhe und unter Belastung statistisch signifikant ($p < 0,001$).

Diese enge Beziehung zwischen Sauerstoffpartialdruck und Pulmonalarterienmitteldruck ist aus pathophysiologischer Sicht interessant, da in allen Fällen - von einer Ausnahme abgesehen - der arterielle Kohlendioxydpartialdruck nicht erhöht war und somit keine Zeichen einer globalen alveolären Hypoventilation bestanden. Die Korrelation kann nicht aus dem von v. Euler und Liljestrand [8] beschriebenen Reflexmechanismus erklärt werden, da die Voraussetzung zu diesem Mechanismus, die alveoläre Hypoxie, nicht erfüllt ist. Es stellt sich deshalb erneut die bisher unbefriedigend geklärte Frage, ob die arterielle oder zentralvenöse Hypoxämie unabhängig von den alveolären Gasspannungen zu einer Drucksteigerung im Lungenkreislauf beitragen kann. Rossier und Bühlmann [6, 19] haben sich wiederholt gegen eine solche Interpretation ausgesprochen. Andere, vor allem anglo-amerikanische Autoren unterstreichen die Bedeutung der Hypoxämie für die Entstehung der pulmonalen Hypertonie [3, 7, 11, 15].

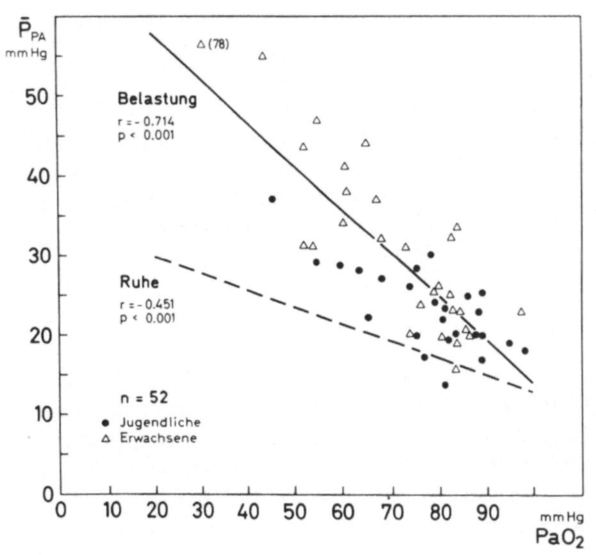

Abb. 2a. Beziehung zwischen arteriellem Sauerstoffpartialdruck (PaO$_2$) und Pulmonalarterienmitteldruck (P̄PA) in Ruhe und unter Belastung. Zur besseren Übersichtlichkeit sind die Werte in Ruhe nicht eingezeichnet, sondern nur durch die Regressionsgerade repräsentiert

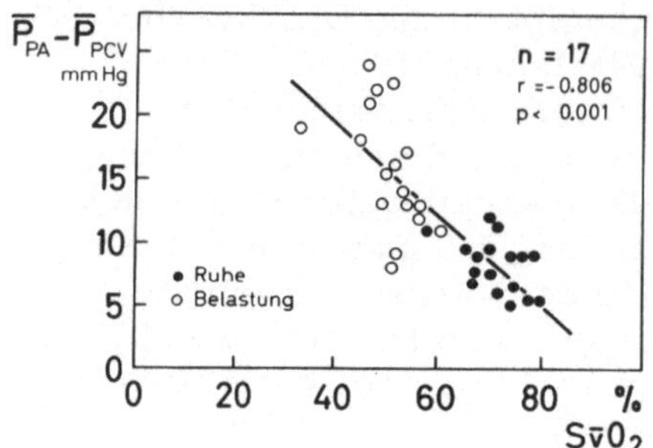

Abb. 2 b. Abhängigkeit des Gradienten zwischen Pulmonalarterienmitteldruck und mittlerem Pulmonalkapillardruck ($\bar{P}_{PA}$ - $\bar{P}_{PCV}$) von der gemischtvenösen Sauerstoffsättigung ($S\bar{v}O_2$) in Ruhe und unter Belastung

In diesem Zusammenhang mag eine weitere Beobachtung an den Skoliose-patienten von Interesse sein. Bei 17 Erwachsenen, bei denen die gemischt-venöse Sauerstoffsättigung bestimmt wurde, fand   sich statistisch eine Abhängigkeit des Druckverhaltens von der Sättigung (Abb. 2 b). Mit ab-nehmender zentralvenöser Sauerstoffsättigung vergrößerte sich der Gradient zwischen Pulmonalarterienmitteldruck und mittlerem Pulmonalkapillardruck. Wie aus Abb. 2 b ersichtlich, läßt sich für die Werte in Ruhe und unter Belastung eine gemeinsame Regressionsgerade errechnen. Der Korrelations-koeffizient ist mit 0,806 erstaunlich hoch (p < 0,001). Dieser Befund ist mit den tierexperimentell gewonnenen Ergebnisse von Boake et al. [3] sowie mit den Mitteilungen von Doyle et al. [7]vereinbar. Er steht jedoch im Widerspruch zu den Beobachtungen, die Widimsky [23] an Tuberkulose-kranken mit Cor pulmonale machen konnte.

SCHLUSSFOLGERUNG

Gesamthaft betrachtet geht aus den eigenen Ergebnissen hervor, daß bei Patienten mit thorakal gefesselter Lunge vielfältige, teils enge Beziehun-gen zwischen den Parametern der Atemfunktion und Hämodynamik be-stehen. Viele dieser Beziehungen mögen Parallelerscheinungen sein, die auf eine gemeinsame "Störgröße" zurückgehen. Es ist vorstellbar, daß die Fesselung der Lunge gleichermaßen zu einer Einschränkung der respira-torischen wie zirkulatorischen Reserven führt. Die Hinwendung verschie-dener Funktionsparameter zum Pathologischen bei körperlicher Belastung unterstreicht das Problem der Reserven, von dem das Funktionsmuster der gefesselten Lunge vorranging bestimmt wird.

LITERATUR

1. Amrein, R., Keller, R., Joos, H., Herzog, H.: Neue Normalwerte für die Lungenfunktionsprüfung mit der Ganzkörperplethysmographie. Dtsch. med. Wschr. 94, 1785 (1969)
2. Bjure, J., Grimby, G., Nachemson, A.: Correction of body height in predicting spirometric values in scoliotic patients. Scand. J. clin. Lab. Invest. 21, 190 (1968)

3. Boake, W.C., Daley, R., McMillan, I.K.R.: Observations on hypoxic pulmonary hypertension. Brit. Heart J. 21, 31 (1959)

4. Briscoe, W.A., DuBois, A.B.: The relationship between airway resistance, airway conductance and lung volume in subjects of different age and body size. J. clin. Invest. 37, 1279 (1958)

5. Bühlmann, A., Schaub, F., Luchsinger, P.: Die Bedeutung des Arbeitsversuches beim Herzkatheterismus für das Studium der Hämodynamik des Lungenkreislaufes und für die Diagnostik der kardialen Rechtsüberlastung. Verh. Dtsch. Ges. Kreislaufforschg. 21, 346 (1955)

6. Bühlmann, A., Schaub, F., Rossier, H.: Zur Ätiologie und Therapie des Cor pulmonale. Schweiz. med. Wschr. 84, 587 (1954)

7. Doyle, J.T., Wilson, J.S., Warren, J.V.: The pulmonary vascular responses to short-term hypoxia in human subjects. Circulation 5, 263 (1952)

8. Euler, von, U.S., Liljestrand, G.: Observations on the pulmonary arterial blood pressure in the cat. Acta physiol. Scand. 12, 301 (1946)

9. Fegler, G.: Measurement of cardiac output in anaesthetized animals by a thermal dilution method. Quart. J. exp. Physiol. 39, 153 (1954)

10. Grueter, H.: Über die ventilatorische Funktion und Elastizität der Lungen bei Skoliose. Verh. Dtsch. Orthop. Ges. 50, 118 (1963)

11. Harvey, R.M., Ferrer, M.I., Richards, D.W., Cournand, A.: Influence of chronic pulmonary disease on the heart and circulation. Amer. J. Med. 10, 719 (1951)

12. Mankin, H.J., Graham. J.J., Schack, J.: Cardiopulmonary function in mild and moderate idiopathic scoliosis. J. Bone Jt. Surg. 46-A, 53 (1964)

13. Meznik, F., Kummer, F.: Skoliose und Lungenfunktion. Z. Orthop. 108, 382 (1970)

14. Meister, R., Heine, J.: Die skoliotische Thoraxdeformität und ihre Auswirkung auf die Lungenfunktion. Prax. Pneumol. 29, 219 (1975)

15. Motley, H.L., Cournand, A., Werkö, L., Himmelstein, A., Dresdale, D.: Influence of short periods of induced acute anoxia upon pulmonary artery pressure in man. Amer. J. Physiol. 150, 315 (1947)

16. Naeye, R.L.: Kyphoscoliosis and cor pulmonale: a study of the pulmonary vascular bed. Amer. J. Path. 38, 561 (1961)

17. Nolte, D.: Der bronchiale Strömungswiderstand im Kindesalter. Klin. Wschr. 46, 783 (1968)

18. Polgar, G., Promadhat, V.: Pulmonary function testing in children. Techniques and standards. Philadelphia-London-Toronto: W.B. Saunders Com. 1971

19. Rossier, P.H., Bühlmann, A.: Cor pulmonale et pathophysiologie alveolaire. Cardiologia (Basel) 25, 132 (1954)

20. Scheier, H.: Skoliose und Lungenfunktion. In: Prognose und Behandlung der Skoliose. Stuttgart: Georg Thieme 1967

21. Westgate, H.D.: Pulmonary function in thoracic scoliosis. Before and after corrective surgery. Minnesota Med. 53, 839 (1970)

22.   Westgate, H. D. , Moe, J. H. : Pulmonary function in kyphoscoliosis
      before and after correction by the Harrington instrumentation method.
      J. Bone Jt. Surg. 51-A, 935 (1969)
23.   Widimský, J. : DerEinfluß der Anoxie auf den kleinen Kreislauf bei
      Lungentuberkulose. In: Cor pulmonale bei Lungentuberkulose.
      J. Widimský, Ed. Jena: Gustav Fischer 1963

Dr.med. R. Meister
Medizinische Universitätsklinik
Westring 3
44 Münster

Pneumonologie Suppl. 1976, 125-132

Interpretation of Pulmonary Function by Means of the Pulmonary Age Equivalent (PAE)

H. Löllgen and F. H. Hertle

Krankenhaus Bethanien für die Grafschaft Moers, Moers and
Deutsche Klinik für Diagnostik, Wiesbaden

Abstract. Most of the cardiopulmonary function data demonstrate an age dependence. Reversing this relationship, and combining several lung function parameters, age can be estimated by a multiple regression equation. This estimated age then can be regarded as a "functional age". In this study, preliminary results of the estimated functional age are given. The equations for this estimation have been developed in a population of healthy subjects and have been applied to groups of smokers, exsmokers, and elder sportsmen. The results demonstrate the validity and sensitivity of the described procedure. Further studies will have to establish the reliability and the limitations of the concept. Main fields of application seem to be epidemiologic surveys and early detection of cardiopulmonary diseases.

Key words: Pulmonary age equivalent - Age dependence - Lung function - Exercise test - Data reduction - Smoking

---

INTRODUCTION

When interpreting pulmonary function analysis, differences of more than twofold standard deviation between the measured data and the mean normal values are taken as pathologic. The final judgment depends on the subjective, descriptive summary of all the normal and pathologic values with special regard to the investigator's experience.

In the last years, methods have been described combining several functional parameters to differentiate between degrees of physical fitness or between health and illness, for example discriminance analysis (Küng et al., 1969; Michaelis, 1972), and factor analysis (Ismail et al., 1965; Israel et al., 1969). Another approach for combining assessment of lung function parameters has been suggested by Lange et al., (1968), the so-called pulmonary age equivalent (PAE).

Recently, the mathematical procedure for the PAE has been developed, and the model has been tested in an epidemiologic study (Lange et al., 1973).

The concept of the pulmonary age equivalent derives from the observation, that most of pulmonary variables demonstrate an age dependence at rest and/

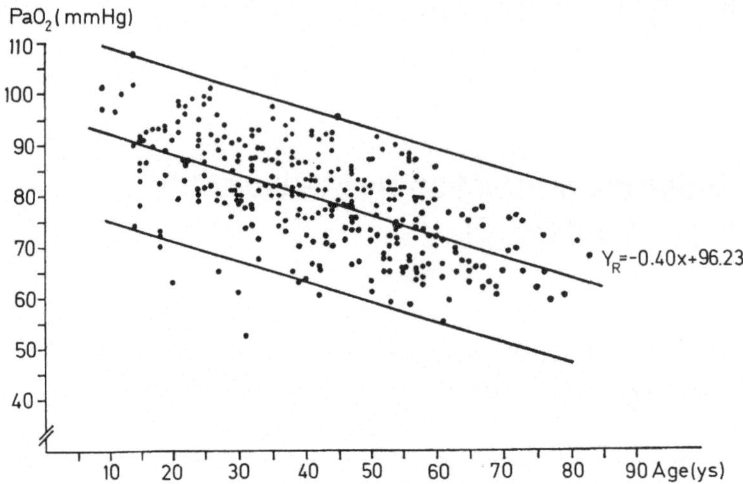

Fig. 1. Age dependence of arterial oxygen partial pressure (from Hertle et al. , 1971)

or at exercise. The same comes true for cardiocirculatory data. This then can be called the cardiopulmonary age equivalent. In this communication, these two terms are used in an identical sense though it should be kept in mind that are differences.

One typical example for the age dependence is shown in Figure 1. Arterial oxygen partial pressure (PaO_2) decreases with increasing age. Reversing the regression equation in Figure 1, that means $x = a \cdot y + b$ instead of $y = a \cdot x + b$ (with age = x and PaO_2 = y), age can be estimated from the measured arterial oxygen partial pressure. This estimation of age then shows a wide variation, which is suggested to become smaller if age is estimated (or calculated) by several age-dependent variables by means of a multiple regression equation. This estimation is assumed to represent the functional age, or, if the calculation is based on lung function data, the pulmonary age equivalent.

In the present study an attempt was made to establish multiple regression equations based on a greater number of cardiopulmonary variables at rest and at exercise. For the evaluation of the data, a group of strictly defined healthy subjects has been investigated in a prospective study. Final the obtained formulas should be applied on a group of smokers, exsmokers, and elderly sportsmen in order to test the discriminatory power of the equations.

MATERIAL

One hundred healthy subjects were examined in this study. Fifty-eight of them fulfilled the criteria given in a negative catalogue, that means they had no diseases of the cardiopulmonary and vascular system at any time before the investigation. Among the resting healthy subjects, there were 18 nonsmoking middle-aged men actively engaged in muscular exercise, 9 healthy exsmokers (no smoking at least for 1 year prior to the examination) and 15 healthy smokers (more than 20 cigarettes at least more than 1 year before the examination).

The subjects for this study were randomly selected by the Bahnarzt (Dr. R. Stufler ✛) of the Deutsche Bundesbahn (Mainz) and sent to the laboratory for further examinations.

METHODS

All subjects gave a detailed family and personal past history and underwent a thorough clinical examination with emphasis on the cardiorespiratory system. A biochemical profile was established from venous blood and revealed normal values in all subjects. Chest X-ray were without pathologic findings. The following examinations were carried out:

Spirometry: open system with a pneumotachograph; airway resistance and intrathoracic gas volume (IGV) by means of a volume constant whole body plethysmograph (Fa. Jaeger, Würzburg); respiratory gas analysis - endtidal and mixed expiratory gas - by mass spectrometry (Fa. Varian MAT, Bremen); (for details see Löllgen et al., 1973); blood gases (Gas Check, Fa. AVL, Linz); the ergometer used was an electrically braked bicycle ergometer (Fa. Jaeger, Würzburg), pedal revolutions were 60 rpm. ECG: at rest and exercise 8-channeled recorder (Minograph Fa. Elema, Sweden). The signals of expiratory partial pressures of O_2 and CO_2 were registered on a UV recorder (Fa. Bell & Howell, Friedberg). From the measured values, other variables, such as $\dot{V}_{O_2}$ have been calculated.

MATHEMATICAL EVALUATION

The mathematical approach has been described in detail by Lange et al. (1973). Therefore the procedure is summarized here. In a first step, a matrix of coefficients of correlation was calculated including anthropometric data and lung function values. A further evaluation was done with the following age-dependent variables: at rest: vital capacity (VC), forced expiratory volume within 1 s ($FEV_{1.0}$), IGV, Pa_{O_2}; at exercise (10 mkp/s): base excess, heart rate and oxygen uptake ($\dot{V}_{O_2}$) and Pa_{O_2}. The age dependence of these values remained significant after eliminating the influence of height and weight arithmetically by means of partial correlation analysis. The obtained relationships proved linear in the normals' group (aged from 22-60 years; $\bar{x}$ = 41 years).

Therefore, there was no need for a transformation of the variables into linearized relationship. However, nonlinear relationships can easily be included after linearization into this method.

As most of the lung function data demonstrate significant relationships to height and weight (Hertle et al., 1971), the used variables had to be standardized according to both of these anthropometric values. This was done by a multiple regression equation, estimating each value by age (x_1), height (x_2), and weight (x_3), and constants (d), (k_1). In general, this equation can be expressed by:

$$y = a_1 x_1 + a_2 x_2 + a_3 x_3 + d \qquad (1)$$

or, for VC, e. g. ,

$$y = 3, 5\ x_1 + 5.\ 09\ x_2 - 3.\ 24 \qquad (2)$$

This can be rearranged to:

$$- 3, 5\ x_1 + k_1 = VC - 5, 09\ x_2 + 3.\ 24 \qquad (3)$$

solving for age, we get:

$$x_1 = 0.\ 31\ VC + 1.\ 57\ x_2 - 1.\ 0 \qquad (4)$$

In the multiple regression equations of the above-mentioned eight variables, the coefficients of weight were almost zero, thus they could be neglected. In equation (4), x_1 is the standardized VC, a term introduced by Lange et al. (1973). However, this "standardized" variable indeed is the estimation of age by means of one variable (in this example VC) and height. Therefore, equation (4) can be rewritten as:

$$\hat{A} = - 0.\ 31\ VC + 1.\ 57\ x_2 - 1.\ 0 \qquad (5)$$

with $\hat{A}$ as a symbol for the estimated age, i. e. , the functional age. After all variables are given by multiple regression equation (if necessary), the modified variables are used to calculate again a multiple regression equation by the method of the last squares to establish formulas for estimating the functional age - or the age equivalent - based on four (6) to eight variables (7). The indices of equations (6) and (7) are as follows:

x_1 = VC (ml); x_2 = $FEV_{1.0}$ (ml); x_3 = IGV (ml); x_4 = Pa_{O_2} (Torr); x_5 = Pa_{O_2} (Torr) (at exercise); x_6 = $\dot{V}_{O_2}$ (ml/min); x_7 = base excess (mEqu/1); x_8 = heart rate (beats/min); y_1 = height (cm); A = age (years).

The formula for the age equivalent, based on four variables at rest is:

$$\hat{A} = 0.\ 028\ x_1 - 0053\ x_2 - 0.\ 027\ x_3 + 0.\ 605\ x_4 - 0.\ 217\ y_1 +$$
$$0.\ 434\ A - 58, 1 \qquad (6)$$

based on four variables at rest and on four variables at exercise, the equation is:

$$\hat{A} = 0.\ 026\ x_1 + 0.\ 027\ x_2 - 0.\ 023\ x_3 + 0.\ 437\ x_4 + 0.\ 38\ x_5 +$$
$$0.\ 423\ x_7 - 0.\ 115\ x_8 - 0.\ 11\ y_1 + 0.\ 57\ A - 46.\ 8$$

Finally, the difference between the chronologic age and the estimated age $(\hat{A})$ is denoted by $\Delta\ \hat{A}$. This difference was assumed to be zero in the normals. This means, according to the underlying concept, that chronologic age and functional or estimated age are indentical.

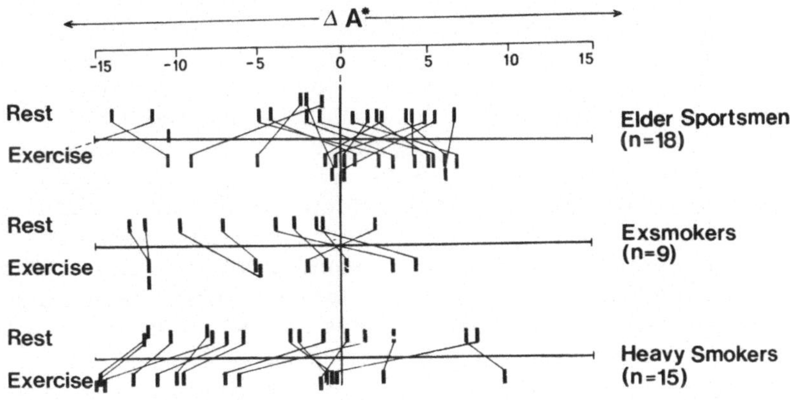

Fig. 2. Bar chart of differences between chronologic age and estimated age ($\Delta \hat{A}$) for three groups. Above the abscissa, values estimated by equation (6), below by equation (7)

RESULTS AND DISCUSSION

The $\Delta \hat{A}$ values obtained by the above-noted formulas are shown in Figure 2. The lines above the abscissa are values of equation (6), the lines below are those of equation (7). The individual values are connected to demonstrate the shift of $\Delta \hat{A}$, when exercise test values are included into the equation.

The corresponding mean values are listed in Table 1. The $\Delta \hat{A}$ values for exsmokers and smokers are shifted to the negative range applying formula (6), whereas the values of the elder sportsmen are about zero. The estimation of $\Delta \hat{A}$ by means of lung function values at rest and exercise [formula (7)] demonstrate that the three groups can be discriminated more exact-

Table 1. Mean values and standard deviation of the $\Delta \hat{A}$ values

	Elder Sportsmen	Ex-smokers	Smokers
At rest	- 0. 6 ± 5. 6	- 6. 5 ± 4. 6	- 3. 4 ± 6. 5
At exercise	- 0. 1 ± 6. 4	- 3. 6 ± 6. 4	- 6. 6 ± 7. 0

130

ly. Figure 2 shows the differences between $\Delta \hat{A}$ values of equation (6) and equation (7). In the smokers' group, the values become more negative, the values of the elderly sportsmen remain unchanged; in the exsmokers, $\Delta \hat{A}$ values even increase. This can be explained by the often seen decrease of ventilatory disturbances at exercise in these subjects. Figure 2 and Table 1 reveal that mean values for $\Delta \hat{A}$ in the physically active subjects do not differ significantly from those of the normals. This can be explained by the fact that pulmonary function is nearly unaffected by physical training (Löllgen et al., 1973); in addition, the submaximal exercise test, used to establish equation (7), may not be sufficiently appropriate to render differing results in trained and untrained subjects. However, when separating normals and smokers, this test procedure yields data which enable a sufficient differentiation of the two groups (Figure 3, Table 2).

The differences of the mean values among the three groups have been tested by means of student's test. The results are listed in Table 2, demonstrating the significant differences. Sportsmen differ from exsmokers in the resting values and from smokers in the exercise data and the difference values. Smokers and exsmokers mainly differ in the different behavior of $\Delta \hat{A}$ at exercise.

The given examples illustrate that estimation of PAE by combining various criteria into a multiple regression equation is possible. The preliminary results point out that influencing factors, e. g. smoking, can be demonstrated by this procedure. Formulas depending on exercise values give additional information and increase the sensibility of the method.

In the above-given equations (6) and (7), A is estimated by several variables including age. This means that $\hat{A}$ cannot be calculated by lung func-

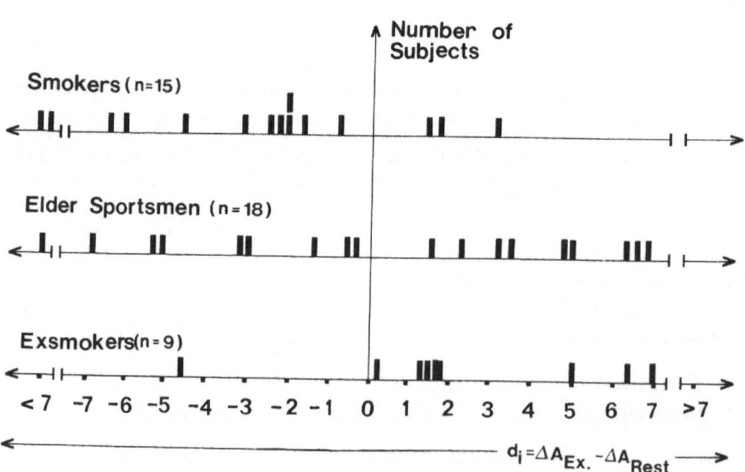

Fig. 3. Bar chart of differences between $\Delta \hat{A}$ values estimated by equation (6) and (7), i. e., (6)-(7). For details see text

Table 2. Levels of statistical significance (Student's test) between the differences of the groups (mean values of Table 1). xx = $p < 0.01$; E = exercise; R = rest

	Exsmokers	Smokers
Elderly Sportsmen		
R	xx	Ø
E	Ø	xx
E - R	Ø	xx
Exsmokers		
R	-	Ø
E	-	Ø
E - R	-	xx

tion data only. Continuing evaluations considering other variables, e. g., $\dot{V}O_{2max}$ or DL_{CO} (Luft, 1973) will show if the coefficient of age can be reduced further.

In addition, it has to be tested in another study if a certain combination of variables, including cardiac function, will enable a differentiation of a cardiac age equivalent from a PAE.

It should be admitted here, that one disadvantage of this model is the lack of age dependence of some variables important in lung function analysis, for example airway resistance. However, such values have to be considered in the conventional way, as no definitive solution for this problem has yet been found.

The advantages of the described model are that such an index is easy to understand, even by nonphysicians, that it combines various criteria with regard to weight of the single variable (lowered or increased by the coefficient). Up to now there are only small experiences with the PAE. The study needed is to apply the formulas on clinical routine. The preliminary results point out that the model functions well in epidemiologic surveys (Lange et al., 1973). In addition, early diagnosis of cardiopulmonary diseases will be another promising field of application.

The authors acknowledge the very careful assistance of Mrs. Friese-Küchler and Mrs. Winkler. The experiments of this study were performed in the II. Med. Klinik and Poliklinik (Mainz) with support of the Deutsche Forschungsgemeinschaft. The statistical evaluation was performed with the help of the Institut für Med. Datenverarbeitung (Prof. Dr. H. J. Lange), Munich, FRG.

REFERENCES

Hertle, F. H. , Goerg, R. , Lange, H. J. : Die arteriellen Blutgaspartialdrucke und ihre Beziehungen zu Alter und anthropometrischen Größen.
Respiration 28, 1-30 (1971)

Ismail, A. H. , Falls, H. B. , MacLeod, D. F. : Development of a criterion
for physical fitness tests from factor analysis. J. Appl. Physiol. 20,
991-999 (1965)

Israel, S. , Thierbach, P. , Israel, G. : Faktorenanalytische Darstellung
von Kennziffern der Herzkreislauffunktion bei Herzen unterschiedlicher
Größe. Med. Sport. (Berlin) 7, 209-213 (1969)

Küng, S. , Müller, H. , Schönholzer, G. : Der Aussagewert spiroergome-
trischer Untersuchungen im Leistungsfähigkeitsspektrum des Menschen.
Schweiz. Zschr. Sportmed. 16, 91-135 (1969)

Lange, H. J. , Hertle, F. H. : Zum Problem der Normalwerte. In:Hertz, C.
W. : Begutachtung von Lungenfunktionsstörungen. Stuttgart: Georg Thieme Verlag 1968

Lange, H. J. , Reiter, R. , Welzl, G. , Neiss, A. : Das Altersäquivalent -
Ein Verfahren zur Datenverdichtung bei der Auswertung multivariater
epidemiologischer Studien. Meth. Inform. Med. 12, 61-67 (1973)

Löllgen, H. , Hertle, F. H. , Stufler, R. : Spirometrische und atemmechanische Meßgrößen und aerobe Kapazität. Med. Sport (Berlin) 13, 211-214
(1973)

Luft, U. C. : Die körperliche Leistungsfähigkeit von Berufspiloten in Abhängigkeit vom Alter. XXI. Int. Kongr. f. Luft- und Raumfahrtmedizin,
München, 1973, Proceedings pp 173-177

Michaelis, J. : Zur Anwendung der Diskriminanzanalyse für die medizinische Diagnostik. Habilitationsschrift, Mainz 1972

Dr. med. H. Löllgen
Laboartorium für Atmung
und Kreislauf
D-4130 Moers

Pneumonologie Suppl. 1976, 133-136

Atemreserve und Arbeitsatemminutenvolumen als atemmechanische leistungsbegrenzende Faktoren

L. Kühner

Thoraxchirurgische Klinik Wehrawald, Todtmoos

Abstract. Considering pulmonary function restrictive factors the reduced or during work premature exhaustion of the respiratory reserve due to a lung disease (mostly restriction) should not be neglected; the ergospirometry - ventilation measuring presumed - showing that a reduced maximum breathing capacity in account of frequently occuring additional pathologically increased respiratory minute volume during work is already exhausted at low watt adjustments. The limit is at about two thirds of the maximum breathing capacity. Frequently, the respiratory reserve can also be exhausted prematurely owing to a pathologically increased respiratory minute volume during work if a normal maximum breathing capacity is available (e. g. in cases of O_2 impaired diffusion or commencing pulmonary emphysema). The conditions of 84 adults, mainly suffering from tuberculosis, are demonstrated. The cases were detected on evaluation of 500 ergospirometries. The capacity of the patients was only 30 watt at highly reduced maximum breathing capacity (25 - 40 1), and of most patients only 50 watt at moderately reduced maximum breathing capacity (40 - 70 1). The majority of a third group with normal maximum breathing capacity but pathologically increased respiratory minute volume during work had a capacity limit of 50 - 75 watt. Distinct alterations of blood gas occured only in one third of the cases, almost each one however showing a decreased pH level.

Key words: Respiratory reserve - Maximum breathing capacity - Respiratory minute - Volume during work - Ergospirometry

Zusammenfassung. Bei den pulmonal leistungsbegrenzenden Faktoren muß auch an eine infolge Lungenerkrankung (vorwiegend Restriktion) verkleinerte oder sich bei Arbeit vorschnell erschöpfende Atemreserve gedacht werden, wobei bei der Ergospirometrie - die Messung der Ventilation ist Voraussetzung - ein herabgesetzter Atemgrenzwert durch das oft noch zusätzlich pathologisch erhöhte Arbeitsatemminutenvolumen schon auf niederen Wattstufen verbraucht ist; die Grenze liegt bei 2/3 des Atemgrenzwertes. Häufig kann die Atemreserve auch durch ein pathologisch erhöhtes Arbeitsatemminutenvolumen allein bei normalem Atemgrenzwert vorzeitig erschöpft sein (z. B. bei O_2-Diffusionsstörung oder beginnendem Lungenemphysem).

Darstellung dieser Verhältnisse an 84 Fällen von vorwiegend tuberkulosekranken Erwachsenen, die sich bei Durchsicht von 500 Ergospirometrien ergeben hatten. Bei stark herabgesetztem Atemgrenzwert (25 - 40 ltr.) wurden nur 30 Watt, bei mittelmäßig herabgesetztem (40 - 70 ltr.) von den meisten nur 50 Watt geleistet. Bei der Mehrzahl einer dritten Gruppe mit normalem Atemgrenzwert, aber pathologisch erhöhtem Arbeitsatemminutenvolumen war die Leistungsgrenze bei 50 bis 75 Watt erreicht. Deutliche Blutgasveränderungen waren nur in 1/3 der Fälle vorhanden, das pH war aber fast in allen Fällen erniedrigt.

Schlüsselwörter: Atemreserve - Atemgrenzwert - Arbeitsatemminutenvolumen - Ergospirometrie

---

Üblicherweise lautet auf die Frage nach dem leistungsbegrenzenden Faktor im Bereich der äußeren Ventilation die Antwort: erhöhte Atemarbeit infolge pathologisch erhöhter Atemwegs- und Lungengewebswiderstände. Eine altbekannte Tatsache, auf die wir hiermit hinweisen wollen, tritt dabei vielleicht manchmal in den Hintergrund, die Tatsache nämlich, daß man bei erhöhter Atemarbeit auch an eine verkleinerte Atemreserve infolge eines verkleinerten Atemgrenzwertes (AGW) oder infolge eines erhöhten Arbeitsatemminutenvolumen (AAMV) denken muß.

Für uns ist in der präoperativen Funktionsanalyse der AGW, und zwar der direkt gemessene, unentbehrlich. Auch das AAMV bedarf in dieser Beziehung einer Aufwertung, da in den letzten Jahren bei der Ergometrie vielfach auf die Messung von Ventilation und Gasaustausch verzichtet wird.

Neben einem verkleinerten AGW kann das AAMV entweder normal oder pathologisch vergrößert sein. In nicht seltenen Fällen - z. B. bei Sauerstoffdiffusionsstörung oder beginnendem Emphysem - ist der AGW hingegen normal und allein das AAMV pathologisch erhöht; hier ist die Atemreserve beim Arbeitsversuch ebenfalls verkleinert und früher erschöpft als beim Atemgesunden.

In all diesen Fällen spielen bei der Verursachung vermehrter Atemarbeit erhöhte Widerstände selbstverständlich immer eine Rolle; es tritt aber hinzu eine verstärkte Inanspruchnahme der Atemmuskulatur durch erhöhte Atemfrequenz und vertiefte Atemexkursionen zur weitestmöglichen Ausschöpfung einer verkleinerten Atemreserve oder, bei erhöhtem AAMV, die Vergrößerung des 3. Faktors in der Gleichung Arbeit = Kraft x Weg.

Erhöhte Atemarbeit führt zur Dyspnoe. Diese tritt auf, wenn 2/3 der Atemreserve durch das AAMV in Anspruch genommen sind (Rossier). Die Dyspnoe führt bei weiterer Arbeitssteigerung auch bald wegen Erschöpfung der Atemreserve zum Arbeitsabbruch. Ein völliges Ausschöpfen der Atemreserve gibt es offenbar nicht. Nach Mellerowicz wird bei maximaler körperlicher Dauerleistung nur mit 60 bis 75% des AGW geatmet.

Der in vorliegender Fragestellung zur Feststellung des AAMV stets erforderliche Arbeitsversuch besteht bei uns zunächst aus einer Wattstufe von
50, evtl. sogar nur 30 Watt, wenn hier die Leistungsgrenze schon erreicht
ist, ggf. aus einer zweiten, höheren Wattstufe, die aber aus Gründen des
nil nocere bei unseren risikobehafteten Patienten immer unter einem Lei-
stungs-Gewichts-Quotienten von 1, 0 liegt.

Das AAMV bei 50 Watt beträgt unserer Erfahrung nach in der Norm
25 bis 35 ltr. ; sein Anstieg bei 2 Wattstufen unter der vorhergenannten
Voraussetzung nicht mehr als 5 ltr. pro 10 Watt.

Wir haben aus unserem Material von ca. 1000 Ergospirometrien 500
Fälle der letzten 5 Jahre hinsichtlich der vorliegenden Fragestellung
durchgesehen und 84 entsprechende Fälle gefunden. Es handelt sich um
erwachsene, meist tuberkulosekranke Patienten, hauptsächlich mit
restriktiver und gemischtförmiger Ventilationsstörung, aber auch um Fälle
mit Emphysem und Diffusionsstörung. Wir haben versucht, die Ergebnisse
kurz und einfach darzustellen.

Als normalen AGW würden wir Werte von 100 ltr. an aufwärts bezeichnen.
Dabei sind keine, jedoch von 80 ltr. nach unten funktionelle Einbußen bzw.
Herabsetzung der Arbeitskapazität zu erwarten. Alle unsere Fälle lagen
unterhalb eines AGW von 80 ltr. Ihre Atemreserve war bei 50 Watt durch
das AAMV um über 50% verbraucht.

Der untere Grenzbereich des AGW liegt zwischen 25 und 40 ltr. Hierunter fallen 19 Patienten. Sie leisten nur noch 30 Watt (mit 3 Ausnahmen);
dabei ist ihr AGW durch das AAMV bereits aufgebraucht. Sie müssen beim
Treppensteigen wegen Dyspnoe im 1. Stockwerk stehen bleiben.

Als mittelmäßig herabgesetzt würden wir einen AGW zwischen 40 und
70 ltr. bezeichnen. Hierunter fallen 44 Patienten, davon 19 mit normalem
und 25 mit zusätzlich erhöhtem AAMV; im Schnitt betrug ihr AGW 61 ltr.

Von diesen 44 Patienten mit mittelmäßig eingeschränkter Atemreserve
war die Leistungsgrenze in 3 Fällen bei 25 bis 30 Watt, in 25 Fällen bei
50 Watt und in 4 Fällen bei 70 bis 75 Watt fast oder ganz erreicht (bei 12
Patienten war sie nicht ausgetestet). Überzeugende Parallelen zwischen
erreichter Leistungsgrenze und Größe des AGW innerhalb des doch relativ
kleinen Bereiches von 30 ltr. (zwischen 40 und 70 ltr.) ließen sich wohl
im Einzelfalle, aber nicht beim Gesamtdurchschnitt finden. Die Atemreserve
war bei Erreichen der Leistungsgrenze im Schnitt um 70% aufgebraucht.

Eine letzte Gruppe von 21 Patienten, teilweise mit nicht obstruktivem
Emphysem und Sauerstoffdiffusionsstörung bei interstitieller Fibrose, zeigt
einen normalen AGW, jedoch beim Arbeitsversuch, der wegen bestehender
Kurzatmigkeit durchgeführt wird, ein teilweise erheblich, im Schnitt bei
50 Watt auf 39 ltr. erhöhtes AAMV und damit ebenfalls eine im Arbeitsversuch eingeschränkte Atemreserve. Bei einzelnen dieser Fälle zeigt
sich das pathologisch erhöhte AAMV erst im 2-Wattstufen-Versuch, wobei
der Anstieg pro 10 Watt oft weit mehr als 5 ltr., im Einzelfall über 10 ltr
betrug.

Infolge der bei Arbeit sich relativ schnell verkleinernden Atemreserve
ist auch in diesen Fällen - die Verhältnisse liegen etwas günstiger als bei
den vorhergehenden Gruppen - die Leistungsgrenze auf unteren Wattstufen

136

bald erreicht. Von den betreffenden 21 Patienten hat einer nur 30 Watt,
drei 50 - 60 Watt, zwölf 70 - 75 Watt und nur einer 90 Watt geleistet
(drei nicht ausgetestet).

Die dargestellten Fälle zeigen, daß eine infolge eines eingeschränkten
AGW verkleinerte oder sich beim Arbeitsversuch infolge eines pathologisch
erhöhten AAMV vorschnell verbrauchende Atemreserve die Leistungsgrenze der betroffenen Patienten deutlich herabsetzt.

Für das Vorliegen eines pulmonalen Limit spricht, daß fast in allen
Fällen (außer drei) die Arbeitspulsfrequenz innerhalb des Normbereiches
der entsprechenden Wattstufe lag. - Deutlichere Blutgasveränderungen,
insbesondere Abfall des O_2-Druckes waren nur in 1/3 der untersuchten
Fälle vorhanden. Das pH allerdings war fast in allen Fällen sauer.

Dr. L. Kühner
Klinik Wehrawald
7867 Todtmoos, Schwarzwald

Pneumonologie Suppl. 1976, 137-143

Der humorale Inter-alpha-trypsininhibitor als Inhibitogen für sekretorische Proteaseinhibitoren. Serumkonzentrationen bei Erwachsenen und bei Kindern mit Atemwegserkrankungen

K. Hochstraßer, B. Rasche, C. Mietens, K. Schorn, C.E. von Pilar und A. Bum

HNO-Klinik der Universität München und Medizinische Abteilung des Silikose-Forschungsinstituts der Bergbau-Berufsgenossenschaft, Bochum, sowie Westfälische Landeskinderklinik Bochum

---

Abstract. The monovalent proteaseinhibitor inter-alpha-trypsininhibitor, present in low activity in human serum, may be the inhibitogen for different secretory, low molecular, polyvalent inhibitors. Kallikreines may be the enzymes liberating these inhibitors. The inhibitogenconcentrations in the serum were measured from adult patients with chronic bronchitis and from children of different age-groups. The adult patients had no deficiencies as consequence of their airway disease. In contrast inhibitogendeficiency was found in the serum of praemature and newborn children with respiratory distress syndroms and infections. The normal production rate of inhibitogen is not yet obtained in these children. Thus an inhibitordeficiency will be the result of a high consumption of inhibitor during inflammation or of an excessive liberation of kallikreines.

Key words: Inhibitogen-Inter-alpha-trypsininhibitor- Secretory inhibitor-Kallikrein-Inflammation - Serum-levels in children and adults

Zusammenfassung. Der schwache monovalente, humorale Proteaseninhibitor Inter-alpha-trypsininhibitor ist als Inhibitogen für verschiedene sekretorische, niedermolekulare, polyvalente Inhibitoren aufzufassen. Kallikreine wirken als inhibitorliberierende Enzyme. Die Inhibitogenspiegel im Serum wurden bei erwachsenen Bronchitikern und Kindern verschiedener Altersstufen bestimmt. Bei den erwachsenen Patienten konnte kein Inhibitogenmangel als Folge der Erkrankung festgestellt werden. Im Gegensatz dazu sind Inhibitogenmangelzustände bei Früh- und Neugeborenen mit Atemnotsyndrom und entzündlichen Erkrankungen sehr häufig. Die Inhibitogenproduktionsrate ist im frühen Kindesalter offensichtlich noch nicht voll ausgeprägt, so daß bei erhöhtem Inhibitorverbrauch oder exzessiver Kallikreinfreisetzung ein Inhibitogenmangelzustand resultiert.

Schlüsselwörter. Inhibitogen -Inter-alpha-trypsininhibitor-
Sekretorische Inhibitoren-Kallikrein-Entzündung - Serumspiegel bei
Kindern und Erwachsenen

EINLEITUNG

Die Sekrete des oberen Respirationstrakts enthalten neben dem säurelabilen,
humoralen $alpha_1$-Antitrypsin einen säurestabilen, niedermolekularen
Proteaseninhibitor (BSI = Bronchialsekretinhibitor) (Hochstraßer et al.
1972). Dieser Hemmstoff bewirkt etwa 70% der antiproteolytischen Aktivität der Sekrete (Reichert et al. , 1972). Das Hemmspektrum ähnelt
dem des $alpha_1$-Antitrypsins. Neben den Pankreasproteasen Trypsin und
Chymotrypsin werden die elastaseähnlichen Proteasen der Granulozyten
besonders stark gehemmt (Hochstraßer et al. , 1972). Ähnlich wie für
$alpha_1$-Antitrypsin (Ohlsson, 1971) konnte auch für diesen Inhibitor nachgewiesen werden, daß er in situ mit Leukozytenelastase Komplexe bildet
(Hochstraßer et al. , 1975). Die Menge von komplexiertem Inhibitor in
den Sekreten korreliert mit der Stärke der entzündlichen Reaktion.

Bei der biochemischen Charakterisierung des BSI stellten wir fest, daß
dieser Hemmstoff mit Antikörpern gegen den humoralen Inter-alpha-
trysininhibitor (im folgenden als ITI bezeichnet) eine Kreuzreaktion zeigt
(Hochstraßer et al. , 1973).

Im Gegensatz zum BSI ist der humorale ITI aber nur ein schwacher
monovalenter Trypsininhibitor; er kommt in den Sekreten nur selten in
nachweisbaren Konzentrationen vor. Auch aufgrund seiner relativ niedrigen
Konzentration im Serum - hier entfallen nur etwa 3% der antiproteolytischen
Aktivität auf diesen Hemmstoff - war eine physiologische Funktion für diesen
Inhibitor bisher nicht bekannt. Infolge der immunologischen Befunde mußten
jedoch enge Beziehungen zwischen dem ITI und dem BSI angenommen werden. Es war neheliegend anzunehmen, daß der offensichtlich leicht sezernierbare BSI aus dem ITI durch einen spezifischen Vorgang entsteht.

Auf Umwegen konnten wir einen offensichtlich allgemeinen Freilegungs-
mechanismus für niedermolekulare und säurestabile Proteaseninhibitoren
aus dem hochmolekularen ITI auffinden. Die auch im Blutplasma und Harn
nachweisbaren säurestabilen Proteaseninhibitoren zeigen nämlich ebenfalls eine immunologische Kreuzreaktion mit dem ITI, obwohl diese Hemmstoffe aufgrund ihres Hemmspektrums und ihres Peptidmusters mit dem
BSI nicht in direkter Beziehung stehen (Hochstraßer et al. , 1974 a). Die
Konzentration des säurestabilen Inhibitors, die im Enteiweißungsüberstand
der Seren bestimmt werden kann, steigt bei Nephropathien unterschiedlicher
Ätiologie stark an (Hochstraßer et al., 1974 b). Diese Beobachtung legte
die Annahme nahe, daß dieser Inhibitor laufend intravasal aus ITI gebildet
und durch die Niere ausgeschieden wird. Wir konnten einen solchen Konzentrationsanstieg der antiproteolytischen Aktivität im Serum durch Vor-
inkubation mit überschüssigem Trypsin simulieren und stellten fest, daß
die freisetzbare Aktivität mit dem ITI-Gehalt der Seren korreliert. Die
chemischen und immunologischen Eigenschaften des durch Trypsin frei-

setzbaren Inhibitors waren identisch mit den Eigenschaften der von uns aus
dem Enteiweißungsüberstand von Serum und Harn durch Affinitätschromato-
graphie isolierten Inhibitoren. Wird jedoch die antiproteolytische Aktivität
aus dem Enteiweißungsüberstand von Serum und Harn mit konventionellen
Methoden angereichert, so findet man bei gleicher immunologischer Kreuzreaktion mit ITI wesentlich höhere Molekulargewichte. Durch Inkubation
dieser Inhibitoren mit Trypsin entstehen jedoch Hemmstoffe mit den gleichen Eigenschaften, wie sie durch Trypsinabbau von ITI erhalten werden.

Die Befunde belegen, daß offensichtlich durch limitierte Proteolyse
aus dem hochmolekularen ITI ein niedermolekularer Inhibitor freisetzbar
ist. Die artifizielle Liberierung mit exogenem Trypsin führt jedoch nicht
zur Bildung eines freien aktiven Inhibitors; es entsteht ein inaktiver Inhi-
bitor-Trypsinkomplex, aus dem der aktive Inhibitor nur durch Denaturie-
rung des Enzymanteils freigesetzt werden kann. Physiologischerweise entsteht jedoch ein aktiver Inhibitor. Als inhibitorliberierende Protease in
vivo war deshalb nur ein Enzym vorstellbar, das weder vom als Inhibitogen
zu bezeichnenden ITI noch vom liberierten Inhibitor gehemmt wird. Als
Proteasen, die aus ITI sezernierbare, niedermolekulare Inhibitoren frei-
setzen, konnten wir die ubiquitär vorkommenden Kallikreine identifizieren
(nähere Angaben dazu siehe Hochstraßer et al., 1972, 1974 a und 1976;
Bretzel und Hochstraßer, 1976).

ERGEBNISSE UND DISKUSSION

Der schleimhautspezifische Bronchialsekretinhibitor BSI ist in den Sekreten
der oberen Luftwege einfach zu bestimmen. Aus bekannten Gründen sind
aber aus chemischen Befunden, erhoben an Sputum, nur bedingt diagnostische
Hinweise abzuleiten. Da offensichtlich ITI als Inhibitogen auch für den Bronchialsekretinhibitor anzusehen ist, versuchten wir, Beziehungen zwischen
Inhibitogen (= ITI)-spiegel im Serum und Erkrankungen der oberen Luftwege
zu finden.

Wir erwarteten zunächst bei erhöhtem Verbrauch von BSI als Folge der
Infektion der oberen Luftwege eine Verminderung des Inhibitogenspiegels
im Serum. Bei 1025 Patienten mit chronischer Bronchitis bestimmten wir
mittels der Elektroimmunodiffusionsmethode die ITI-Serumspiegel. Im ge-
samten Kollektiv fanden wir nur 3 Fälle mit einem um 50% erniedrigten
Inhibitogenspiegel. Diese Patienten zeigten jedoch eine zusätzliche schwere
Leberdystrophie mit eingeschränkter Proteinsynthese. Der Vergleich der
Inhibitogenspiegel dieses Kollektivs mit einem gesunden Kontrollkollektiv
zeigte keine signifikante Abweichung. Berücksichtigt man die relativ große
Fehlerbreite der immunologischen Bestimmungsmethode, so kann unter
Vorbehalt eine geringe durchschnittliche Erhöhung des Inhibitogenspiegels
bei den Bronchitikern angenommen werden. Eine individuelle Bestimmung
des Inhibitogenspiegels hat nach unseren bisherigen Ergebnissen keinen dia-
gnostischen Wert. Offensichtlich führt gesteigerter Verbrauch von BSI zu
keiner Verminderung des Inhibitogenspiegels im Serum (Rasche et al. 1975).
Erhöhter Inhibitogenverbrauch scheint durch Erhöhung der Inhibitogenproduktion bei den hier zur Untersuchung gelangten Patienten kompensiert zu

140

werden. Ein Hauptziel dieser Untersuchungen war es, einen hereditären
Inhibitogenmangel ähnlich dem $alpha_1$-Antitrypsinmangel zu finden. Ein
hereditärer Inhibitogenmangel müßte im Bronchialbereich ähnliche pathologische Zustände hervorrufen wie der $alpha_1$-Antitrypsinmangel in der
Lunge.

Aufgrund der bisherigen Befunde und der in der Einleitung kurz referierten Ergebnisse glauben wir, daß ein hereditärer Inhibitogenmangel bei
Erwachsenen nicht gefunden werden wird; er würde den Ausfall des antiproteolytischen Systems nicht nur in den Schleimhäuten der oberen Luftwege, sondern auch der harnbereitenden und ableitenden Systeme bedeuten.
Wir nehmen deshalb an, daß ein hereditärer Inhibitogenmangel einen Letalfaktor darstellen würde, zumal wir Hinweise besitzen, daß auch noch andere
sekretorische Inhibitoren aus ITI freigesetzt werden können.

Aus diesem Grund bestimmten wir die Inhibitogenspiegel bei Kindern
verschiedener Alterstufen ohne Erkrankungen und mit entzündlichen Erkrankungen verschiedener Ätiologie. Bereits beim bis jetzt untersuchten
Patientenkollektiv stellten wir altersabhängig Inhibitogenmangelzustände
mit hohem Prozentanteil fest; die Befunde sind in der Tabelle 1 zusammengestellt. Bei allen Patienten wurden die $alpha_1$-Antitrypsinspiegel im
Serum mitbestimmt, aber kein Fall von hereditärem Mangel gefunden. Auffallend ist zunächst der hohe Prozentsatz von Inhibitogenmangelzuständen
(65%) bei Neugeborenen mit Atemnotsyndrom und entzündlichen Erkrankungen bei gleichzeitig voll ausgebildeter Proteasenhemmkapazität im
Serum (beruhend auf $alpha_1$-Antitrypsin). Eine relativ hohe Häufigkeit von
Inhibitogenmangel ist bei Neugeborenen mit etwa 40% feststellbar, während

Tabelle 1. Altersabhängige Verteilung von Inhibitogenmangelzuständen bei
Atemwegserkrankungen und anderen entzündlichen Vorgängen

| Alter | n | Inhibitogen | | %Anteil |
		normal	erniedrigt	erniedrigt
Frühgeb.	30	11	19	65
0-2 Mon.	87	53	34	39
3 Mon. - 2 Jahre	140	121	19	13
3-15 Jahre	145	138	7	5
20-70 Jahre Bronchitiker	1025	1025	3	0,03
0-2 Mon. gesund	22	22	1	5
3 Mon. - 2 Jahre	35	35	1	3

normal   = 80 - 130% eines Vergleichsserumpools
erniedrigt = 10 - 76% eines Vergleichsserumpools

ein Kollektiv von gesunden Neugeborenen nur etwa in 4% der Fälle ITI-
Mangel zeigte. In der Altersgruppe von 3 Monaten bis 2 Jahren ist ein
Inhibitogenmangel mit etwa 13% noch recht häufig, im Vergleichskollektiv
fanden wir nur bei einem der Probanden ITI-Mangel. Auch in der Gruppe
der 3 bis 15-jährigen Patienten fanden wir immerhin noch Mangelzustände
mit einer Häufigkeit von 5%. Im Gegensatz dazu fanden wir bei dem großen
Kolletiv von erwachsenen Bronchitikern praktisch keine Inhibitogenmangelzustände. Exakte Angaben über die Häufigkeit von Atemwegserkrankungen
bzw. deren Beteiligung bei am Krankheitsgeschehen ablaufenden Vorgängen
können noch nicht gemacht werden. Bei diesem Stadium der Untersuchungen
bieten sich für das Zustandekommen von Inhibitogenmangelzuständen zwei
Hypothesen an, die auch gleichzeitig zutreffen können. Die hohe Häufigkeit
des Inhibitogenmangels bei Frühgeborenen berechtigt zu der Annnahme,
daß die Inhibitogenproduktion noch verlangsamt abläuft. Ein erhöhter Inhibitorverbrauch wirkt sich dann durch eine starke Verminderung des Inhibitogenspiegels im Serum aus. Der hohe Anteil von Inhibitogenmangelzuständen bei kranken Neugeborenen und die niedrige Mangelhäufigkeit bei gesunden Neugeborenen kann mit den beiden Hypothesen zwanglos erklärt
werden.

Aufgrund neuerer Untersuchungen wissen wir, daß Inhibitogenmangelzustände durchaus auch bei Erwachsenen auftreten können; in diesen Fällen
sind jedoch schwere Entzündungen verschiedener Ursache der auslösende
Faktor. Der hohe lokale Inhibitorverbrauch bei Bronchitikern führt offensichtlich nicht zu Inhibitogenmangelzuständen.

Durch die weitere Untersuchung des Systems Inhibitogen-Inhibitor-
liberatoren glauben wir eine allgemein gültige Möglichkeit zur Diagnostik
verschiedener entzündlicher Erkrankungen zu finden. Bei der Freisetzung
säurestabiler Inhibitoren aus ITI durch Kallikrein in vitro entstehen zusätzlich zwei noch nicht näher charakterisierte säurelabile ITI-Derivate.
Diese Derivate sind auch physiologischerweise und mit stark erhöhter
Konzentration im Serum bei entzündlichen Erkrankungen nachzuweisen,
wobei die immunelektrophoretischen Bilder auf einen erhöhten Umsatz
von Inter-alpha-trypsininhibitor bei Entzündungsvorgängen hindeuten.

Untersuchungen, inwieweit diese Konzentrationserhöhungen mit verschiedenen Erkrankungen korrelieren, sind im Gange.

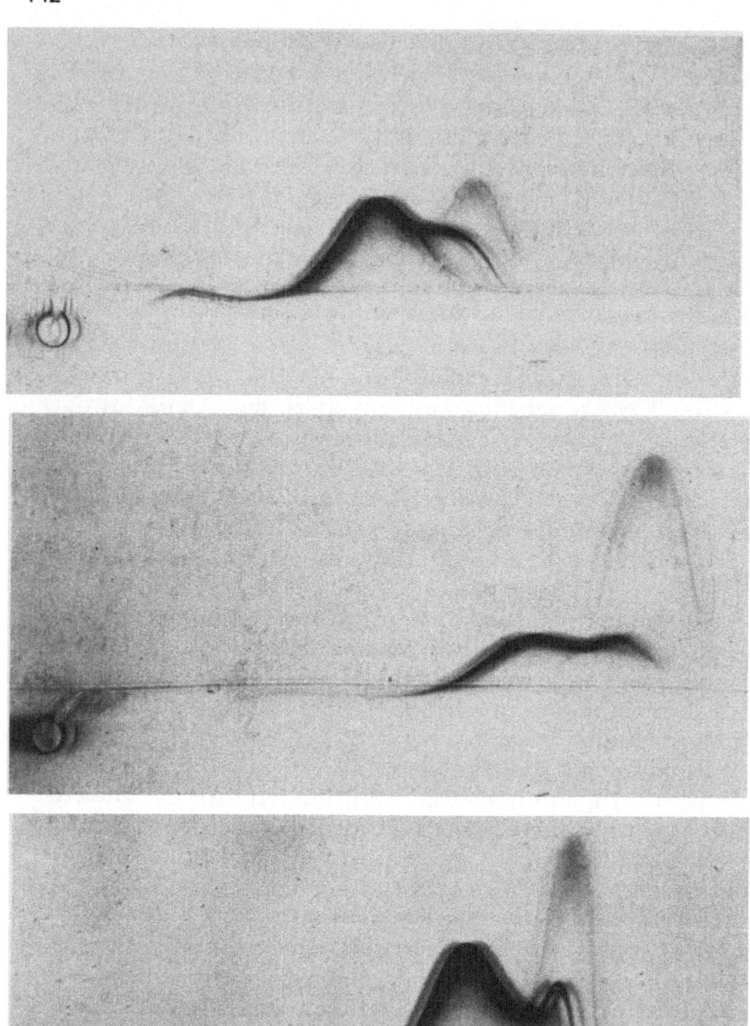

Abb. 1. Zweidimensionale Immunelektrophorese von a. Kindlichem Normalserum. b. Serum eines Kindes mit Mucoviscidose, ITI-Mangel mit Erhöhung
eines Derivates. c. Serum eines Patienten mit chronisch obstruktiver
Bronchitis ohne ITI-Mangel und mit Erhöhung der Derivate (Erwachsenen-
Normalserum wie a). 1. Fraktion: Inter-alpha-trypsininhibitor (ITI)
2. und 3. Fraktion: ITI-Derivate

LITERATUR

Bretzel, G., Hochstraßer, K.: Liberation of acid stable proteinase inhibitors
from the inter-alpha-trypsininhibitor by the action of kallikrein.
Z. physiol. Chem. 357, 487 (1976)

Hochstraßer, K., Reichert, R., Schwarz, S., Werle, E.: Isolierung und
Charakterisierung eines Proteaseninhibitors aus menschlichem
Bronchialsekret. Z. physiol. Chem. 353, 221 (1972)

Hochstraßer, K., Reichert, R., Heimburger, N.: Antigenic relationship
between the human bronchial mucus inhibitor and plasma inter-alpha-
trypsininhibitor. Z. physiol. Chem. 354, 923 (1973)

Hochstraßer, K., Feuth, H., Hochgesand, K.: Proteinase inhibitors of
the respiratory tract: Studies on the structural relationship between
acid stable inhibitors present in the respiratory tract, plasma and
urine. Bayer Symposium V, Proteinase Inhibitors, p. 111, Berlin-
Heidelberg-New York: Springer Verlag 1974 a

Hochstraßer, K., Feuth, H., Fall, O., Kemkes, B.: Säurestabile
Proteaseninhibitoren im Blutplasma bei verschiedenen Nephropathien.
Klin. Wschr. 52, 1018 (1974 b)

Hochstraßer, K., Schorn, K., Rasche, B., Lemparth, K., Raffelt, CH.:
Characterisation of masked specific proteinase inhibitor from bronchial
secretions in purulent sputum as complex with leucocytic proteinases.
Pneumologie 152, 15 (1975)

Hochstraßer, K., Bretzel, G., Feuth, H., Hilla, W., Lempart, K.:
The inter-alpha-trypsininhibitor as precursor of the acid stable
proteinase inhibitors in human serum and urine. Z. physiol. Chem. 357,
153 (1976)

Ohlsson, K.: Interaction between human or dog leucocytic proteases and
plasma protease inhibitors. Scand. J. Clin. Lab. Invest. 28, 225
(1971)

Rasche, B., Hochstraßer, K., Marcic, I., Ulmer, W.T.: Schleimhautspezifische Proteaseinhibitoren im Bronchialschleim bei schwerer
chronisch obstruktiver Bronchitis und bei $alpha_1$-Antitrypsinmangel-
syndrom. Respiration 32, 340 (1975)

Reichert, R., Hochstraßer, K., Conradi, G.: Untersuchungen zur
Proteasenhemmkapazität des menschlichen Bronchialsektrets.
Pneumologie, 147, 13 (1972)

Prof. Dr. K. Hochstraßer
HNO Klinik der Universität
Pettenkoferstraße 4a
8000 München - 2

Dr. B. Rasche
Silikose- Forschungsinstitut
der Bergbau-Berufsgenossenschaft
Hunscheidtstraße 12
4630 Bochum

Pneumonologie Suppl. 1976, 145-152

Akupunktur bei Bronchialobstruktion –
Bodyplethysmographische Meßergebnisse

D. Berger und D. Nolte

Forschungsanstalt für Erkrankungen der Atmungsorgane und Innere
Abteilung II des Städtischen Krankenhauses Bad Reichenhall
(Leitender Arzt: Prof. Dr. D. Nolte)

Acupuncture in Bronchial Obstruction - Bodyplethysmographic Measurements

Abstract. In 12 patients with reversible bronchial obstruction the effects
of acupuncture (45 tests altogether) on airway resistance have been investigated. In 9 patients there was a significant decrease of airway resistance
10 min, 1 h and 2 hrs after the end of acupuncture. The lowest level for
airway resistance (70, 1% of control value) was reached during the first
hour after acupuncture. The possibility of a merely suggestive effect
could be excluded, because "placebo-acupunctures" did not change airway
resistance significantly. The comparison with a parasympatholytic acting
drug as a metered aerosol (Atrovent ®) demonstrated that acupuncture had
a somewhat weaker bronchospasmolytic effect. 3 patients showed after
repeated acupunctures no reaction whatever.

Zusammenfassung. An zwölf Patienten mit reversibler Bronchialobstruktion wurde mit der Methode der Bodyplethysmographie der Effekt
von insgesamt 45 Akupunkturen auf die Atemwegs-Resistance untersucht.
Neun Patienten zeigten zehn Minuten, eine Stunde und zwei Stunden nach
der Akupunktur eine statistisch signifikante bronchospasmolytische Wirkung. Der niedrigste Wert wurde eine Stunde nach Akupunktur erreicht
und betrug 70, 1% des Ausgangswerts. Ein Suggestiveffekt konnte ausgeschlossen werden: "Placeboakupunkturen" zeigten keine signifikanten
Änderungen der Resistance. Zum Vergleich durchgeführte Untersuchungen
mit einem parasympathikolytisch wirkenden Dosieraerosol (Atrovent®)
ergaben eine etwas stärkere Abnahme der Resistance als unter Akupunktur.
Drei von zwölf Patienten zeigten unter mehrfach durchgeführten Akupunkturen keine Reaktion.

Zahlreiche Untersuchungsergebnisse der letzten Jahre zeigen immer
deutlicher, welch dominierende Rolle Reflexmechanismen in der Regulation des Bronchialmuskeltonus spielen (Übersicht bei [20]).
Dies trifft in besonderem Maße für die afferent und efferent über den

Vagus verlaufenden nozizeptiven Reflexe zu [17]. Darüberhinaus gibt es
aber zweifellos auch extrapulmonale Reize, die den Bronchialmuskeltonus
beeinflussen können [9]. Vor diesem Hintergrund sind die Akupunkturver-
suche zu sehen, über die im folgenden berichtet werden soll.

Wir gingen davon aus, daß Stiche von Akupunkturnadeln ebenfalls als
extrapulmonaler Reiz in Frage kommen; tatsächlich wurde von öster-
reichischen Autoren ein Effekt der Akupunkturbehandlung auf die
Atmung behauptet [2, 4]. Eine Wirkung auf den Bronchialmuskeltonus war
nach unserer Meinung am ehesten dann zu erwarten, wenn die Nadeln in
den bekannten pulmonalen Reflexzonen der Haut, den Head' schen Zonen,
plaziert würden. Ob sich ein solcher Effekt mit Hilfe eines von der Mitarbeit des Patienten unabhängigen Lungenfunktionsparameters wirklich
objektivieren läßt, haben wir mit Hilfe der bodyplethysmographischen
Methode zu klären versucht.

Wir konzentrierten uns zunächst bewußt auf den akuten Effekt
einer Akupunkturbehandlung. Dieses Versuchsmodell bot unter anderem
den Vorteil, Effekte von bronchospasmolytisch wirkenden Pharmaka als
Vergleichsgröße gegenüber einem etwaigen Akupunktureffekt heranziehen
zu können.

METHODIK

a) Bodyplethysmographie: Es wurde ein volumenkonstantes Gerät
der Fa. Jaeger, Würzburg, verwendet ("Bodytest"). Methodische Einzelheiten können früheren Publikationen entnommen werden [6, 14, 16].

b) Akupunktur: Es wurden jeweils neun verschiedene Punkte ver-

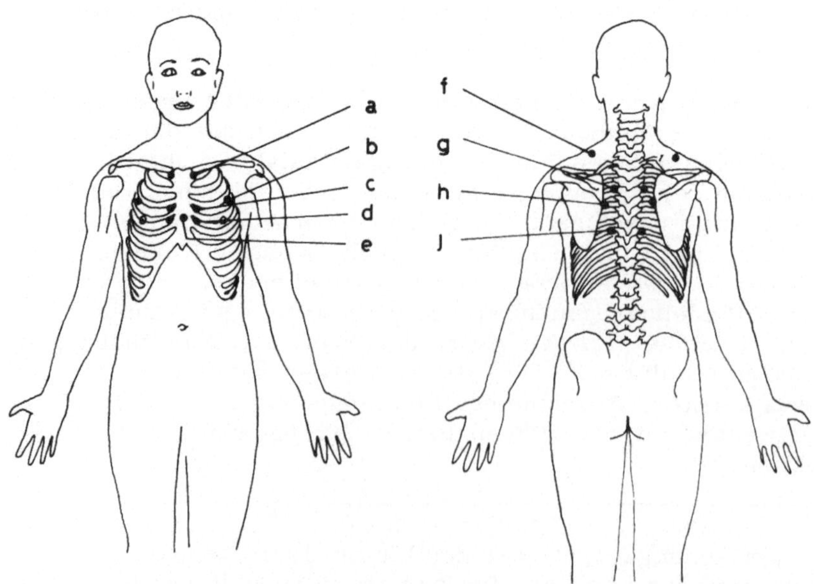

Abb. 1. Lokalisation der verwendeten Akupunkturpunkte

wendet, deren Lokalisation aus Abb. 1 hervorgeht. Die Einstichtiefe betrug
dorsal bis zu 3,5 cm, ventral (abhängig von der Stärke des Unterhautfett-
gewebes) etwa 2 cm. Verwendet wurden chinesische Stahlnadeln mit einer
Länge von 1" bzw. 1 1/2". Die Akupunktur wurde am sitzenden Patienten
vorgenommen und dauerte insgesamt etwa 20 Minuten; von Zeit zu Zeit
wurden die einzelnen Nadeln mit der Hand gedreht [3, 13, 21] .

Um einen eventuellen Suggestiveffekt erfassen zu können, wurden außerdem sogenannte Placeboakupunkturen vorgenommen. Dabei wurden Stellen
an der Außenseite des Ober- und Unterarmes, an der Vorderseite des
Oberschenkels oberhalb des Knies und an der lateralen Seite des Oberschenkels verwendet. Diese Stellen sind aufgrund der bis heute vorliegenden
Erfahrungen für die Akupunktur bei Atemwegserkrankungen ungeeignet.

c) Untersuchungen: An zwölf Patienten mit einem durchschnittlichen
Alter von 50 Jahren (15 bis 73 Jahre) wurden insgesamt 45 Akupunkturen
durchgeführt. Die Patienten hatten eine mittelgradige Bronchialstruktion,
die aufgrund von Vorversuchen gut pharmakodynamisch beeinflußbar war.
Hinweise für infektiöse Herde ("Foci"), die eine Akupunkturbehandlung
hätten stören können, ergaben sich nicht. Der Ausgangswert für die Atemwegs-Resistance betrug im Mittel $7,6 \pm 2,3$ cm $H_2O/1/s$. Nach der Akupun-
tur fanden jeweils drei Kontrollmessungen statt, und zwar nach zehn Minuten,
nach einer Stunde und nach zwei Stunden.

Fünf Patienten dieses Kollektivs bekamen außerdem Placebo-Akupunkturen.
Bei sechs Patienten wurde zum Vergleich ein anticholinergisch wirkendes
Dosier-Aerosol getestet (Atrovent®, Firma Boehringer, Ingelheim; Dosis
2 Hübe zu 0,02 mg).

ERGEBNISSE

Von den zwölf Patienten reagierten neun nach der Akupunktur mit einem
Abfall der Atemwegs-Resistance. Sieben Patienten zeigten diesen Effekt
regelmäßig bei jeder einzelnen Sitzung. Zwei Patienten bildeten insofern
eine Ausnahme, als der Resistance-Abfall erst bei der zweiten und dann
bei allen weiteren Akupunkturen zu beobachten war.

Bei drei Patienten mit insgesamt 15 Einzelakupunkturen zeigte die
Resistance keine Änderung oder sogar einen leichten Anstieg. Diese drei
Patienten wurden als "non-responder" angesehen.

Um die neun "responder" miteinander vergleichen zu können, wurde der
jeweilige Ausgangswert für die Resistance gleich 100% gesetzt; dies ist auch
bei der Prüfung von Bronchospasmolytika ein geläufiges Vorgehen [18].

Die Ergebnisse sind in Abb. 2 graphisch dargestellt und mit den jeweiligen
Ergebnissen nach Placeboakupunktur und nach Behandlung mit Atrovent®
verglichen. Die Abnahme der Atemwegs-Resistance (R) betrug im Mittel
nach zehn Minuten 24,1%, nach einer Stunde 29,9% und nach zwei Stunden
27,4%. Die Änderungen gegenüber dem Ausgangswert sind nach dem t-Test
(Paarvergleich) mit einer Irrtumswahrscheinlichkeit $p < 0,005$ signifikant.
Dagegen unterscheiden sich die drei Mittelwerte zehn Minuten, eine Stunde
und zwei Stunden nach Akupunktur nicht signifikant voneinander.

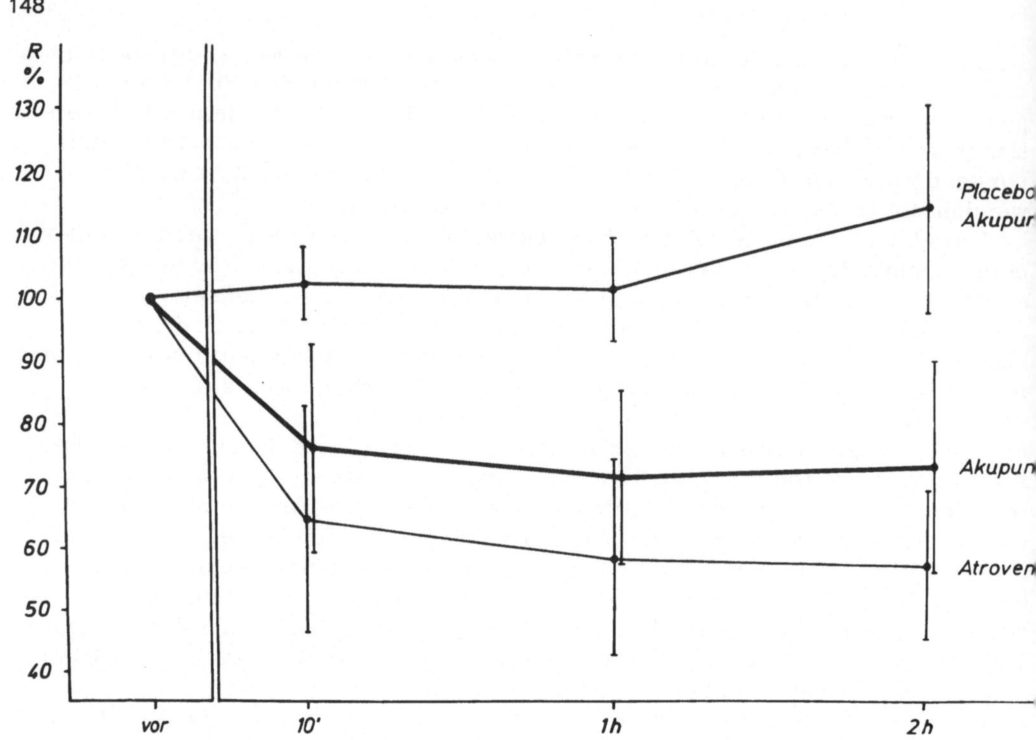

Abb. 2. Verhalten der Resistance unter Akupunktur, Placeboakupunktur und Behandlung mit Atrovent®

Die Mittelwerte nach Placeboakupunktur stiegen um 2, 3% (zehn Minuten), 1% (eine Stunde) bzw. 13, 9% (zwei Stunden) gegenüber dem Ausgangswert, an, die Veränderungen sind jedoch nicht statistisch signifikant.

Ein Vergleich zwischen der Placeboakupunktur und der Akupunktur mit Hilfe des t-Tests für unabhängige Stichproben ergibt für alle drei Kontrollen (zehn Minuten, eine Stunde und zwei Stunden) einen statistisch hochsignifikanten Unterschied mit $p < 0,005$.

Die ebenfalls in Abb. 2 dargestellten Mittelwerte der pharmakodynamischen Versuche mit dem Parasympathikolytikum Atrovent® ergaben im Mittel eine Resistance-Abnahme um 35, 3% nach 10 Minuten, um 41, 6% nach einer Stunde und um 42, 9% nach zwei Stunden. Diese Veränderungen sind ebenfalls statistisch signifikant ($p < 0,05$; t-Test, Paarvergleich). Aus Abb. 2 scheint der Trend hervorzugehen, daß der Atrovent® -Effekt stärker ist als der Akupunktureffekt. Der Unterschied zwischen den jeweiligen Mittelwerten ließ sich aber nicht mit einer ausreichend kleinen Irrtumswahrscheinlichkeit nachweisen ($p < 0, 1$; t-Test bei unabhängigen Stichproben).

DISKUSSION

In der Literatur gibt es bereits Beobachtungen, wonach sich die Lungen-
funktion durch Akupunktur beeinflussen lassen soll [2, 4]. Die eigenen Untersuchungen erbringen nunmehr einen objektiven Beweis dafür, daß es bei
Patienten mit Asthma bronchiale gelingt, mit Hilfe der Akupunktur den
Atemwegswiderstand zu senken. Dieses Ergebnis ist jedoch nicht bei allen
Patienten reproduzierbar; in der vorliegenden Studie zeigte jeder vierte
Patient keinen sicheren Effekt. Die bronchospasmolytische Wirkung ist
bereits zehn Minuten nach der Akupunktur vorhanden und hält mit Sicherheit zwei Stunden lang an. Da spätere Kontrollmessungen nicht durchge-
führt wurden, kann die Frage nach der Dauer des Akupunktureffekts im
Augenblick noch nicht beantwortet werden. Die Abnahme der Atemwegs-
Resistance entspricht mit der Größenordnung von 25 bis 30% nicht ganz
den Werten, wie sie aus pharmakodynamischen Versuchen bekannt sind [15].
Der direkte Vergleich zwischen der Akupunkturwirkung und dem Effekt
des parasympatholytisch wirkenden Dosieraerosols Atrovent® zeigt
- wahrscheinlich infolge der geringen Fallzahl - keinen statistisch sicheren
Unterschied. Aus Abb. 2 geht hervor, daß die pharmakodynamische Bronchospasmolyse mit Atrovent® eher stärker ist als die mit der Akupunktur er-
reichbare Bronchospasmolyse.

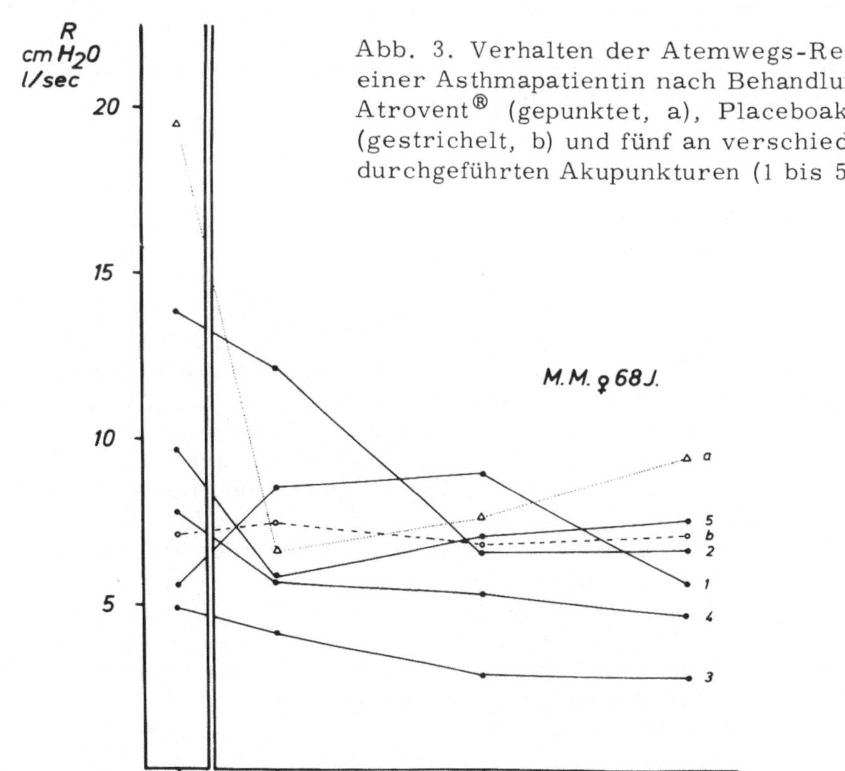

Abb. 3. Verhalten der Atemwegs-Resistance bei
einer Asthmapatientin nach Behandlung mit
Atrovent® (gepunktet, a), Placeboakupunktur
(gestrichelt, b) und fünf an verschiedenen Tagen
durchgeführten Akupunkturen (1 bis 5)

Wie kann man sich die Akupunkturwirkung auf die Atemwegs-Resistance erklären? Es liegt nahe, zunächst an einen Suggestiveffekt zu denken. In Analogie zu dem bei Arzneimittelprüfungen geläufigen Placeboversuch haben wir uns bemüht, diese Frage mit Hilfe einer "Placeboakupunktur" zu beantworten. Hierzu wurden versuchsweise Akupunkturpunkte im Extremitätenbereich gewählt, die nach vorliegenden Erfahrungen für die Akupunktur bei Atemwegserkrankungen bedeutungslos sind. Das Ergebnis war insofern überraschend, als alle Patienten subjektiv eine Besserung ihrer Atembeschwerden angaben, objektiv aber in keinem einzigen Fall eine Abnahme der Atemwegs-Resistance nachzuweisen war. Dieses Ergebnis läßt den Schluß zu, daß der bronchospasmolytische Effekt der Akupunktur kein Suggestiveffekt sein kann.

Unklar ist ein Phänomen, das am Beispiel der Abb. 3 dargestellt ist: Die erste Akupunktur führte bei einer 68-jährigen Patientin paradoxerweise zu einem Anstieg des Atemwegswiderstandes, sämtliche weiteren Akupunkturen (2 bis 5 in Abb. 3) hatten dann aber den erwarteten bronchospasmolytischen Effekt. Zum Vergleich sind in Abb. 3 auch die Ergebnisse der Placeboakupunktur (kein Effekt) und des pharmakodynamischen Versuchs mit Atrovent® (starke bronchospasmolytische Wirkung) mit dargestellt.

Solange es keine allgemeingültige naturwissenschaftliche Erklärung für die Wirkungsweise der therapeutisch angewandten Akupunktur gibt, läßt sich auch die spezielle Frage nach dem Mechanismus des bronchospasmolytischen Effekts kaum beantworten. Denkbar ist eine Verbindung zwischen bestimmten Hautzonen und der glatten Bronchialmuskulatur über einen kutiviszeralen Reflex. Dies würde eine Umkehrung des viszerokutanen Reflexes darstellen, der in Form der Hyperalgesie in den Headschen Hautzonen und ähnlich auch als vermehrte Spannung und Druckschmerzhaftigkeit im Bereich der von Mackenzie [11] beschriebenen Muskelzonen immer wieder demonstriert werden kann. Die der Lunge zugeordneten Segmente sind C3 und C4 und Th3 bis Th9 [7,8]. Entsprechend wurden auch für unsere Versuche Akupunkturpunkte gewählt, die sich innerhalb dieser Segmente befanden.

Während der Beweis für einen Reflexweg von der Haut oder von der Skelettmuskulatur zu den glatten Muskelfasern der Bronchien und Bronchiolen noch aussteht, konnte in Tierversuchen von verschiedenen Autoren für andere Organsysteme - etwa für den Magen-Darm-Trakt - ein kutiviszeraler Reflex nachgewiesen werden [1,12,19]. Wurden z.B. die zugeordneten Dermatome durch Wärme oder andere hyperämisierende Maßnahmen gereizt, so kam es zu einer Vasodilatation und zu einer verstärkten Bewegung der korrespondierenden Magen-Darm-Abschnitte. Umgekehrt führten Kälte- und Schmerzreize zu Vasokonstriktion und Abnahme der Peristaltik. Diese Effekte waren auch nach Dezerebrierung des Versuchstieres nachweisbar, weshalb es sich um einen rein spinalen Reflex handeln muß [10].

Unsere Ergebnisse reichen nicht aus, um damit für oder gegen eine Außenseitermethode plädieren zu können. Eine bronchospasmolytische Wirkung der Akupunktur im akuten Experiment kann nicht mehr bezweifelt werden, jedoch geht gleichzeitig aus unseren Experimenten hervor, daß zwei Atemzüge aus einem Dosier-Aerosol nicht nur bequemer, sondern auch wirksamer sind.

LITERATUR

1. Baumann, W. : Über thermometrische Untersuchungen im Zwölffinger-
    darm und der Leber und den segmental zugeordneten Dermatomen.
    Münch. med. Wschr. 96, 605 (1954)
2. Bergsmann, O. : Objektivierung der Akupunktur als Problem der
    Regulationsphysiologie. Heidelberg: F. Haug 1974
3. Bischko, J. : Einführung in die Akupunktur. Heidelberg: F. Haug 1970
4. Bischko, J. : Akupunktur. 13. Tagung der Österr. Gesellschaft für
    Lungenerkrankungen und Tuberkulose 1975
5. Dittmar, F. : Die kutiviszerale Reflexbahn, Acta neuroveg. (Wien) 8,
    183 (1953)
6. DuBois, A. B. , Botelho, S. Y. , Comroe, J. H. : A new method for
    measuring airway resistance in man using a bodyplethysmograph:
    values in normal subjects and patients with respiratory disease. J.
    clin. Invest. 35, 327 (1956)
7. Hansen, K. , Schliack, H. : Segmentale Innervation. Stuttgart:
    Georg Thieme 1962
8. Head, H. : Die Sensibilitätsstörungen der Haut bei Viszeralerkrankun-
    gen. Berlin: Hirschwald 1898
9. Josenhans, W. T. , Melville, G. N. , Ulmer, W. T. : The effect of
    facial cold stimulation on airway conductance in healthy man. J.
    Physiol. Pharmacol. 47, 453 (1969)
10. Kuntz, A. , Haselwood, L. A.: Cutaneo-viszeral vasomotor reflexes in
    the cat. Proc. Soc. exp. Biol. (N. Y.) 43, 517 (1940)
11. Mackenzie, J. : Krankheitszeichen und ihre Auslegung. Würzburg:
    Kabitzsch 1917
12. Molander, C. O. : Physiological basis of heat. Arch. phys. Ther.
    (Lpz.) 22, 335 (1941)
13. Nghi, Nguyen van: Pathologie der Energetik in der chinesischen
    Medizin. Uelzen: Medizin. Literar. Verlagsgesellschaft 1975
14. Nolte, D. : Moderne Lungenfunktionsdiagnostik bei obstruktiven Atem-
    wegserkrankungen: die Ganzkörperplethysmographie. Med. Welt N. F.
    48, 2746 (1967)
15. Nolte, D. : Das Verhalten von Atemwegs-Resistance und intrathorakalem
    Gasvolumen nach Inhalation eines Hydroxyphenyl-Derivates des Orcipre-
    nalin (Th 1165a). Respiration 27, 396 (1970)
16. Nolte, D. : Bodyplethysmographie. Diagnostik 6, 379 (1973)
17. Nolte, D. : Pathogenese und Therapie der Bronchokonstriktion. Med.
    Welt (N. F.) 26, 639 (1975)
18. Nolte, D. , Ulmer, W. T. , Krieger, E. : Lungenfunktionsuntersuchun-
    gen zur bronchospasmolytischen Wirkung der Beta$_2$-Adrenergika
    Salbutamol, Terbutalin und NAB 365 (Doppelblindversuch). Arznei-
    mittel-Forsch. 24, 858 (1974)
19. Sielaff, H. J. : Untersuchungen über die Motilität und kutiviszerale
    Reflexerregbarkeit des menschlichen Dünndarms. Z. ges. exp.
    Med. 120, 585 (1953)

152

20.   Ulmer, W. T. , Islam, M. S. , Bakran, I. : Untersuchungen zur Ursache
       der Atemwegsobstruktion und des überempfindlichen Bronchialsystems.
       Dtsch. med. Wschr. 96, 1759 (1971)
21.   Wancura, I. , König, G. : Neue chinesische Akupunktur. Wien:
       Maudrich 1975

Professor Dr. D. Nolte
Städtisches Krankenhaus
8230 Bad Reichenhall
Riedelstraße 5

DISKUSSION

G. Fuhrmann, München: Atrovent[®] soll überwiegend vagolytisch wirken,
seinen Effekt aber nur bei einem Teil der Patienten mit reversibler
Bronchialobstruktion entfalten.

Haben alle erfolgreich mit Akupunktur behandelten Kranken auf
Atrovent[®] therapeutisch angesprochen? Wenn ja, glauben Sie, daß sich
die Akupunktur für Personen mit vagolytisch therapierbarer Bronchialobstruktion besonders eignet?

D. Nolte, Bad Reichenhall: Alle akupunktierten Patienten haben auf Atrovent[®]
mit einer Abnahme des bronchialen Strömungswiderstandes reagiert. Der
Rückschluß, daß das Ansprechen auf ein Vagolyticum einen Erfolg bei der
Akupunktur verspricht, kann aus unseren Untersuchungen jedoch nicht gezogen werden.

Pneumonologie Suppl. 1976, 153-159

Protektive Medikamentenwirkung bei antigen induziertem Bronchialasthma

M. Debelic, B. Wüthrich und P. Radielovic

Asthma- und Allergieklinik der Hochgebirgsklinik Davos-Wolfgang und
Dermatologische Universitätsklinik Zürich

Protective Drug Effect in Antigen-induced Bronchial Asthma

Abstract. A classic antihistamine (HS 592, Clemastine), a new antiallergic which is also characterised by the additional property of inhibiting histamine release (HC 20-511) and a mast cell stabiliser (DSCG) were compared with regard to their protective effect in antigen-induced bronchial asthma by means of the inhalation antigen provocation test. In 24 patients suffering from extrinsic bronchial asthma the best protection was achieved with HC 20-511, followed by DSCG and HS 592. In view of the small number of patients no statistically significant differences could be demonstrated.

Key words: Antihistamine - Antiallergic - DSCG - Bronchial provocation test - Asthma

Zusammenfassung. Ein klassisches Antihistaminikum (HS 592, Clemastin), ein neuartiges Antiallergikum mit zusätzlicher histaminfreisetzungshemmender Wirkung (HC 20-511) sowie ein Mastzellenstabilisator (DNCG) wurden mittels des inhalativen Antigen-Provokationstests auf ihre protektive Wirkung bei Antigen-induziertem Bronchialasthma untersucht. Bei 24 Patienten mit exogen allergischem Bronchialasthma zeigte HC 20-511 die beste protektive Wirkung, gefolgt von DNCG und HS 592. Bedingt durch die kleine Fallzahl konnte statistisch kein gesicherter Unterschied festgestellt werden.

Im Gegensatz zur allergischen Rhinitis und zur Urticaria werden Antihistaminika in der Behandlung des Bronchialasthmas kaum angewendet. Das dürfte vor allem daran liegen, daß diese Medikamente als Histaminantagonisten schon sehr lange bekannt sind und die Kenntnis ihrer Unwirksamkeit im Asthmaanfall auf alten, rein praktischen Erfahrungen beruht.

Außerdem entbehrt die klinische Anwendung von Antihistaminika beim Bronchialasthma weitgehend exakter experimenteller Grundlagen. Nachdem wir heute eine Fülle von neuen Erkenntnissen über die Pathomechanismen des Bronchialasthmas besitzen, erschien es uns wertvoll, die Wirkung von Antihistaminika bei antigeninduziertem Asthma mittels des inhalativen Provokationstests zu prüfen.

Bisher wurden nur vereinzelte Antihistaminika auf ihre protektive

Wirkung mit Hilfe des bronchialen Antigentests untersucht [2, 3, 8].
Sie haben sich als teilweise bzw. gut wirksam erwiesen, erlangten aber
bisher keine größere Bedeutung in der praktischen Asthmabehandlung [9].

GEPRÜFTE MEDIKAMENTE

In einer Doppelblindpilotstudie mit Plazebo konnte gezeigt werden, daß be-
stimmte Antihistaminika bei vorausgegangener oraler Verabreichung den
allergischen Bronchospasmus gut hemmen. Wir haben vergleichsweise
folgende protektive Wirkungen untersucht:
a) ein bekanntes Antihistaminikum - HS 592 (1-Methyl-2- [2' -(α-methyl-
   p-chlor-benzhydryloxy)-äthyl]-pyrrolidin-hydrogenfumarat, Clemastin,
   Tavegyl),
b) ein neuartiges Antiallergikum - HC 20-511 (4-(1-Methyl-4-piperidyli-
   den)-4H-benzo [4, 5] cyclohepta [1, 2-b] thiophen-10-(9H)-on-hydrogen-
   fumarat, Ketotifen, Zaditen®)
   und
c) ein bekannter Mastzellenstabilisator - DNCG (Dinatrium cromoglyci-
   cum, Intal®, Lomudal®, Cromolyn®).
Aus den tierexperimentellen und pharmakodynamischen Untersuchungen
geht hervor, daß sich dieses neuartige Antiallergikum klar von den klassischen Antihistaminika unterscheidet. Im Gegensatz zu Clemastin hemmt
HC 20-511 die kutane anaphylaktische Reaktion am Tier, bzw. zeigt eine
dosisabhängige Hemmung vom Histaminliberator 48/80. Ebenso wurde nachgewiesen, daß HC 20-511 die zyklische Phosphodiesterase aus den perito-
nealen Mastzellen, Lunge und Herz hemmt [10].

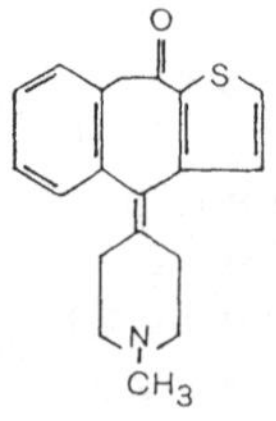

Abb. 1. Strukturformel von HC 20-511

METHODIK

Die Versuchsanordnung enthielt drei inhalative Provokationstests mit einem
Antigen, das bei der Hauttestung eine starke Reaktion auslöste und möglicherweise anamnestisch als Ursache der asthmatischen Beschwerden erkannt wurde. Der erste Test erfolgte ohne Prämedikation und war jeweils
mäßig bis stark positiv. Danach nahm der Proband 3 Tage HS 592 oder
HS 20-511 2 x 1 Kapsel tägl. im Doppelblindversuch ein. Anschließend
erfolgte die zweite inhalative Provokation mit dem gleichen Antigen und in
gleicher Dosierung wie im ersten Versuch. Nach einer Pause von 1 bis
2 Tagen Inhalation von DNCG mittels Spinhalers 4 mal 1 Kapsel täglich über

3 Tage mit darauffolgendem inhalativem Bronchialtest wie in den ersten
beiden Versuchen. Die Kontrollmessungen der Lungenfunktion erfolgten
5, 15, 20 und 30 Minuten nach der Antigeninhalation.

Der inhalative Antigen-Provokationstest wurde nach der Methode von
Debelic [5] durchgeführt. Nach Ermittlung der Leer- und Kontrollwerte
(Inhalation einer Kontrollösung ohne Antigen) inhaliert der Patient bis zu
1 ml einer standardisierten Allergenlösung. Die Messung der Lungenfunktion erfolgt spirographisch (Vitalograph). Der Test wird als positiv angesehen, wenn der Abfall der Einsekundenkapazität (FEV_1) nach der Antigeninhalation mehr als 20% von den Ausgangs- oder Kontrollwerten beträgt [5].

Die prophylaktische Wirkung der Medikamente wurde bei 24 Patienten
mit gesichertem exogen-allergischen Bronchialasthma (Anamnese, positive Haut- und Provokationstests, Immunglobulin E) untersucht. HS 592
und HC 20-511 wurden von jeweils 12 Patienten in einem Doppelblindver-
fahren eingenommen, DNCG anschließend in offener Versuchsanordnung
von allen 24 Kranken inhaliert. An Antigenen wurden 8 mal Hausstaub,
13 mal Hausstaubmilbe Dermatophagoides pt., 2 mal Schimmelpilzsporen
und 1 mal Katzenhaare angewandt.

ERGEBNISSE

Die Ergebnisse sind als Wiedergabe von Mittelwerten auf Abb. 2 zusammengefaßt. Der Abfall von FEV_1 nach Antigeninhalation war ohne Prämedikation am größten. Nach vorausgegangener Einnahme der drei Medikamente
waren die Reduktionen der FEV_1-Werte deutlich kleiner, wobei HC 20-511
und DNCG etwa im gleichen Bereich lagen, während HS 592 etwas schlechter abschnitt. Da die FEV_1^- Ausgangswerte jedoch unterschiedlich sind,
gewinnt man über die protektive Wirkung der einzelnen Medikamente einen
besseren Eindruck, indem man die prozentuellen Abfälle von FEV_1 als
Mittelwerte vergleicht (Abb. 3). Dabei fällt auf, daß die relativen
FEV_1-Abfälle nach den Medikamentengaben deutlich kleiner als ohne
Prämedikation sind.

Die Analyse der einzelnen Ergebnisse zeigt, daß das gleiche Medikament
bei dem einen Kranken eine gute, bei dem anderen eine partielle oder keine
Schutzwirkung vor dem antigeninduzierten Bronchospasmus bietet. Dabei
bestand keine feste Beziehung unter den Medikamenten. Bei ein und dem-
selben Patienten konnte eines der Medikamente einen guten Schutz aufbauen,
während das andere die protektive Wirkung völlig verfehlte. An einigen
Patienten wurde ein guter Schutz durch beide Medikamente festgestellt.

Falls man eine Beschränkung des FEV_1-Abfalls unter 20% des Ausgangswertes vor der Provokation als ausreichende protektive Wirkung
betrachtet, so liegt der Schutz aller drei Medikamente zwischen 50 und
100% der Fälle (Tabelle 1). Die kleinste protektive Wirkung gewährleistet
HS 592, die beste HC 20-511, DNCG liegt dazwischen. Allerdings muß
betont werden, daß bei Errechnung der Signifikanz mittels des U-Tests
zwischen den 3 Medikamenten keine gesicherten Unterschiede bestehen.

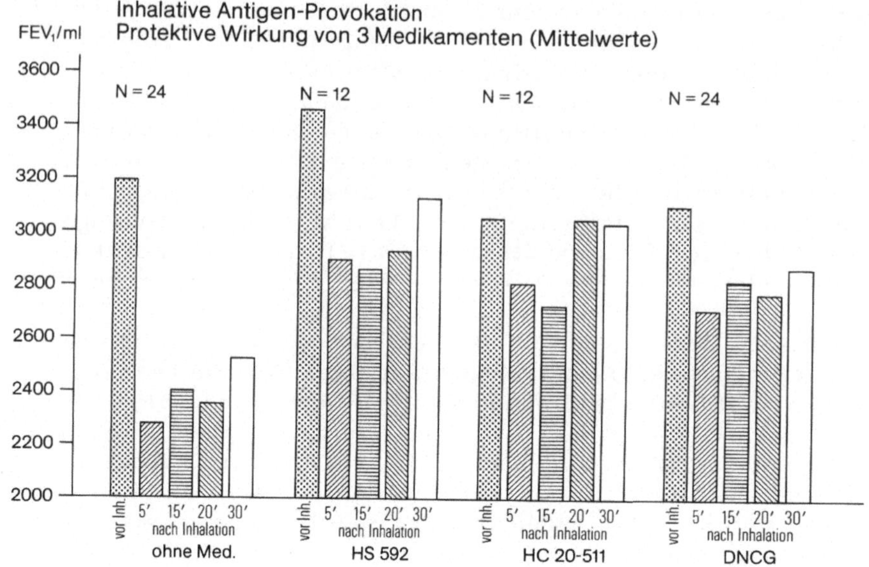

Abb. 2. Absolute FEV_1-Mittelwerte vor und nach inhalativer Antigenprovokation ohne vorausgegangene Medikamenteneinnahme (erste Säulengruppe) und nach Einnahme von HS 592, HC 20-511 und DNCG (zweite bis vierte Säulengruppe)

Tabelle 1. Übersicht der medikamentösen Schutzwirkung auf den inhalativen Antigenprovokationstest bei vorausgegangener oraler Einnahme von HS 592 und HC 20-511 bzw. nach der Inhalation von DNCG. Eine protektive Medikamentenwirkung wird angenommen, wenn der FEV_1-Abfall nach der bronchialen Provokation unter 20% gegenüber dem Ausgangswert liegt

nach Medikament	Patientenzahl	Patienten mit FEV_1-Abfall < 20%		
		Minuten nach Provokation		
		5'	15'	30'
HS 592 (Clemastin)	12	8 (66%)	6 (50%)	9 (75%)
HC 20-511	12	12 (100%)	10 (83%)	9 (75%)
DNCG	24	19 (79%)	18 (75%)	18 (75%)

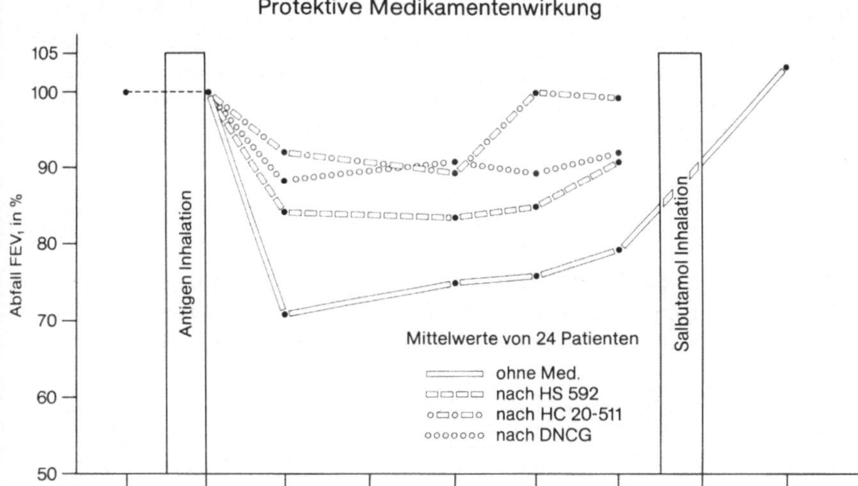

Abb. 3. Mittelwerte der Einsekundenkapazität (FEV_1) vor und nach inhalativen Antigenprovokationstests ausgedrückt in Prozenten des Ausgangswertes vor der Antigeninhalation (100%)

Somit ist es auch bei der relativ kleinen Probandenzahl nicht möglich, von einer überragend besseren Wirkung des einen gegenüber den anderen Medikamenten zu sprechen.

DISKUSSION

Mit dieser Untersuchung konnten wir zeigen, daß die geprüften Substanzen bei prophylaktischer Gabe eine eindeutige protektive Wirkung auf auf den antigenprovozierten Bronchospasmus beim Menschen ausüben. Diese Schutzwirkung ist etwa der des Mastzellenstabilisators DNCG gleichwertig, wobei aber offenbar in der Wirkung der einzelnen Wirkstoffe deutliche Unterschiede bestehen. HC 20-511 erwies sich als wirksamer als HS 592, was sowohl in dem kleineren prozentualen Abfall der FEV_1-Mittelwerte nach der Antigeninhalation (Abb. 2 und 3) als auch in der absoluten Zahl der geschützten Einzelfälle zum Ausdruck kommt (Tabelle 1).

Die protektive Wirkung von DNCG in unserem Krankengut entspricht im wesentlichen den Untersuchungsergebnissen anderer Autoren [3, 4, 6, 9, 11, 12, 14]. Allerdings erlaubt die Versuchsanordnung keine Aussage über die protektive Wirkungsdauer der einzelnen Medikamente oder den therapeutischen Effekt bei bestehendem Bronchospasmus.

Der Wirkungsmechanismus der oral verabreichten Substanzen wird mit großer Wahrscheinlichkeit ein anderer als der des DNCG sein. Unseres Erachtens handelt es sich unter anderem um eine Blockade der spezifischen histaminergischen H_1 oder H_2 Rezeptoren [7]. Daß die Schutzwirkung

der geprüften Substanzen nicht vollständig ist, läßt sich ohne Schwierigkeiten mit der Vielfältigkeit der die Bronchospastik auslösenden Faktoren
(Histamin, SRS, ECF-A, PAF, PGF_a, cholinerge Mechanismen etc) erklären [1, 13]. Die Problematik erfordert zweifellos weitere immunologische, pharmakologische und klinische Untersuchungen.

LITERATUR

1. Austen, K. F. , Orange, R. P. : Bronchial asthma: The possible role
   of chemical mediators of immediate hypersensitivity in the pathogenesis of subacute chronic disease. Amer. Rev. Resp. Dis. 112, 423
   (1975)
2. Batchelor, J. F. , Garland, L. G. , Green, A. F. , Hughes, D. T. D. ,
   Follenfant, M. J. , Gorvin, J. H. , Hodson, H. F. , Tateson, J. E. :
   Doxantrazole, an antiallergic agent orally effective in man. Lancet
   1975 II, 1169
3. Booij-Noord, H. , Orie, N. G. M. , Berg, W. Chr. , de Vries, K. :
   Protection tests on bronchial allergen challenge with disodium
   cromoglycate and thiazinamium. J. Allergy 46, 1 (1970)
4. Booij-Noord, H. , Orie, N. G. M. , de Vries, K. : Immediate and late
   bronchial obstructive reactions to inhalation of house dust and
   protective effects of disodium cromoglycate and prednisolone.
   J. Allergy Clin. Immunol. 48, 344 (1971)
5. Debelic, M. : Ein einfacher und registrierbarer inhalativer Provoka-
   tionstest. Acta allerg. (Kbh) 23, 103 (1968)
6. Engström, I. : Inhibition of the bronchial reaction induced by allergen
   inhalation in children. Respiration 27, Suppl. 357 (1970)
7. Fleisch, J. H. , Kent, K. M. , Cooper, Th. : Drug receptors in smooth
   muscle. In: Asthma, Physiology, Immunopharmacology and Treatment.
   K. F. Austen and L. M. Lichtenstein, Eds. New York, San Francisco,
   London: Academic Press 1973
8. Herxheimer, H. : Antihistamines in bronchial asthma. Brit. Med. J.
   1949 II, 901
9. Kuschinsky, G. : Arzneimittel gegen Asthma bronchiale. Dtsch.
   Ärzteblatt 72, 213 (1975)
10. Martin, U. : Persönliche Mitteilung
11. Pepys, J. , Hargreave, F. E. , Chan, M. , McCarthy, D. S. : Inhibi-
    tory effects of disodium cromoglycate on allergen-inhalation tests.
    Lancet 1968 II, 134
12. Schultze-Werninghaus, G. , Schwarting, H. -H. : Die protektive Wir-
    kung von Dinatrium cromoglicicum im inhalativen Antigen-Provoka-
    tionstest bei Bäckerasthma. Pneumonologie 151, 115 (1974)
13. Ulmer, W. T. : Pathphysiologische Grundlagen obstruktiver Atem-
    wegserkrankungen. Dtsch. med. Wschr. 100, 1575 (1975)

14. Wüthrich, B.: Inhibitorischer Effekt von Dinatrium cromoglicicum
(Lomudal) auf die inhalative Antigenprovokation beim atopischen
Asthma bronchiale im einfachen Blindversuch. Schweiz. med.
Wschr. 101, 1034 (1971)

Dr. M. Debelic
Asthma- und Allergieklinik
CH-7299 Wolfgang - Davos
Schweiz

Pneumonologie Suppl. 1976, 161-169

Broncholytic and Protective Effects of Antiallergic Drugs in Allergen Inhalation Tests

G. Schultze-Werninghaus, E. Gonsior, and J. Meier-Sydow

Klinikum der Johann Wolfgang Goethe-Universität Frankfurt am Main
Zentrum der Inneren Medizin, Abteilung für Pneumologie

Abstract. Bronchial provocation tests are an appropriate in vivo model for studies of bronchodilators and antiallergic compounds. Curative as well as protective effects can be studied. Bronchial obstruction is most sensitively measured by body plethysmography as specific airway resistance (SR_{aw}) or specific airway conductance (SG_{aw}). Of spirometric values the forced expiratory volume in the first second (FEV_1) is recommended, as it correlates best with SR_{aw}.

A comparative study of fenoterol, salbutamol, aminophylline, and ipratropiumbromide (Sch 1000) is presented as an example of bronchodilator trials. The drugs were applied in clinical dosages. A rank order of broncholytic potency was found: fenoterol = salbutamol > ipratropiumbromide > aminophylline.

Protective drugs require a more extensive mode of trial. Such a study is presented by an example of sodium cromoglycate, which offers significant protection in experimental bronchial asthma.

Zusammenfassung. Inhalative Antigenprovokationsproben sind als in-vivo Modell zur Erprobung bronchospasmolytisch und antiallergisch wirksamer Substanzen geeignet. Sowohl kurative als auch protektive Substanzeffekte können geprüft werden. Als geeignete Obstruktionsmaße werden die Spezifische Resistance (SR_{aw}), die Spezifische Conductance (SG_{aw}) und mit Einschränkungen die Einsekundenkapazität (FEV_1) empfohlen. Als Beispiel einer Broncholytika-Erprobung werden vergleichende Untersuchungen mit Fenoterol, Salbutamol und Iprotropiumbromid (jeweils per inhalationem) und Aminophyllin (i. v.) mitgeteilt. Die Substanzen wurden in den klinischen üblichen Dosierungen angewendet. Es ergab sich eine Rangfolge der bronchospasmolytischen Wirkung: Fenoterol = Salbutamol > Ipratropiumbromid > Aminophyllin. Protektive Substanzen erfordern eine umfangreichere Versuchsanordnung. Eine solche wird am Beispiel von Dinatrium cromoglicicum gezeigt, das einen signifikanten Schutz bei experimentellem Bronchialasthma bietet. Die vorgelegten Untersuchungen demonstrieren die Eignung der inhalativen Antigenprovokationsprobe zur Pharmaka-Erprobung und geben darüber hinaus Hinweise für Ursachen und Therapie der Bronchialobstruktion.

Bronchial provocation tests have been used for trials of bronchodilators or antiallergic drugs for about 30 years (Schiller and Lowell, 1947). Accuracy, reliability, and reproducibility of this in vivo model has improved with the development of better devices and criteria for the assessment of bronchial obstruction.

METHODS

Body plethysmography, which demands the least cooperation by the patient, is now generally accepted as the best routine method for lung function tests. We have used specific airway resistance (SR_{aw}) as the best plethysmographic parameter (Lloyd and Wright, 1963) to correct the airway resistance (R_{aw}) in respect of thoracic gas volume, i. e. , age and height (Briscoe and DuBois, 1958; Doershuk et al. , 1974).

The best correlation of plethysmographic and spirometric values has been determined for SR_{aw} and forced expiratory volume in the first second (FEV_1) (Quanjer et al. , 1971). This has been proved using allergen inhalation tests (Gonsior et al. , 1974).

As criteria for a positive inhalation test we use a rise of SR_{aw} above 20 cmH_2O x s - the "dyspnea threshold" (Meier-Sydow, 1967) as well as a rise of at least 50% from the baseline values (Gonsior, in preparation).

The exact dosage of the inhalant - antigen or compound - is essential for satisfactory reproducibility of the tests. We use a conventional nebulizer (Heyer, Bad Ems) with a flow of 8 1 per min. For the dosage we take not only the concentration of the inhalant into account, but also the total inhaled amount of antigen, estimated by weighing the nebulizer on a precision balance before and after inhalation. Certain losses of substance are inevitable. The inhalation test is stopped if the patient feels a slight to moderate dyspnea, i. e. , if the SR_{aw} reaches a value between 20 and 60 cmH_2O x s.

With the method described above we tested a number of bronchodilators in patients with extrinsic allergic bronchial asthma. In no case was a patient under therapy during the trial.

As an example of a trial on broncholytic effects in bronchial provocation tests we present a comparative study of fenoterol (Th 1165 a, Berotec®), salbutamol (Sultanol®, Ventolin®) ipratropiumbromide (Sch 1000, Atrovent®), and aminophylline (Euphyllin®). Fenoterol (1. 25 mg), salbutamol (1. 25 mg), and ipratropiumbromide (0. 1 and 0. 25 mg) were tested as a respirator solution (1 ml 0. 9% sodium chloride).Aminophylline was applied as an intravenous injection (0. 24 g in 3 min).

Plethysmographic measurements were carried out prior to and after control inhalation with the diluent, after antigen inhalation, and up to 150 min after application of the bronchodilator. Variations in the above test intervals between some substances were necessary for technical reasons.

Fenoterol, aminophylline, and ipratropiumbromide were tested in 10 patients, respectively, salbutamol in 20 patients. There was no significant difference between the groups in respect to baseline values and antigen effects, so that collective comparison was possible (see Fig. 2). For comparative reasons we recorded the course of bronchial provocation tests in 15 patients having no inhaled compound.

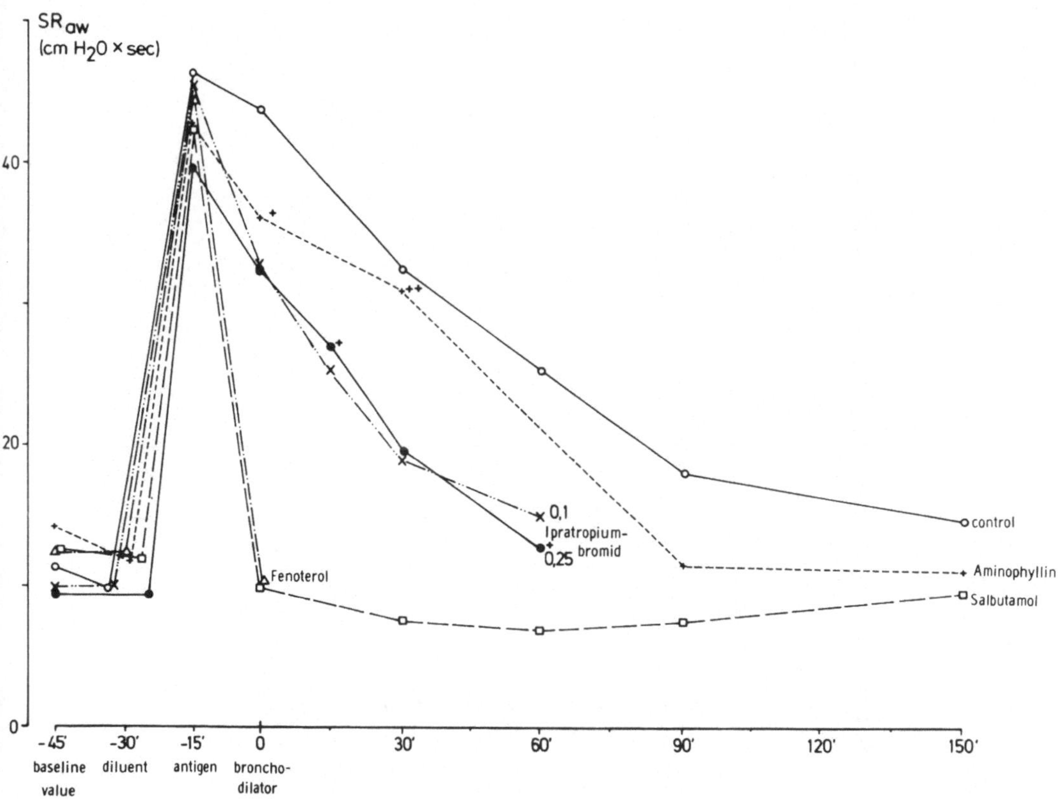

Fig. 1. Comparison of broncholytic effects in antigen-induced bronchial obstruction. Mean values of specific airway resistance SR_{aw} (cmH_2O x s). (Fenoterol, iprotropiumbromide, aminophylline: n = 10, salbutamol: n = 20, control: n = 15)

RESULTS

Fig. 1. presents the mean values for the complete test showing effects recorded up to 150 min after bronchodilation. Fig. 2 shows the immediate broncholytic effects of the tested compounds. Fenoterol and salbutamol have an immediate and complete broncholytic effect (see Tables 1 and 2). Ipratropiumbromide is only a weak bronchodilator. No difference in effect can be seen between 0.25 mg and 0.1 mg. Intravenous application of amino-phylline has no broncholytic potency at all in this trial (Schultze-Werning-haus et al., 1975).

These results indicate that betastimulants can be regarded as the therapy of choice in moderate allergic asthma. No significant difference was seen between fenoterol and salbutamol. Ipratropiumbromide represents no alternative. It should be mentioned, however, that we made a further study with ipratropiumbromide in patients with considerably elevated base-

Table 1. Comparison of broncholytic effects in antigen-induced bronchial obstruction. Mean values $\bar{x}$ and standard errors $s_{\bar{x}}$ of specific airway resistance SR_{aw} ($cmH_2O \times s$)

		Control (without bronchodilator)	Fenoterol	Salbutamol	Aminophylline	Ipratropiumbromide 0.1	0.25
		n = 15	n = 10	n = 20	n = 10	n = 10	n = 10
Baseline value (after diluent)	$\bar{x}$	9.9	12.2	11.5	11.8	10.0	9.5
	$s_{\bar{x}}$	1.3	1.5	0.9	1.1	1.0	0.8
Antigen	$\bar{x}$	46.2	44.4	42.9	42.6	45.3	39.6
	$s_{\bar{x}}$	10.4	6.2	4.8	5.9	11.6	4.8
Bronchodilation o'	$\bar{x}$	43.6	10.2	9.6	36.0[+]	32.8	32.4
	$s_{\bar{x}}$	9.5	1.2	1.5	7.5	9.6	5.1
30'	$\bar{x}$	32.3	-	7.6	30.9[++]	19.0	19.7[+]
	$s_{\bar{x}}$	8.2	-	1.1	9.8	5.3	4.5
60'	$\bar{x}$	25.3	-	6.9	-	14.9	14.7[+]
	$s_{\bar{x}}$	6.7	-	1.0	-	2.3	2.4
90'	$\bar{x}$	18.0	-	7.5	11.6	-	-
	$s_{\bar{x}}$	3.9	-	1.1	0.9	-	-
150'	$\bar{x}$	14.7	-	9.6	11.2	-	-
	$s_{\bar{x}}$	2.6	-	0.7	3.0	-	-

+ = Frequency of further bronchodilations

Table 2. Significance of broncholytic tests in antigen-induced bronchial obstruction (Wilcoxon test)

a) Test for significant bronchodilation (specific airway resistance SR_{aw} after antigen inhalation compared with SR_{aw} after bronchodilation)

Compound	Bronchodilation
Control (without bronchodilator)	not significant
Fenoterol	significant
Salbutamol	significant
Aminophylline	significant
Ipratropiumbromide 0.1 mg	significant
Ipratropiumbromide 0.25 mg	significant

b) Test for complete bronchodilation (SR_{aw} after diluent compared with SR_{aw} after bronchodilation)

Compound	Bronchodilation
Control (without bronchodilator)	incomplete
Fenoterol	complete
Salbutamol	complete
Aminophylline	inconplete
Ipratropiumbromide 0.1 mg	incomplete
Ipratropiumbromide 0.25 mg	incomplete

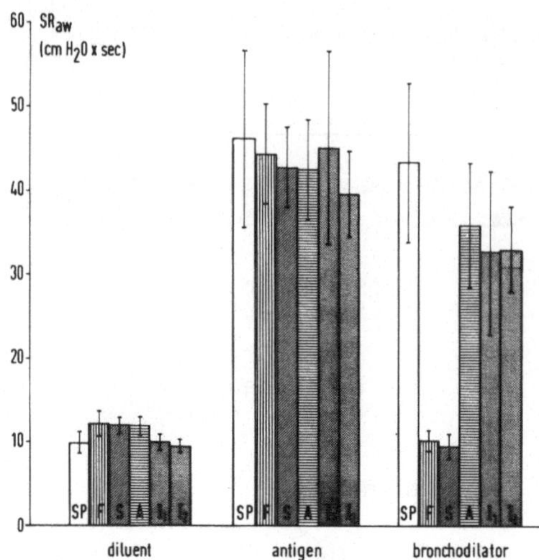

Fig. 2. Effect of antigen inhalation and broncholytic action of a number of compounds (immediate effects). Mean values $\bar{x}$ and standard errors $s_{\bar{x}}$ of specific airway resistance SR_{aw}

SP = Spontaneous course of bronchial provocation tests
F = Fenoterol
S   = Salbutamol
A = Aminophylline
I_1 = Ipratropiumbromide (Sch 1000)0. 1 mg
I_2 = Ipratropiumbromide (Sch 1000)0. 25 mg

line values (mean value 23. 2 cmH_2O x s SR_{aw}). These patients reached a mean value of 41. 5 cmH O x s SR_{aw} as did the other groups (mean value about 40. 0 cmH_2O x s). In this group ipratropiumbromide (0. 25 mg) seemed to be a suitable bronchodilator, as it led to a mean SR_{aw} of 26. 5 cmH_2O x s, i. e. , SR_{aw} reached the baseline values immediately after inhalation of the drug. This suggests a predominantly vagally mediated etiology of the bronchial obstruction in these cases unlike the patients with normal baseline values. This confirms other authors (Kersten, 1974) who found beneficial effects with atropine derivates.

In the light of the broad clinical application of aminophylline the poor broncholytic action of a single dose given intravenously, was unexpected. However, this finding has been also confirmed by other authors (Podlesch and Ulmer, 1966), whereas its beneficial effects, when given as intravenous infusion, in severe asthma, are generally accepted. This has recently been stressed by several authors (Mitenko and Ogilvie, 1973; Nicholson and Chick, 1973).

Following this presentation of bronchodilators only a short review on protective antiallergic compounds in bronchial provocation tests can be given, using an example of a study with sodium cromoglycate (DSCG). Fifteen patients with extrinsic allergic bronchial asthma were submitted to three identical tests with a 48-h interval between each test. Bronchial obstruction was measured as FEV_1. Provocation tests A and C (Fig. 3, Table 3) served as controls. Test B was done following inhalation of 20 mg DSCG with the spinhaler. A significant protection could be demonstrated (Fig. 3) (Schultze-Werninghaus and Schwarting, 1974).

Protection tests are methodologically more complicated than bronchodilator tests, as several control tests are essential. Multiple allergen inhalations without test substance are necessary to detect a possible alteration of bronchial reaction or lasting substance effects. This is underlined in the presented study where we found a reduced antigen effect in test C compared with test A.

From our results we conclude the applicability of bronchial provocation tests for trials of bronchodilators and protective antiallergic drugs, if a reliable and sensitive method is applied. A number of further questions could only be touched upon, e. g. , the clinical relevance of such studies and the pharmacologic aspects of bronchial obstruction.

Bronchial provocation tests are suitable for extrinsic allergic asthma attacks. However, we want to stress that a generalization of the results obtained by this model is not possible, as different conditions are present in other kinds of bronchial obstruction, e. g. , chronic obstructive lung disease or status asthmaticus.

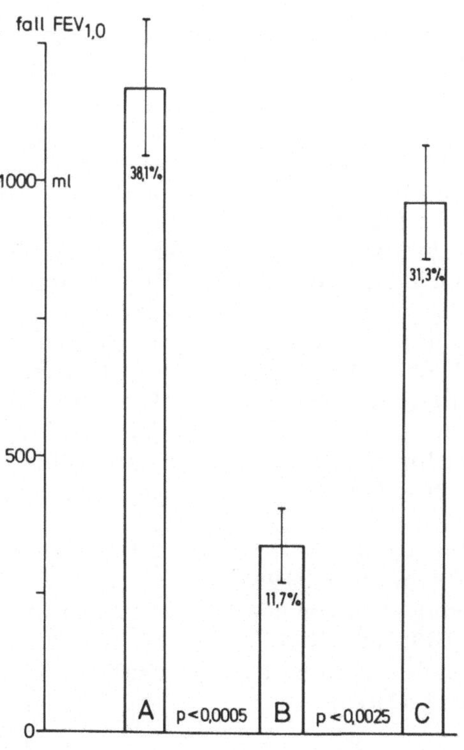

Fig. 3. Effect of sodium cromoglycate in allergen inhalation tests. Identical test A and C without DSCG. Test B with prior inhalation of 20 mg DSCG. Test intervals 48 h. Fall in FEV_1 (absolute values on y-axis, percentage on top of columns)

Table 3. Protective effect of sodium cromoglycate (DSCG) in antigen-induced bronchospasm. Mean values $\bar{x}$ and standard errors $s_{\bar{x}}$ of maximal fall in FEV_1 within 30 min after bronchial provocation test
N = 15

	Test A Antigen without DSCG	Test B Antigen with prior inhalation of 20 mg DSCG	Test C Antigen without DSCG
Fall in FEV_1/ml	1165. 3 $\pm$ 126. 7	341. 3 $\pm$ 67. 3	959. 3 $\pm$ 102. 9
(ml)			
(%)	38. 7	13. 6	31. 1
Significance	< 0. 0005	< 0. 0025	
P	> 0. 05		

REFERENCES

Briscoe, W.A. , DuBois, A.B. : The relationship between airway resistance, airway conductance and lung volume in subjects of different age and body size. J. clin. Invest. 37, 1279 (1958)

Doershuk, C.F. , Fisher, B.J. , Matthews, L.W. : Specific airway resistance from the perinatal period into adulthood. Amer. Rev. Resp. Dis. 109, 452 (1974)

Gonsior, E. , Krüger, M. , Meier-Sydow, J. : Comparison of different methods in bronchial antigen challenge. Allergy 74. Proc. Europ. Congr. Allergy Clin. Immunol. , London 1974, p. 343. London: Pitman 1975

Kersten, W. : Protektive Wirkung von Ipratropium-bromid (Sch 1000) bei akuten Bronchokonstruktionen durch Allergeninhalationen. Respiration 31, 412 (1974)

Meier-Sydow, J. : Die exspiratorische Atemgeschwindigkeit bei Bronchialobstruktion. Habilitationsschrift, Frankfurt, 1967

Mitenko, P.A. , Ogilvie, R.I. : Rational intravenous dose of parenteral theophylline. New Engl. J. Med. 183, 600 (1973)

Nicholson, P.P. , Chick, T.W. : A re-evaluation of parenteral aminophylline. Amer. J. Resp. Dis. 108, 241 (1973)

Quanjer, Ph. H. , de Pater, L. , Tammeling, G. J. : Plethysmographic eval-
uation of airway obstruction, p. 116. Leusden: Netherlands Asthma
Fund 1971
Podlesch, I. , Ulmer, W. T. : Die Wirkung der intravenösen Euphyllin-In-
jektion auf Strömungswiderstand, Strömungsgeschwindigkeit, intraalve-
oläre Druckdifferenzen, funktionelles Residualvolumen und arterielle
Blutgase bei chronisch-obstruktiven Atemwegserkrankungen. Beitr.
Klin. Tuberk. 133, 49 (1966)
Schiller, I. W. , Lowell, F. C. : The effect of drugs in modifying the response
of asthmatic subjects to inhalation of pollen extracts as determined by
vital capacity measurements. Ann. Allergy 5, 564 (1947)
Schultze-Werninghaus, G. , Schwarting, H. -H. : Die protektive Wirkung
von Kinatrium cromoglicicum im inhalativen Antigen-Provokationstest
bei Bäckerasthma. Pneumonologie 151, 115 (1974)
Schultze-Werninghaus, G. , Gonsior, E. , Thiel, C. , Kroidl, R. , Meier-
Sydow, J. : Vergleichende Untersuchungen über die Wirkung von Fenoterol, Aminophyllin und Salbutamol bei antigeninduzierter Bronchialobstruktion. Therapiewoche 25, 40, 5727 (1975)

Dr. Gerhard Schultze-Werninghaus
Zentrum Innere Medizin
Abteilung Pneumologie
Theodor Stern Kai 7
6000 Frankfurt/Main 70

Pneumonologie Suppl. 1976, 171-175
by Springer-Verlag 1976

Die Beeinflussung des Plasmas cAMP durch inhalative und parenterale β_2-adrenerge Stimulatoren

P. Endres, K.H. Schnabel und R. Ferlinz

Abteilung für Pneumologie, Universitätsklinikum Mainz

Abstract. Regarding observations of a decreased urinary cAMP after adrenergic stimulation in asthmatics we examimed comparing endobronchial resistance and plasma cAMP. The changes of resistance after erbutalin s.c., salbutamol p.inh. and fenoterol p.inh. were all in the same range, but cAMP increased differently. Also in normal persons there was the same cAMP increase. It is estimated, that the plasma cAMP origin after adrenergic stimulation is not the lung.

Key words: Plasma cAMP - β-adrenerge Stimulation

Zusammenfassung. Nach früheren Untersuchungen soll bei Asthmatikern im Urin die cAMP Vermehrung nach adrenerger Stimulation vermindert sein. Wir haben daher vergleichend endobronchialen Widerstand und Plasma cAMP untersucht. Die Resistanceveränderungen nach Terbutalin s.c., Salbutamol per inh. und Fenoterol p.inh. waren alle in der gleichen Größenordnung, während sich die cAMP Anstiege unterschieden. Auch bei Normalpersonen fand sich ein gleichsinniger Anstieg. Es wird vermutet, daß das ausgeschüttete Plasma cAMP nicht aus der Lunge stammt.

Das zyklische Adenosinmonophosphat - auch cAMP genannt - gilt als intrazellulärer Mediator verschiedener Hormonwirkungen [6]. Adrenalin und andere adrenerge Substanzen führen zu einer Stimulation der Adenylzyklase, die eine Vermehrung des intrazellulären cAMP zur Folge hat. Hierfür wird der β-adrenerge Anteil verantwortlich gemacht [6].

Im Rahmen der Regulation des bronchialen Muskeltonus wird eine cAMP Vermehrung als ursächlich für eine Bronchospasmolyse und eine cAMP Verminderung als ursächlich für eine Bronchokonstriktion angesehen [5]. So soll bei Asthmatikern mit gestörter bronchialer Muskelmotorik die cAMP Vermehrung nach adrenerger Stimulation unterbleiben [1].

Ziel unserer Untersuchung war zu prüfen, ob cAMP Verhalten und Bronchomotorik durch verschiedene β 2 Stimulatoren unterschiedlich beeinflußt wurden. Da zwischen intra- und extrazellulärem Raum ein Gleichgewicht

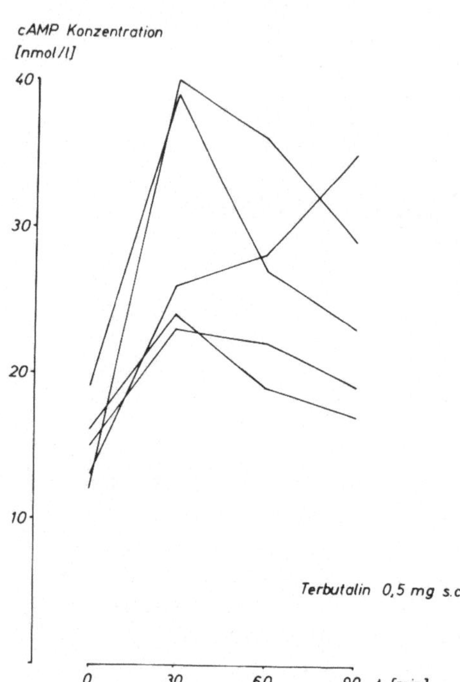

Abb. 1. Plasma cAMP Konzentrations-
verlauf bei 5 gesunden Probanden nach
Terbutalin 0,5 mg s.c.

angenommen wird [2] und sich bisherige Untersuchungen zum Teil auf Befunde im Urin stützen [1] , haben wir die cAMP Bestimmungen im Plasma
durchgeführt. Sie erfolgte mittels einer Proteinbindungstechnik, die von
Gilman [3] entwickelt und von Tovey [7] und Mitarbeitern modifiziert wurde.
Als Kriterium des bronchialen Muskeltonus wurde die Veränderbarkeit des
ganzkörperplethysmographisch gemessenen endobronchialen Widerstandes
herangezogen.

Zunächst haben wir bei 5 Probanden ohne bronchiale Obstruktion vor
und halbständig nach 1/2 mg Terbutalin subkutan Blutproben untersucht.
Die normalen Ausgangswerte der cAMP Konzentration von 15 ± 3 nmol/l
veränderten sich durch Terbutalin signifikant. Nach 30 Minuten erreichten
die Werte die doppelte Höhe und fielen insignifikant nach 60 und nach 90
Minuten um 13 und 19% ab (Abb. 1).

Bei 3 weiteren Patienten haben wir gleichzeitig aus der Arteria
femoralis und einer Armvene vor und 30 Minuten nach 1/2 mg Terbutalin
subcutan Blutentnahmen vorgenommen. Vor der Injektion waren keine
arteriovenösen Differenzen nachweisbar, nach der Injektion war in allen
3 Fällen in der Armvene ein höherer cAMP-Spiegel als in der Arterie
(Abb. 2).

Bei 12 Patienten bestimmten wir simultan Atemwegs-Resistance und
cAMP-Konzentration vor und 30 Minuten nach 1/2 mg Terbutalin subcutan.
Der endobronchiale Widerstand fiel signifikant um 16% ab, während die
normale cAMP-Ausgangskonzentration signifikant um 80% zunahm und

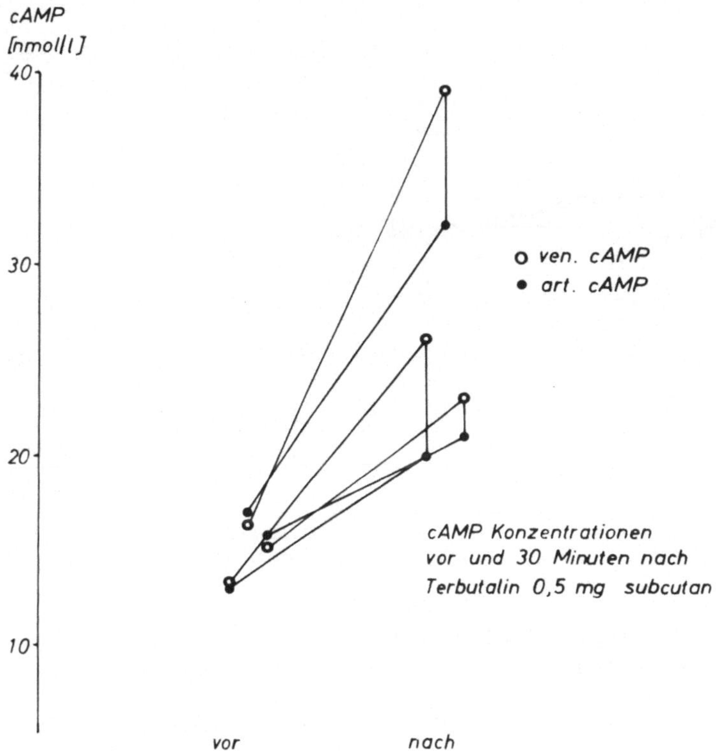

Abb. 2. Plasma cAMP Konzentration in Arterie und Vene vor und
30 Minuten nach Terbutalin 0,5 mg s.c.

somit ein gleiches Verhalten aufwies, wie bei den normalen Probanden.
Bei Betrachtung der Einzelfälle zeigt sich, daß die cAMP Veränderungen
unabhängig vom Ausgangs- oder Endwert der Resistance waren.

Auch nach Inhalation von 0,3 mg Salbutamol aus einem Taschendosier-
aerosol kam es bei 12 Patienten innerhalb von 10 Minuten zu einer signifikanten Besserung der Resistance um 24% und zu einem geringen, jedoch
signifikanten Anstieg der normalen cAMP Konzentration um 18%. Im Vergleich zu Terbutalin subcutan ist die Resistanceveränderung in der gleichen
Größenordnung und die cAMP Veränderung deutlich geringer.

Fenoterol führte nach Inhalation von 0,6 mg Substanz bei 9 Probanden
zu einem Abfall der Resistance um 30%, während der cAMP Spiegel aus
dem Normbereich um 56% anstieg. Im Vergleich zu den beiden anderen
Substanzen ist die Resistanceveränderung annähernd gleich, während die
cAMP Veränderungen in der Größenordnung von Terbutalin subcutan liegt
(Abb. 3).

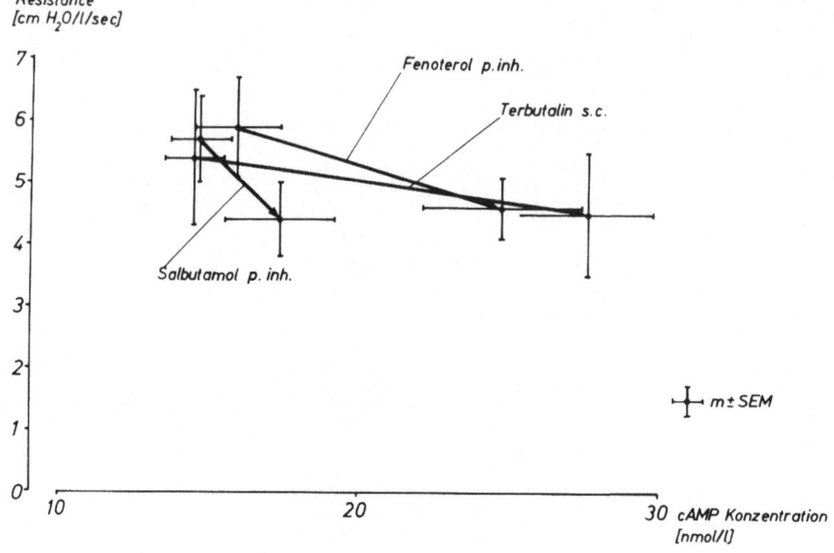

Abb. 3. Resistance- und Plasma cAMP Veränderungen nach verschiedenen β_2 adrenerg wirksamen Substanzen

DISKUSSION

Da sowohl bei Normalpersonen als auch bei Patienten mit Bronchospasmus keine wesentlichen Unterschiede des Plasma cAMP Gehaltes nach Terbutalin zu beobachten waren, ist eine Diskrepanz zwischen den hypothetischen erniedrigten intrazellulären [5] und gemessenen erhöhten extrazellulären cAMP Spiegel zumindestens bei Patienten mit Bronchokonstriktion anzunehmen. In Analogie dürfte dies auch für Salbutamol und Fenoterol gelten. Bei annähernd gleicher Bronchodilatation war eine deutliche cAMP Differenz nach diesen Substanzen vorhanden. Die arteriovenöse Differenz nach Terbutalin läßt eine Ausschüttung des cAMP aus anderen Organen oder der Muskulatur annehmen [4]. Dieser Frage werden wir uns weiter widmen.

Der schnelle Anstieg der cAMP Konzentration nach Inhalation spricht für eine Resorption und systemische Wirkung. Die Ursache der cAMP Unterschiede nach Salbutamol und Fenoterol ist vermutlich in einer unterschiedlichen systemischen Wirkung zu sehen, da die Bronchspasmolyse annähernd gleich war. Hierfür spricht auch das annähernd gleiche Verhalten des cAMP und der Resistance nach Terbutalin und Fenoterol trotz unterschiedlicher Applikation.

LITERATUR

1. Bernstein, R.A., Linarelli, L., Facktor, M.A., Friday, G.A.,
    Drash, A.L., Firemann, Ph.: Decreased urinary adenosine 3' 5'
    monophosphate (cyclic AMP) in asthmatics. J. Lab. Clin. Med. 80,
    772-779 (1972)
2. Gerbitz, K.D., Wieland, O.H.: Extrazelluläre zyklische Nukleotide:
    Vorkommen, Analytik und diagnostische Bedeutung. Z.Klin.Chem.
    11, 224-232 (1973)
3. Gilman, A.G.: A protein binding assay for adenosine 3' 5' cyclic
    monophosphate. Proc. Nat. Acad. Sci 67, 305-312 (1970)
4. Liljenquist, J.E., Bomboy, D.J., Lewis, St.B., Sinclair Smith, B.C.,
    Felts, Ph.W., Lacy, W.W., Crofford, O.B., Liddle, G.W.:
    Effect of glucagon on net splanchnic cyclic AMP Production in normal
    and diabetic men. J. Clin. Invest. 53, 198-204 (1974)
5. Murad, F.: Beta-blockade of epinephrin-induced cyclic AMP formation
    in heart, liver, fat and trachea. Biochim. Biophys. Acta 304, 181-187
    (1973)
6. Schultz, G., Hardman, J.G., Sutherland, E.W.: Cyclic nucleotides
    and smooth muscle function. In: Asthma. Hsg. V.F.R. Austen und
    L.W. Lichtenstein, S. 123-137. New York, San Fancisco, London:
    Academic Press 1973
7. Tovey, K.G., Oldham, K.G., Whelan, J.A.M.A.: A simple direct
    assay for cyclic AMP in plasma and other biological samples using
    an improved competetive protein binding technique. Clin. Chim. Acta
    56, 221-234 (1974)

Dr.P. Endres
Abteilung für Pneumologie
Universitätsklinikum
Langenbeckstrasse 1
D-6500 Mainz

Pneumonologie Suppl. 1976, 177–182

Die theoretische Ventilationsleistung der Lunge, Diagrammdarstellung. Vergleich mit der physiologischen Interpretation

Peter-Paul Heusinger

Bergbau-Forschung, Essen

Abstract. The ventilation power of the lung to overcome friction and elasticity consists of an irreversible component which is to be found in the pressure-volume diagram and of a reversible component which is to be found in the pressure-flow diagram. The effective power which results, is a measure for part of the metabolic losses due to the ventilation mechanism. In physiology, the components of ventilation work are interpreted together in the pressure-volume diagram.

Key words: Irreversible, reversible, effective power –
            Metabolic losses.

Starting point of the following considerations is a general thorax-pleura-lung model (Fig. 1). Functionally, the thorax represents the active drive mechanism, the pleura the neutral transmission mechanism, and the lung the passive ventilation mechanism. The thorax is supplied with chemical energy and transfers it into mechanical work and into metabolic losses. The mechanical conversion of energy by friction is irreversible and the conversion by elasticity is reversible. According to this principal divi-

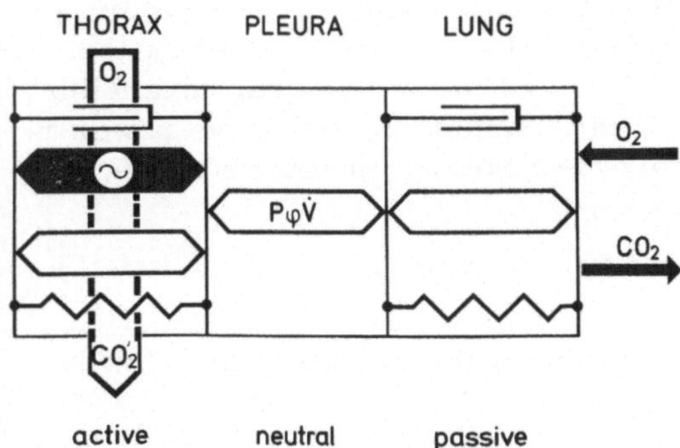

Fig. 1. General model

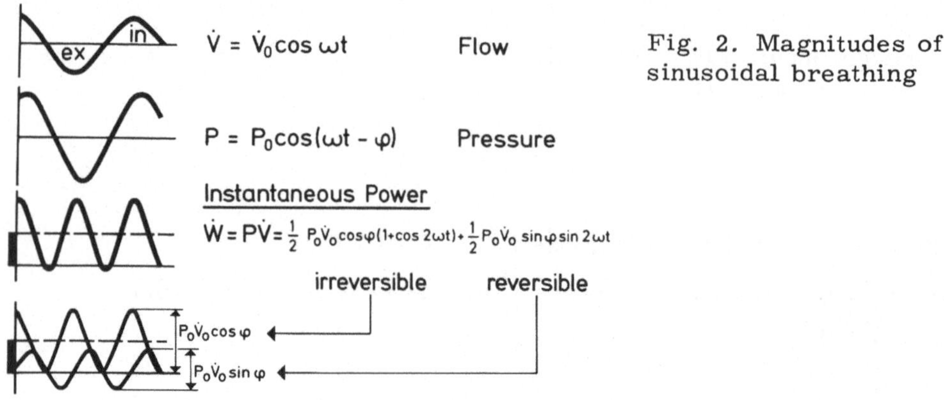

Fig. 2. Magnitudes of sinusoidal breathing

sion, work or the work in a time unit, i. e., the power, is divided into two components excluding each other. The effective power resulting therefrom is the equivalent for the metabolic losses, multiplied by the efficiency. In this model, we differ between the inner power of the thorax and the power transmitted by the pleura to the lung: the ventilation power proper. It comes to bear by the oscillatory pressure P and flow $\dot{V}$ in the pleural periphery. Due to the complexity of friction and elasticity, pressure and flow have a phase lag φ.

The most simple mathematical arrangement is made with the idealized sinusoidal breathing (Fig. 2).

$$\dot{V} = \dot{V}_0 \cos \omega t \qquad P = P_0 \cos(\omega t - \varphi) \qquad \omega = 2\pi f$$

The product of pressure and flow gives the instantaneous power.

$$\dot{W} = P\dot{V} = \frac{1}{2}P_0\dot{V}_0 \cos \varphi (1 + \cos 2\omega t) + \frac{1}{2}P_0\dot{V}_0 \sin \varphi \sin 2\omega t$$

The separation into a cosinus term and into a sinus term gives us the instantaneous irreversible and the instantaneous reversible power. This is due to the phase angle which becomes zero with an only irreversible conversion of energy by friction and which amounts to $\pi/2$ with an only reversible conversion of energy by elasticity. This can be seen also by the development in time: On the average, the sinus term is zero and the cosinus term equal to the mean value of the instantaneous power.

The amplitudes of the two terms can be understood as complementary projections of the distance $1/2\ P_0\dot{V}_0$ under the phase angle φ. So Figure 3 shows the representation of the components of the effective power as the geometrical sum of the integral irreversible and of the integral reversible power. This is confirmed by the general definition of the effective power as the product of the effective values of the power factors pressure and flow:

$$\dot{W}_{eff} = P_{eff}\dot{V}_{eff} = \sqrt{\frac{1}{T}\int_0^T P^2 dt \ \frac{1}{T}\int_0^T \dot{V}^2 dt} \qquad T = \frac{1}{f}$$

In the sinus case we obtain the square relation of the representation of the components as follows:

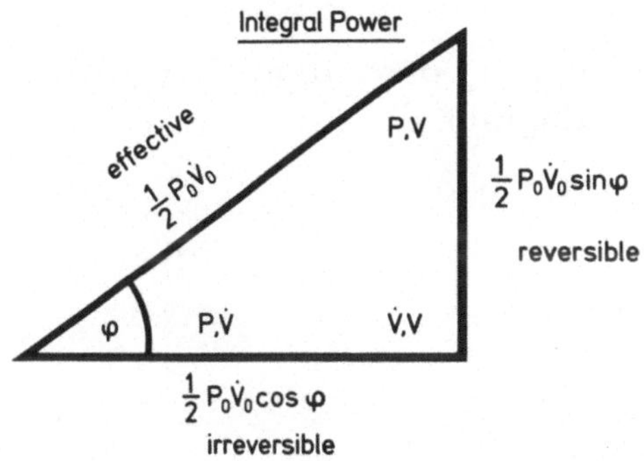

Fig. 3. Geometric composition of integral power

$$\dot{W}^2_{eff} = (\tfrac{1}{2}P_0\dot{V}_0 \cos\varphi)^2 + (\tfrac{1}{2}P_0\dot{V}_0 \sin\varphi)^2 = (\tfrac{1}{2}P_0\dot{V}_0)^2.$$

Beside the integral term for the effective power, we can give also the following general integral term for the irreversible power in the meaning of the mean power:

$$\dot{W}_{irr} = \frac{1}{T}\int_0^T P\dot{V}dt.$$

In this form $\dot{W}_{eff}$ and $\dot{W}_{irr}$ apply to the real nonsinusoidal breathing, too. The mutual exclusivity of irreversible and reversible power demands generally the vertical placement of the components to each other or their square relation. Therefore we find for the integral reversible power:

$$\dot{W}_{rev} = \frac{1}{T}\sqrt{\int_0^T P^2 dt \int_0^T \dot{V}^2 dt - (\int_0^T P\dot{V}dt)^2}.$$

The representation of the integrals by areas leads, by means of mathematical transformations, to the graphical method where, in addition to P and $\dot{V}$, their time integrals $\int Pdt = Q$ and $\int \dot{V}dt = V$ are used, too. The combinations of these magnitudes in pairs produce, in carthesian coordinates, closed cyclic diagrams, the areas of which are proportional to the derived magnitudes.

$$P^2_{eff} = \frac{1}{T}\int_0^T P^2 dt \equiv f\oint PdQ \triangleq fA_{PQ}$$

$$\dot{V}^2_{eff} = \frac{1}{T}\int_0^T \dot{V}^2 dt \equiv f\oint \dot{V}dV \triangleq fA_{\dot{V}V}$$

$$\dot{W}_{irr} = \frac{1}{T}\int_0^T P\dot{V}dt \equiv f\oint PdV \triangleq fA_{PV}$$

$$\dot{W}_{rev} = \sqrt{P^2_{eff}\dot{V}^2_{eff} - \dot{W}^2_{irr}} \triangleq f\sqrt{A_{PQ}A_{\dot{V}V} - A^2_{PV}}.$$

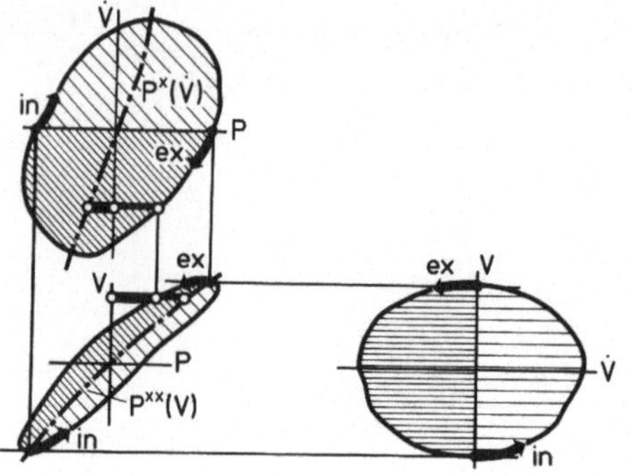

Fig. 4. P-V, P-V̇, V̇-V
diagram

Instead of the complicated relation for the reversible power, we can
also use approximately a simple sinus relation which leads to the power-
flow diagram.

$$\overset{\cdot}{W}_{rev \atop sin} = \frac{1}{2\pi} \int\limits_{o}^{T} P\ddot{V}dt \qquad \ddot{V} = \frac{d\dot{V}}{dt}$$

$$\overset{\cdot}{W}_{rev} \approx \frac{1}{2\pi} \oint Pd\dot{V} \cong \frac{1}{2\pi} A_{P\dot{V}} \ .$$

The representation in closed diagrams has the advantage of a clearer interpretation (Fig. 4). The extent of nonsinusoidal breathing can be seen by the
deviation from the elliptical shape. Whereas, with sinusoidal breathing,
there is proportionality between the irreversible pressure term and the
flow as well as between the reversible pressure term and the volume, it is
probable at nonsinusoidal breathing that the irreversible pressure term is
at least an exclusive function of the flow and that the reversible pressure
term is an exclusive function of the volume. [1]

$$P_{sin} = R\dot{V} + \frac{1}{C} V = P_{irr \atop sin} + P_{rev \atop sin} \qquad\qquad resistance\ R,\ compliance\ C$$

$$P(\dot{V},V) = P^*(\dot{V}) + P^{**}(V) = P_{irr} + P_{rev}.$$

As flow and volume are related to each other infinitesimally, the pressure
relation can be stated indentically for the P-V̇ diagram and the P-V diagram.

$$P(\dot{V}) = P^*(\dot{V}) + P^{**}(\int \dot{V}dt)$$

$$P(V) = P^*(\frac{dV}{dt}) + P^{**}(V)$$

It is borne in mind that V̇ and V have, on the average, a phase lag against
each other by a quarter period, so we find two things:

---

[1] The term of acceleration of mass is neglected. If it would be taken into
consideration, the further would become somewhat complicated but, after
all, realizable.

1. As synchronous functions, $P^*(\dot{V})$ in the pressure-flow diagram and $P^{**}(V)$ in the pressure-volume diagram, represent the separating lines of the cyclic diagrams.

2. As functions with phase lag, $P^*(dV/dt)$ in the pressure-volume diagram and $P^{**}(\int \dot{V}\,dt)$ in the pressure-flow diagram represent the pressure sections between the separating line and the diagram line.

Thus, the P-V diagram only includes irreversible pressure sections and the P-$\dot{V}$ diagram only reversible pressure sections and hence the separate representation of power components is expressed graphically, too.

In contrast, in conventional physiology, the work per cycle, i.e., power multiplied by cycle time, and its components are represented together in the P-V diagram (Campbell).

The elastic work is interpreted as an area between the elastic separating lines or limited by the volume axis. In fact, this is the elastic energy of the final position of the volume compared with the initial position or the working capacity but not the elastic work during a cycle. The discrepancy becomes clear, if the elastic work is calculated from the compliance and the effective flow. In the sinus case, we then obtain a factor π, compared with a factor <2, when calculated from the P-V diagram.

As negative work, the outer area between the diagram line and the volume axis is represented and is then interpreted as the not converted elastic energy or as a work absorbed by the thorax associated with metabolic losses. This interpretation should be objected to, however — and this concerns both the negative work and the elastic work — that the relation between work and metabolic losses must not be reversed in such a way that only a reasonable division of areas is associated with the phases of breathing. Instead the metabolic losses are consistent with the effective work by the principle of division between irreversibility and reversibility in the same way as with the power, from the P-V diagram and the P-$\dot{V}$ diagram. In other words: The integral $\int P\,dV$ is not sufficient for the definition of cyclic work under consideration of metabolic losses.

Dipl. Phys. Peter-Paul Heusinger
Bergbau-Forschung Essen
Frillendorfer Strasse 351
4300 Essen 13

DISCUSSION

U. Schmidt, Moers: It appears to me very important according to your explanations that in describing breathing work we no longer take into consideration the areas of the P-V diagram, but also those of the P-$\dot{V}$ diagram, because "reversible" is the last section only in the physical sense; physiologically compression work is not "free".

You have calculated the equations by postulating sinusoidal curves. But don't your results also hold for the irregular forms of breathing of our patients since you start from area integrals?

P. Heusinger, Essen: The equivalent of metabolic losses developed for reversible ventilation wirk is, in physiologic as well as in physical meaning, irreversible. In an analogous, exclusively physical, periodically working system, too, additional irreversible losses would arise in the energy source (thorax) in case reversible work is performed in the energy consumer (lungs).

The physiologic, metabolic losses, though, contain besides the equivalent for effective — irreversible and reversible — work, also amounts for chemical processes, which carry out no work.

Sinusoidal breathing allows for a particularly simple, mathematical arrangement into irreversible and reversible components. The integral term itself is interpretative of the general validity for the real, irregular forms of breathing. A limitation certainly holds for the integral of reversible work:

$$\frac{1}{\omega} \oint P\,d\dot{V}$$

It can, however, be substituted by the mathematical expression:

$$\sqrt{\oint P\,dQ \oint \dot{V}\,dV - \left(\oint P\,dV\right)^2} \qquad Q = \int P\,dt$$

The integrals contained therein again represent the area contents of closed diagrams. Wierich's explanations have in an example made clear the difference between conventional sinus methods and the integration methods reported on here.

Pneumonologie Suppl. 1976, 183-191

Die Ventilationsleistung isolierter Lungen in verschiedenen Lebensaltern unter Berücksichtigung verschiedener Auswertungsmethoden, speziell unter Anwendung der Methode nach Heusinger[*]

W. Wierich

Aus dem Institut für Pathologie der Ruhr-Universität Bochum
(Lehrstuhl I: Prof. Dr. med. W. Hartung)

Abstract. By measurements of the power required for the ventilation
of isolated human autopsy lungs of different ages an agespecific pattern
analogous to clinical data could be established. Considering the per cent
energy consumption an optimum during early to medium adulthood has
been found.

From the methodical point of view the two different formulae of Cook
and of Heusinger have been applied and their respective results compared.
There were considerable differences, presumably due to alinearities and
deviations from the sinus type of induced ventilatory movements even
in morphologically normal lungs. The use of the more exact method of
Heusinger should be preferred, particularly in the analysis of diseased
lungs.

Key words: Postmortal lung function - Mechanics of breathing -
Ventilatory work of breathing - Locus diagram

Zusammenfassung. Die spezifische Ventilationsleistung von Lungen
aus unterschiedlichen Lebensaltern wurde durch Beatmung der Lungen im
künstlichen Thorax gemessen. Dabei konnten in Analogie zu klinischen
Messungen alterstypische Veränderungen festgestellt werden. Sowohl für
die Leistungswerte als auch für den prozentualen Energieverbrauch der
Atemmuskulatur am Gesamtenergieumsatz läßt sich ein Optimum im
mittleren Erwachsenenalter annehmen.

Die Berechnung der Ventilationsleistung erfolgte einerseits unter Anwendung einer von Cook angegebenen Formel, zum anderen wurde sie nach
der physikalisch exakten Methode nach Heusinger berechnet. Dabei fanden
sich erhebliche Differenzen, die auf alineare Atemgesetze und Abweichungen
der Atemgrößen von sinusförmigem Verlauf zurückzuführen sind. Bei

---

* Mit Unterstützung des Ministers für Wissenschaft und Forschung des
  Landes Nordrhein-Westfalen.

vertretbarem Mehraufwand scheint die von Heusinger angegebene Methode
geeignet zu sein, besonders im Falle pathologischer Atembedingungen,
eine genaue Berechnung atemmechanischer Parameter zu ermöglichen.

In den vorangegangenen Beiträgen und Diskussionen über die Ventilationsleistung und die Leistungsbreite der Lungen wurde eine Einflußgröße, das
Lebensalter, deutlich. Durch Analysen der mechanischen Lungenfunktion
isolierter Lungen konnten wir dies bestätigen.

METHODIK

Die Durchführung der Messungen im künstlichen Thorax erfolgte im wesentlichen nach der von Hartung et al. angegebenen Methode [15, 16, 17, 24,
25]. Die Lungen wurden mittels einer einfachen Kolbenpumpe beatmet,
deren Hubvolumen stufenlos verstellbar war. Die Beatmungsfrequenz konnte
zwischen 5/min und 12O/min variiert werden. Die Beatmung erfolgte entsprechend früheren Untersuchungen im Bereich der FRC mit einem Atemzugvolumen von etwa 1O% der TLC [24, 25] . Die Meßgrößen wurden simultan registriert und gleichzeitig auf Magnetband gespeichert (Universal-Meß-
anlage ifd, Mülheim).

Für die Berechnung der Ventilationsleistung werden in der Literatur
unterschiedliche Formeln angegeben [8, 2O, 21, 23]. Derartige Formeln
sind i.a. nur für den Fall sinusförmiger Atmung und linearer Atemgesetze
gültig. Die von uns angewendete, von Cook entwickelte, übliche Formel
zur Berechnung der Ventilationsleistung $\dot{W}$ ($=\Delta P \times AMV \times O,6$) setzt
Sinusatmung, lineare Atemgesetze und ein empirisch ermitteltes, konstantes
Verhältnis zwischen den Reibungselementen und der Elastizität voraus [8].

Hinweise auf alineare Gesetzmäßigkeiten der Lungenmechanik sowie Ansätze entsprechender Berechnungsmethoden finden sich in neuerer Literatur vereinzelt [1, 11, 2O, 22]. Heusinger hat derartige Ansätze zusammengefaßt und eine umfassende, physikalisch exakte Methode zur Lungenfunktionsanalyse auch für den Fall alinearer Gesetzmäßigkeiten und nicht sinusförmiger Atmung erarbeitet [13, 14]. Wir haben diese Methode zu Ver-
gleichszwecken neben der Formel von Cook angewendet.

Die gesamte Ventilationsleistung (effektive Leistung) $\dot{W}_Z$ sowie deren
reversible Komponente der Elastizität $\dot{W}_X$ und deren irreversible Komponente der Reibung $\dot{W}_R$ ergeben sich nach Heusinger aus den Flächen der
Umlaufdiagramme $\oint pdV$, $\oint pd\dot{V}$ und $\oint \dot{V}dV$. Bei vertretbarem Zeitaufwand
ist die Flächenberechnung mechanisch mittels eines Planimeters möglich
und wurde bei klinischen Messungen bereits vereinzelt durchgeführt
[3, 11]. Bei Untersuchungen an isolierten Lungen mit der Möglichkeit
vielfältiger Variationen der Atembedingungen und gleichzeitiger Messung
mehrerer alveolärer bzw. intrapulmonaler Drucke aus unterschiedlichen
Lungenabschnitten ist der Zeitaufwand erheblich. Die Möglichkeit der
on-line-Auswertung mit einem geeigneten Rechner, unmittelbar während
der Messung, bringt erhebliche Vorteile.

Um exakte Werte aus den Umlaufdiagrammen zu gewinnen, muß sehr
sorgfältig auf den Dämpfungsgrad einzelner Elemente der Versuchsanord-

nung geachtet werden, da bereits geringe Phasenverschiebungen zu erheblichen Fehlern der Meßergebnisse führen können. Um besonders bei hohen Atemfrequenzen Fehler durch ungenügende Einstellzeiten des x-y-Schreibers zu vermeiden, reduzieren wir bei der Registrierung der Umlaufdiagramme die Geschwindigkeit des Magnetbandes um den Faktor 0,25.

ERGEBNISSE

In Abb. 1 sind die gemessenen Werte der spezifischen effektiven Ventilationsleistung $\dot{W}_Z$/ml der Lungen eines 3 Monate alt gewordenen Kindes, eines 36 Jahre alt gewordenen Mannes und eines 79 Jahre alt gewordenen Mannes mit senil-atrophischem Emphysem (Alterslunge) dargestellt. Die gestrichelten Säulen entsprechen den jeweiligen Werten bei Ruheatemfrequenz, die bei dem Kind mit 40/min, im übrigen mit 15/min angesetzt wurde.

Dieser Wert sinkt von etwa 160 g cm min^{-1} bei dem Kind auf 100 g cm min^{-1} im mittleren Erwachsenenalter ab und steigt im höheren Alter auf etwa 130 g cm min^{-1} wieder an. Nach dem Ergebnis weiterer, hier noch nicht verwerteter systematischer Messungen kann ein Optimum zwischen 20. und 35. Lebensjahr angenommen werden.

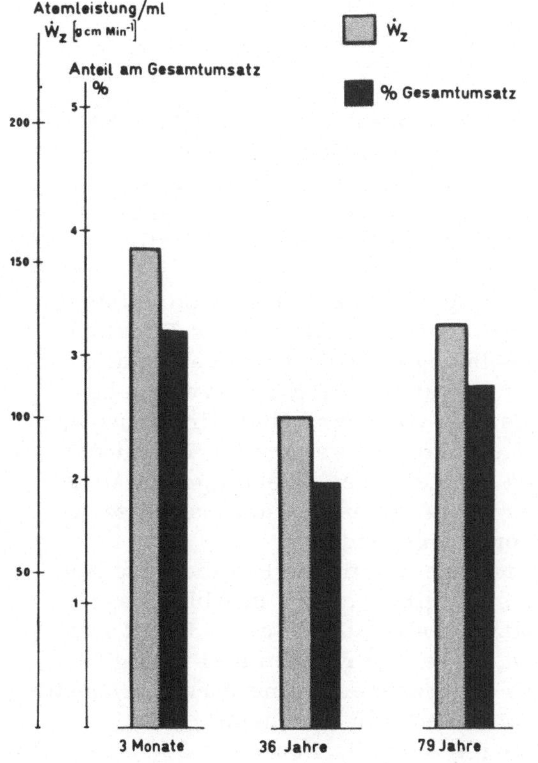

Abb. 1. Spezifische effektive Ventilationsleistung (Atemleistung/ml) sowie deren prozentualer Anteil am Gesamtumsatz in verschiedenen Lebensaltern. Vgl. Text

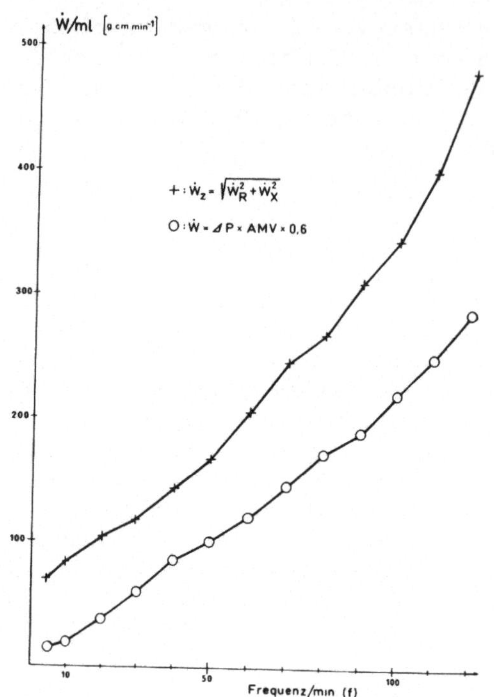

Abb. 2. Beziehung zwischen spezifischer Ventilationsleistung und Atemfrequenz. Errechnete Werte nach Cook (o) und nach Heusinger (+)

Die Ventilation erfordert einen bestimmten prozentualen Anteil der Energie des Grundumsatzes. Unter Berücksichtigung von Literaturangaben über unterschiedliche Wirkungsgrade der Atemmuskulatur in verschiedenen Lebensaltern[5, 6, 7, 12, 19] ergeben sich die in Abb. 1 als schwarze Säulen eingezeichneten Werte. Auch hier zeigt sich ein Optimum im mittleren Lebensalter.

Die im künstlichen Thorax gemessene spezifische Ventilationsleistung ist im Falle des 36 Jahre alt gewordenen Mannes in Abb. 2 als Funktion der Frequenz wiedergegeben. Die Berechnung erfolgte einerseits nach konventioneller Methode (o), zum anderen wurden die Effektivwerte berechnet (+). In beiden Fällen ist, abgesehen von sehr hohen Frequenzen, eine etwa proportionale Zunahme der Leistung mit steigender Frequenz deutlich. Die konventionell errechneten Werte liegen allerdings im Mittel um mehr als 50% unter den Effektivwerten. Auch in den anderen Altersstufen ergaben sich Differenzen gleicher Größenordnung.

Schlüsselt man diese Effektivwerte in ihre elastische Komponente $\dot{W}_X$ und ihre Reibungskomponente $\dot{W}_R$ auf, so ergibt sich die in Abb. 3 a-c wiedergegebene Beziehung zur Frequenz. In allen drei Fällen findet sich nur in einem verhältnismäßig niedrigen, etwa der ruhigen und mäßig beschleunigten Atmung entsprechenden Frequenzbereich eine direkt proportionale, etwa lineare Beziehung der Komponenten zur Frequenz.

Bei mittleren und hohen Atemfrequenzen wird die Zunahme der elastischen Leistungskomponente $\dot{W}_X$ geringer und geht schließlich in eine umgekehrt proportionale Beziehung zur Frequenz über. Bei der kindlichen Lunge und

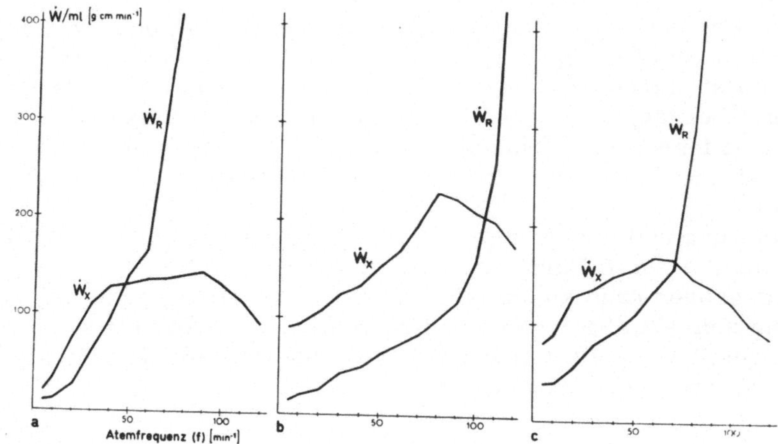

Abb. 3. Beziehung zwischen Atemfrequenz und den Leistungskomponenten in verschiedenen Lebensaltern; a: 3 Monate alt gewordenes Kind; b: 36 Jahre alt gewordener Mann; c: 79 Jahre alt gewordener Mann, Vgl. Text

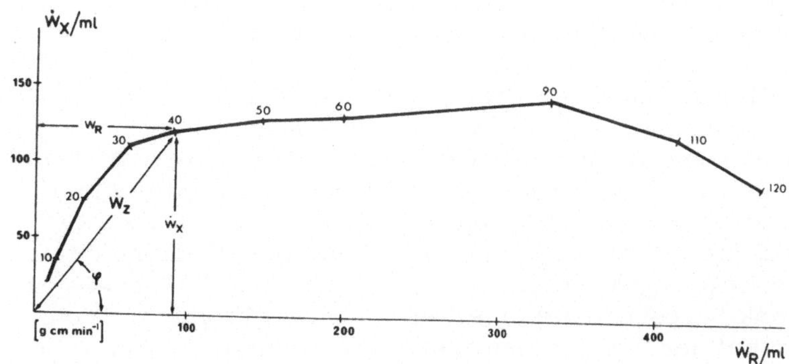

Abb. 4. Leistungsortskurve der spezifischen Leistungswerte im Falle des 3 Monate alt gewordenen Kindes. Laufparameter: Atemfrequenz.
Die Gesamtleistung $\dot{W}_Z$, ihre Komponenten $\dot{W}_X$ und $\dot{W}_R$ sowie die Phasenverschiebung φ sind bei gleicher Teilung der Ordinaten, hier für die Frequenz von 40/min eingezeichnet, direkt ablesbar

der Alterslunge ist dies schon bei vergleichsweise niedriger Frequenz der
Fall. Die Reibungskomponente $\dot{W}_R$ zeigt hingegen bei hohen Atemfrequenzen einen zunehmend steileren Anstieg; die kindliche Lunge und die Alterslunge zeigen diesen Übergang ebenfalls, aber schon bei vergleichsweise
niedriger Frequenz. Diese beiden Lungen lassen weiterhin bei sehr niedriger Frequenz (5-15/min) ebenfalls einen alinearen Verlauf der Reibungskomponente erkennen.

Die effektive Leistung und ihre Komponenten lassen sich beim Vorliegen
alinearer Gesetzmäßigkeiten in Form von Ortskurven darstellen.
Neben den Leistungsgrößen kann aus dieser Art der Darstellung auch die
Phasenverschiebung γ direkt abgelesen werden. In Abb. 4 ist die Orts-
kurve für den Fall des 3 Monate alt gewordenen Kindes wiedergegeben, als
Laufparameter wurde die Frequenz gewählt.

DISKUSSION

Altersabhängige Veränderungen der Lungenmechanik sind aus klinischen
Untersuchungen und aus histomechanischen Messungen an isolierten Lungen
bekannt[2,4,8,9,10]. Für die fötale Lunge und die Lunge des Neugeborenen
konnten wir am isolierten Organ die normale und gestörte Entwicklung der
Lungenmechanik untersuchen[18,24,25].

Die in der vorliegenden Untersuchung gezeigten Veränderungen der Ventilationsleistung mit dem Lebensalter stimmen im wesentlichen mit klinisch-
en Angaben überein. Im Vergleich zu den optimalen Werten des mittleren
Erwachsenenalters ist die Ventilationsleistung beim Kind durch höhere
Reibungswiderstände und höhere elastische Widerstände größer. Im Alter
ist der Wiederanstieg der Ventilationsleistung vorwiegend Ausdruck höherer
Reibungswiderstände.

Nach konventioneller Methode ermittelte klinische Werte der Ventilationsleistung unter Ruhebedingungen liegen etwa 50% über unseren an isolierten
Lungen ermittelten Werten. Diese Differenz dürfte sich im wesentlichen
daraus ergeben, daß in die Messungen im künstlichen Thorax die Widerstände der oberen Luftwege nicht eingehen.

Die Tatsache, daß die mittels der physikalisch exakten Methode errechneten effektiven Leistungswerte im Mittel um mehr als 50% über den
nach der Formel Cook berechneten Werte liegen, beruht in erster Linie
darauf, daß der Verlauf der Atemgrößen trotz sinusförmiger Vorgabe des
Druckverlaufes durch die Atempumpe Abweichungen von der Sinusform
zeigte. Auch die nachgewiesenen alinearen Beziehungen der Leistungskomponenten gehen als Fehler in die formelmäßige Rechnung ein.

Das unerwartete alineare Verhalten der elastischen Komponente erklärt sich wohl überwiegend aus dem mathematisch-theoretischen Ansatz.
In diesem Ansatz ist nämlich auch die i. a. vernachlässigte Masseträgheit
enthalten. Sie hat ein umgekehrtes Vorzeichen und kann eine Abnahme der
elastischen Komponente mit steigender Frequenz bewirken, im Bereich
der Resonanzfrequenz der Lunge würde diese Komponente gleich Null.
Auch inhomogene Ventilation ist als Ursache der Alinearität dieser Komponente zu berücksichtigen.

Bei der kindlichen Lunge und der Alterslunge fand sich im niedrigen Frequenzbereich ein alinearer Verlauf der Reibungskomponente. Die Analyse anderer Meßgrößen sowie theoretische Überlegungen, die sich im Modellversuch beweisen ließen, ergaben, daß dies auf eine Veränderung der normalerweise etwa kreisförmigen Geometrie der Atemwege zurückzuführen ist [24]. Bei geringen Strömungen und Drucken kommt es zu einer elliptischen Verformung der in der kindlichen Lunge noch nicht, bzw. im Alter durch nachlassende Verspannung im Lungengerüst nicht mehr regelrecht stabilisierten Atemwege. Da der Strömungswiderstand bei gleicher durchströmter Fläche im elliptischen Atemweg höher ist als im kreisförmigen, ergibt sich die nachgewiesene Alinearität. Der im oberen Meßbereich beobachtete, bei jeweils unterschiedlicher Frequenz einsetzende alineare Verlauf der Reibungskomponente ist Folge turbulenter Strömungsform. Der Übergang in diese Strömungsform erfolgt in der kindlichen Lunge und der Alterslunge bei deutlich geringerer Frequenz als im mittleren Erwachsenenalter. Mangelhaft stabilisierte Atemwege in Verbindung mit kleinen Bronchialquerschnitten beim Kind und Unregelmäßigkeiten der Bronchialwege im Alter sind hier als wesentliche Ursache anzusehen.

Wie bereits die Messung anderer atemmechanischer Parameter zeigte [24,25], ergibt auch die Messung der effektiven Leistung und ihrer beiden Komponenten, daß für die Lungenmechanik keineswegs lineare Gesetzmäßigkeiten angenommen werden können. Die Berechnung der Ventilationsleistung mittels vereinfachter Formeln muß somit zwangsläufig zu falschen Ergebnissen führen. In vivo ist dieser Fehler sicher größer als bei den Messungen im künstlichen Thorax, weil u. a. die Abweichungen von der Sinusform erheblicher sind und der Atemzeitquotient nicht gleich eins ist.

Die Anwendung der etwas differenzierteren, physikalisch exakten Berechnungsmethode nach Heusinger erscheint somit besonders unter pathologischen Atembedingungen gerechtfertigt.

LITERATUR

1. Albright, C. D. , Bondurant, S. : Respiratory frequency and pulmonary mechanics. J. clin. Invest. 44, 1362-1370· (1965)
2. Avery, M. E. : The lung and its disorders in the newborn infant. Philadelphia, London, Toronto: W. B. Saunders Company 1968
3. Börngen, U. : Normalwerte der ventilatorischen Atemarbeit. Respiration 33, 22-35 (1976)
4. Briscoe, W. A. , Dubois, A. B. : Relationship between airway resistance, airway conductance, and lung volume in subjects of different age and body size. J. clin. Invest. 37, 1279 (1958)
5. Campbell, E. J. M. , Westlake, E. K. , Cherniak, R. M. : Simple methods of estimating oxygen consumption and efficiency of the muscles of breathing. J. appl. Physiol. 11, 303 (1957)
6. Campbell, E. J. M. : The respiratory muscles and the mechanics of breathing. London: Lloyd-Luke Ltd. 1958

7. Comroe, J., Forster, R., Dubois, A., Briscoe, W., Carlsen, E.:
    Die Lunge., Klinische Physiologie und Lungenfunktionsprüfungen.
    Stuttgart: F.K. Schattauer-Verlag 1964

8. Cook, C.D., Sutherland, J.M., Segal, S., Cherry, R.B., Mead, J.,
    McIlroy, M.B., Smith, C.A.: Mechanics of respiration in newborn
    infants. J. clin. Invest. 36, 440-448 (1957)

9. Cook, C.D., Helliesen, P.J., Agathon, S.: Relation between
    mechanics of respiration, lung size and body size from birth to young
    adulthood. J. appl. Physiol. 13, 349 (1958)

10. Frank, N.R., Mead, J., Ferris, B.G.: The mechanical behavior
    of the lungs in healthy elderly persons. J. clin. Invest. 36, 1680-1687
    (1957)

11. Galgóczy, G., Hantos, Z., Mándi, A.: Relationship between the flow-
    resistive work of breathing and the airway resistance. Pneumonologie
    150, 311-318 (1974)

12. McGregor, M., Becklake, M.R.: The relationship of oxygen cost of
    breathing to respiratory mechanical work and respiratory force.
    J. clin. Invest. 40, 971 (1961)

13. Heusinger, P.P.: Zur Theorie der Atemmechanik. Respiration 28,
    306 (1971)

14. Heusinger, P.P.: Die Atemmechanik in komplexer Darstellung.
    Lineare Theorie, Lungenfunktionsmodelle, nichtlineare Theorie.
    Respiration 30, 12 (1973)

15. Hartung, W.: Untersuchungsmethoden an Lungen und Thorax zur
    postmortalen Analyse der Atmungsfunktion. Ergeb. allg. Path. path.
    Anat. 43, 121 (1963)

16. Hartung, W., Büttinghaus, W.: Messungen der dynamischen Volumen-
    dehnbarkeit isolierter menschlicher Lungen. Med. Thorac. 24, 348
    (1967)

17. Hartung, W.: Post-mortem correlates of pulmonary function. In:
    The lung. Int. Acad. Path. Monogr. No 8. Baltimore: Williams &
    Wilkins 1968

18. Hartung, W., Carmanns, B., Wierich, W.: Ventilationsmechanik
    der Lungen von Neugeborenen mit und ohne hyaline Membranen.
    Pneumologie 144, 191 (1971)

19. Millahn, H.P., Eckermann, P.: Der Energieverbrauch der Atmung
    Klin. Wschr. 42, 722-725 (1964)

20. Otis, A.B., McKerrow, C.B., Bartlett, R,A., McIlroy, M.B.,
    Mead, J., Selverstone, N.J., Radford, E.P.: Mechanical factors of
    pulmonary ventilation. J. appl. Physiol. 8, 427-443 (1956)

21. Otis, A.B.: The work of breathing. In: Handbook of Physiology.
    Sec. III. Vol. I, 463. Baltimore: Williams & Wilkins Co. 1964

22. Smidt, U., Muysers, K.: Kritische Betrachtungen zu den methodischen
    Grundlagen der Ganzkörperplethysmographie. Respiration 25, 116
    (1968)

23. Ulmer, W.T., Reichel, G., Nolte, D.: Die Lungenfunktion.
    Stuttgart: Georg Thieme Verlag 1970

24. Wierich, W. : Histomechanische Untersuchungen zum Atemnotsyndrom des Neugeborenen unter Berücksichtigung der Gesetze der Schwingungslehre. Inaugural-Dissertation, Münster 1974
25. Wierich, W. : Untersuchungen zur Atemmechanik von Früh.- und Neugeborenen. I. Statische Messungen an isolierten Lungen. II. Dynamische Messungen an isolierten Lungen. Respiration (im Druck)

Dr. med. Walter Wierich
Institut für Pathologie
der Ruhr-Universität
Postfach 102148
D-4630 Bochum 1

Pneumonologie Suppl. 1976, 193-200

Kontinuierliche Messung des gemischt-venösen Sauerstoffpartialdrucks mittels einer Katheterlektrode

G. Goeckenjan, P. Schneider und J. Heidenreich

I. Medizinische Klinik A und Frauenklinik der Medizinischen Einrichtungen der Universität Düsseldorf

---

Abstract. A method for continuous long term measurement of mixed-venous oxygen pressure by means of a catheter electrode is described. Preliminary results in 6 patients show a good correlation to discontinuous measurements with a Radiometer electrode (r = 0,95, S. E. E. = ± 1,9 mm Hg). Provided the electrode is calibrated every 3 hours the average deviation of the electrode reading compared with the discontinuous measurement is less than 10%. Changes in the mixture of venous blood coming from the superior and inferior Vena cava as well as variations in the position of the electrode may simulate real alterations of mixed-venous oxygen pressure. The influence of a changing arterial oxygen pressure and of short term hemodynamic effects on mixed-venous oxygen pressure is demonstrated in some examples. Essentially the importance of this method is to show short term changes of mixed-venous oxygen pressure.

Key words: Mixed-venous oxygen pressure - Continuous PO_2-measurement - O_2-catheterelectrode - Intensive care monitoring.

Zusammenfassung. Es wird eine Methode zur kontinuierlichen Langzeitmessung des gemischt-venösen Sauerstoffpartialdrucks mittels einer Katheterelektrode beschrieben. Erste Erfahrungen mit dieser Messung an insgesamt 6 Patienten zeigen eine gute Korrelation mit diskontinuierlich gewonnenen Vergleichswerten (r = 0,95, Standardschätzfehler ± 1,9 mm Hg). Bei etwa 3-stündlicher Nacheichung der Elektroden ist mit einer mittleren Abweichung des Elektrodenmeßwertes vom diskontinuierlichen Vergleichswert um weniger als 10% zu rechnen. Die kontinuierliche Messung des rechtsatrialen Sauerstoffpartialdrucks ist problematisch, da wechselnde Mischungsverhältnisse des venösen Blutes aus oberer und unterer Hohlvene sowie geringe Lageänderungen der Meßsonde tatsächliche Änderungen des gemischt-venösen Sauerstoffpartialdrucks vortäuschen können. Der Einfluß von Änderungen des arteriellen Sauerstoffpartialdrucks und von kurzfristigen Änderungen der Hämodynamik auf den gemischt-venösen Sauerstoffpartialdruck wird an Beispielen demonstriert. Die Bedeutung dieser Methode liegt insbesondere in der Darstellung kurzzeitiger Änderungen des gemischt-venösen Sauerstoffpartialdrucks.

Schlüsselwörter: Gemischt-venöser Sauerstoffpartialdruck - kontinuierliche PO_2-Messung - O_2-Katheterelektrode - Intensivüberwachung.

Der gemischt-venöse Sauerstoffpartialdruck kann als Nettoeffekt der Inter-
aktion des respiratorischen und cardialen Systems im Hinblick auf die Ge-
websoxygenation betrachtet werden [6]. In den letzten Jahren entwickelte
polarographische Sauerstoffelektroden [1, 5] ermöglichen die kontinuierliche Langzeitmessung dieses Parameters. Ziel dieser Arbeit ist die Beschreibung des von uns angewendeten Verfahrens der kontinuierlichen Messung des gemischt-venösen PO_2 und die Mitteilung erster Erfahrungen mit
dieser Methode.

METHODIK

Bei 3 auf der Intensivstation behandelten Patienten wurde über einen zu
Infusionszwecken applizierten Subklaviakatheter bzw. über einen Armve-
nenkatheter eine von der Firma Roche, Basel, entwickelte Sauerstoffelek-
trode unter Röntgen-Bildverstärker-Kontrolle in den rechten Vorhof eingeführt. Es handelt sich um eine modifizierte Clark-Elektrode, die 0, 9
mm stark ist und in einem Polyäthylenschlauch eine Kathode aus Silber
und eine Anode aus Silber-Silberchlorid mit einer gepufferten Elektrolyt-
lösung enthält [1, 5]. Die 90%-Ansprechzeit beträgt nach unseren Messungen durchschnittlich 81 Sekunden [2]. Die von uns verwandte Elektrode ist
ein nicht im Handel erhältlicher Prototyp.

Bei 3 weiteren Patienten, bei denen eine Überwachung des pulmonal-ar-
teriellen Druckes durchzuführen war, wurde eine längere Elektrode im Lu-
men eines 2 mm starken Cardioflexkatheters[1] über eine Armvene bzw.
eine Vena subclavia in die Pulmonalarterie eingeschwemmt. Dabei über-
ragt der flexible Sauerstoffkatheter den äußeren Katheter um etwa 4-5 cm.
Die Lokalisation der Katheterlage erfolgt mittels Druckregistrierung. Eine röntgenologische Kontrolle war in diesen Fällen nicht erforderlich. Die
Einführung des kombinierten Katheters in die Pulmonalarterie war - offenbar infolge der guten Flexibilität des führenden Sauerstoffkatheters - rasch
möglich. Bedrohliche Herzrhythmusstörungen oder sonstige Komplikatio-
nen wurden durch diese Untersuchung nicht hervorgerufen.

Die Eichung erfolgte in vivo jeweils mit dem elektrischen Nullpunkt und
einem diskontinuierlich mit einer Clark-Elektrode der Firma Radiometer
gewonnenen Meßwert. Zu diesem Zweck wurden über den äußeren Katheter Blutproben aus dem Bereich der Elektrodenmessung entnommen.

Neben der kontinuierlichen Messung des gemischt-venösen Sauerstoffpartialdrucks wurde gleichzeitig eine kontinuierliche Messung des arteri-

---

[1] Hersteller: Vygon, Aachen.

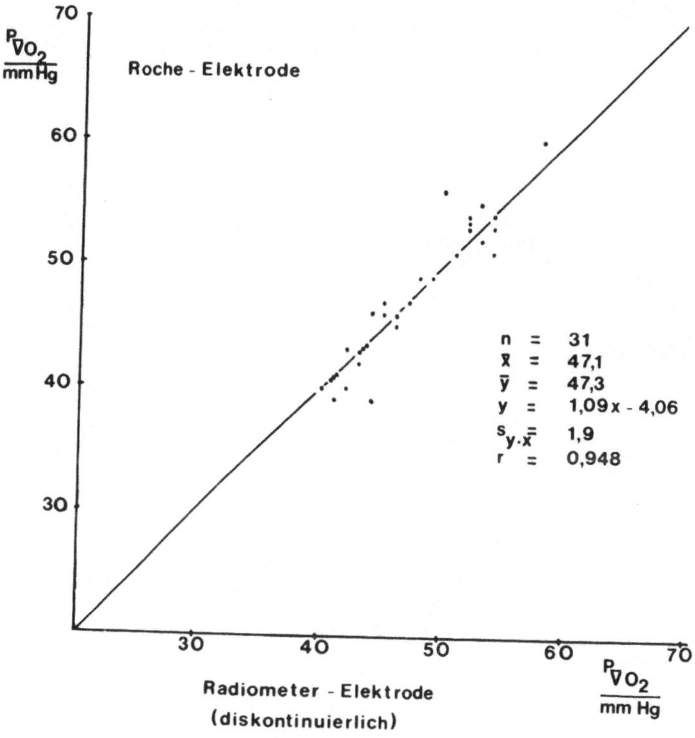

Abb. 1. Korrelation zwischen den Meßwerten der Roche-Katheterelektro-
de und diskontinuierlichen PO_2-Messungen mittels einer Radiometer-Elek-
trode

ellen Sauerstoffpartialdrucks mit einer IBC-Elektrode[2] durchgeführt. Die
Dauer der rechtsatrialen Messungen betrug 2-45 Stunden, die Dauer der
pulmonalarteriellen Messungen 13-68 Stunden.

ERGEBNISSE UND DISKUSSION

Abb. 1 zeigt die Korrelation zwischen den mit der Roche-Katheterelektro-
de bestimmten gemischt-venösen Meßwerten und diskontinuierlichen PO_2-
Messungen mittels einer Radiometerelektrode. Berücksichtigt wurden nur
Meßwerte innerhalb von 3 Stunden nach vorangegangener Eichung. Es findet sich eine gute Korrelation zwischen den Elektrodenmeßwerten und den
Werten der Vergleichsmessung mit einem Standardschätzfehler von etwa
4%. Bei Langzeitmessungen über mehr als 4 Stunden ließ sich eine globale
in-vivo-Drift der Elektrodenmeßwerte von durchschnittlich ± 2, 9%/Stunde

---

[2]Hersteller: International Biophysics Corp. , Irvine (Calif.) USA. Vertrieb
 in der Bundesrepublik Deutschland: Sandoz AG. , Medizintechnik, Nürnberg

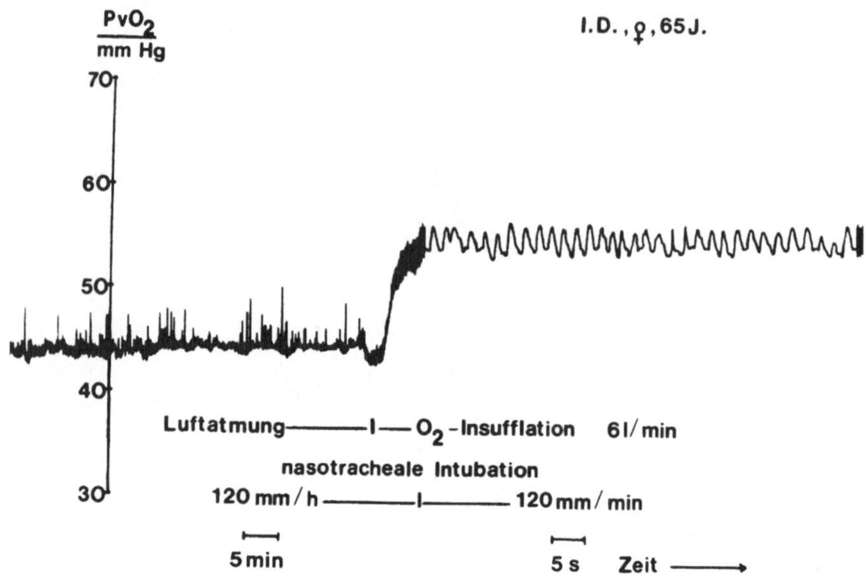

Abb. 2. Kontinuierliche PO_2-Messung im rechten Vorhof beim Übergang von Luftatmung auf Sauerstoffinsufflation. S. Text

(minimal 1, 34%/Stunde, maximal 5, 0%/Stunde), entsprechend $\pm$ 1, 3 mm Hg/Stunde errechnen. Aus diesen Werten folgt, daß bei kontinuierlichen Messungen des venösen Sauerstoffpartialdrucks mit der genannten Elektrode kurzfristige, d. h. etwa 3-stündliche Nacheichungen erforderlich sind, wenn die mittlere Abweichung des Meßwertes unter 10% gehalten werden soll.

Abb. 2 zeigt den kontinuierlich rechtsatrial gemessenen Sauerstoffpartialdruck bei Luftatmung und nach Sauerstoffinsufflation bei einer 65-jährigen soporösen Patientin, die an einer tuberkulösen Meningo-Enzephalitis litt. Die O_2-Elektrode wurde in den unteren Teil des rechten Vorhofs gelegt. Während unter Luftatmung nur geringe Schwankungen des O_2-Partialdrucks beobachtet werden, die auf Änderungen der Mischungsverhältnisse im rechten Vorhof, möglicherweise auch auf Bewegungsartefakte zurückzuführen sind, fallen nach Sauerstoffeinmischung, ohne daß sonstige Bedingungen geändert wurden, stärkere atemsynchrone Schwankungen des Sauerstoffpartialdrucks auf, die am ehesten auf eine Zunahme der O_2-Partialdruck-Differenz zwischen oberer und unterer Hohlvene mit atemsynchron schwankender Durchmischung des zentralvenösen Blutes im rechten Vorhof zurückzuführen sind. Bei Berücksichtigung der relativ langen Ansprechzeit der PO_2-Elektrode ist anzunehmen, daß die tatsächlichen PO_2-Schwankungen wesentlich stärker waren, als durch die Elektrodenmessung wiedergegeben wurde. Eine Verursachung dieser Veränderungen durch Bewegungsartefakte im rechten Vorhof ist nicht ausgeschlossen, jedoch weniger wahrscheinlich. Weitere Messungen haben beim Rückzug der O_2-Elektrode aus dem unteren Bereich des rechten Vorhofs in den oberen

Anteil unter Luftatmung Anstiege des Sauerstoffpartialdrucks um bis zu 7 mm Hg ergeben. Diese Änderungen sind durch die bekannten Differenzen zwischen oberer und unterer Hohlvene bedingt, die im Schock verstärkt auftreten [3]. Obwohl bei diskontinuierlicher Messung wiederholt eine gute Übereinstimmung der rechtsatrialen und der pulmonalarteriellen Werte des Sauerstoffpartialdrucks bzw. der Sauerstoffsättigung gezeigt wurde [3, 7, 8], müssen wir aus unseren Beobachtungen schließen, daß die kontinuierliche Messung des Sauerstoffpartialdrucks im rechten Vorhof problematisch ist, da geringe Lageänderungen der Meßsonde und wechselnde Durchmischverhältnisse Veränderungen hervorrufen können, die oft von einer echten Änderung des gemischt-venösen Sauerstoffpartialdrucks schwer zu unterscheiden sind.

Abb. 3 zeigt den kontinuierlich gemessenen arteriellen und pulmonalarteriellen Sauerstoffpartialdruck bei einer 18-jährigen Patientin mit ei-

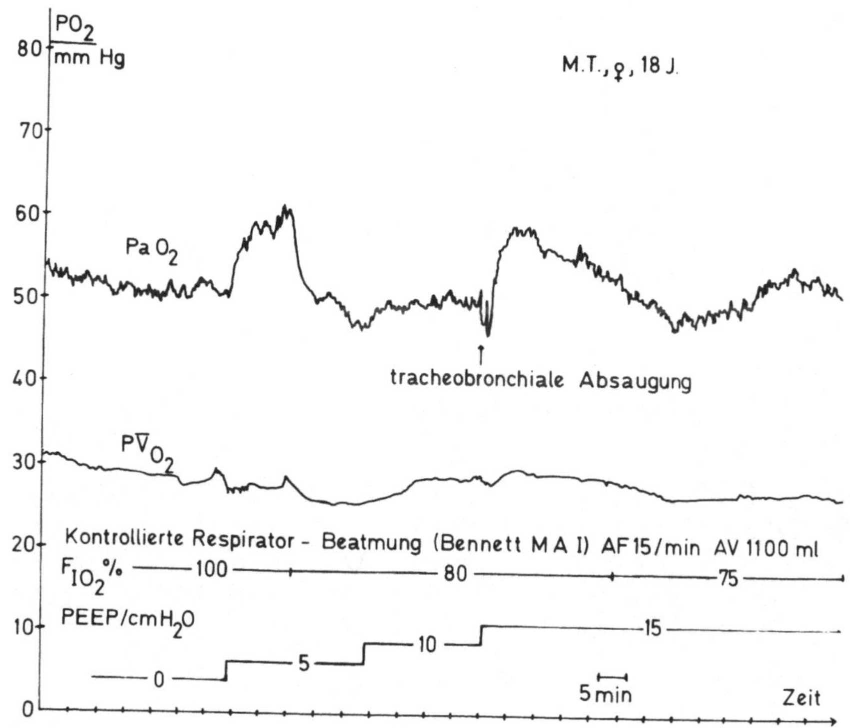

Abb. 3. Kontinuierliche Messung des arteriellen Sauerstoffpartialdrucks (PaO$_2$) und des gemischt-venösen Sauerstoffpartialdrucks P$_{\bar{V}}$O$_2$) unter Respiratorbeatmung bei wechselnden Beatmungsbedingungen (s. Text)

ner Meningo-Enzephalitis, einer schweren Bronchopneumonie und einer Kreislaufinsuffizienz. Unter einer kontrollierten Respiratorbeatmung mit reinem Sauerstoff liegen die arteriellen Sauerstoffpartialdrucke zunächst gering über 50 mm Hg, die gemischt-venösen knapp unter 30 mm Hg. Durch eine PEEP-Beatmung mit endexspiratorischen Drucken bis 15 cm H_2O gelingt es, den arteriellen Sauerstoffpartialdruck kurzfristig anzuheben und die erforderliche inspiratorische O_2-Konzentration auf 75% zu reduzieren. Die Anstiege des arteriellen Sauerstoffpartialdrucks gehen mit einer nur geringen Beeinflussung des gemischt-venösen O_2-Partialdrucks einher. Kurzdauernde Senkungen des arteriellen Sauerstoffpartialdrucks wie z. B. infolge der Unterbrechung der Respiratorbeatmung bei tracheobronchialer Absaugung, führen nur zu geringen Senkungen des gemischt-venösen Sauerstoffpartialdrucks.

Demgegenüber zeigen rasche Veränderungen der Hämodynamik oft ausgeprägtere Reaktionen des gemischt-venösen PO_2, wobei unter der Voraus-

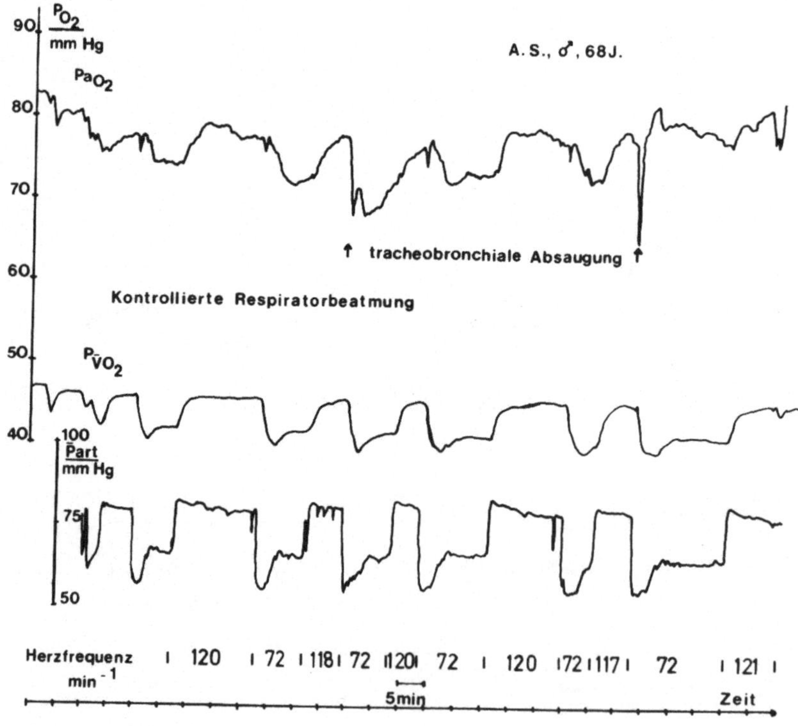

Abb. 4. Kontinuierliche Messung des arteriellen Sauerstoffpartialdrucks (PaO_2), des gemischt-venösen Sauerstoffpartialdrucks ($P_{\bar{v}}O_2$) und des arteriellen Mitteldrucks ($\bar{P}art$) unter Respiratorbeatmung bei Änderungen der Hämodynamik. S. Text

setzung einer konstanten Sauerstoffaufnahme und eines konstanten arteriellen Sauerstoffgehalts eine enge Korrelation zwischen dem gemischt-venösen Sauerstoffpartialdruck und dem Herzzeitvolumen besteht.

Abb. 4 zeigt das Verhalten des gemischt-venösen Sauerstoffpartialdrucks bei einem 68-jährigen Patienten, der wegen einer hypoxischen Hirnschädigung nach einem Kreislaufstillstand beatmet werden mußte und infolge eines intermittierenden AV-Blocks rasch aufeinander folgende Wechsel der Herzfrequenz zwischen einem Schrittmacherrhythmus mit einer Frequenz von 70/min und einem Sinusrhythmus mit einer Frequenz um 120/min bot. Entsprechend dem Anstieg der Herzfrequenz, bzw. dem damit verbundenen Anstieg des Herzzeitvolumens und des kontinuierlich registrierten arteriellen Mitteldrucks kommt es zu deutlichen synchronen Anstiegen des gemischt-venösen Sauerstoffpartialdrucks. Außerdem fällt auf, daß auch der arterielle Sauerstoffpartialdruck dem gemischt-venösen gleichgerichtete Schwankungen zeigt, die allerdings weniger deutlich ausgeprägt sind.

Die Bedeutung der kontinuierlichen Messung des gemischt-venösen Sauerstoffpartialdrucks liegt insbesondere in der Darstellung und Klärung kurzzeitiger Schwankungen dieser Meßgröße, wie sie durch kurzfristige Änderungen der Hämodynamik und der Ventilation hervorgerufen werden können. Ob dieser Methode eine Bedeutung für die Routineüberwachung von Intensivpatienten zukommt, müssen weitere Untersuchungen zeigen. Denkbar wäre der Einsatz in der Überwachung von Patienten mit Herzinfarkt, insbesondere im cardiogenen Schock, wobei besonders die Wirkung von Behandlungsmaßnahmen durch die kontinuierliche Verlaufsbeobachtung besser beurteilt werden könnte. Außerdem kann diese Methode Hinweise auf den Sauerstofftransport bei Wechsel verschiedener Beatmungsformen [4, 9] geben. Durch weitere Untersuchungen wäre zu klären, ob die kontinuierliche Messung des gemischt-venösen Sauerstoffpartialdrucks Vorteile gegenüber der kontinuierlichen Messung der gemischt-venösen Sauerstoffsättigung mittels Fiberoptik-Katheters bietet.

LITERATUR

1. Eberhardt, P., Fehlmann, W., Schiebli, R., Büsser, E.: Kontinuierliche PO_2-Messung mittels intravasaler Sonden. Verh. Dtsch. Ges. Biomed. Techn. 15.-17.5.1974, Hannover
2. Goeckenjan, G., Schneider, P., Heidenreich, J.: Kontinuierliche PO_2-Überwachung mittels intravasaler Sauerstoffelektroden. Dtsch. med. Wschr. 101 (1976)
3. Lee, J., Wright, F., Barber, R., Stanley, L.: Central venous oxygen saturation in shock: a study in man. Anesthesiol. 36, 472-478 (1972)
4. Lutch, J.S., Murray, J.F.: Continuous positive pressure ventilation: Effects on systemic oxygen transport and tissue oxygenation. Ann. Intern. Med. 76, 193-202 (1972)
5. Mindt, W.: Sauerstoffsensor für in vivo-Messung. Dtsch. Ges. Biomed. Techn. 24.-25.5.1973, Erlangen

6. Mithoefer, J. C. , Holford, F. D. , Keighley, J. F. H. : The effect of oxygen administration on mixed venous oxygenation in chronic obstructive pulmonary disease. Chest 66, 122-132 (1974)
7. Scheinman, M. M. , Brown, M. A. , Rapaport, E. : Critical assessment of use of central venous oxygen saturation as a mirror of mixed venous oxygen in severely ill cardiac patients. Circulation 40, 165-172 (1969)
8. Schröder, H. H. , Schmidt, K. , Beckmann, O. W. : Die Beurteilung des gemischt-venösen Sauerstoffpartialdrucks zur Beurteilung der Herzleistung insbesondere beim kardiogenen Schock. Intensivmed. 12, 133-146 (1975)
9. Schulz, V. , Schnabel, K. H. , Erdmann, W. : Beatmung mit positivem end-exspiratorischem Druck - funktionsdiagnostische Untersuchungen und klinische Erfahrungen. Intensivmed. 12, 153-164 (1975)

Dr. G. Goeckenjan
I. Medizinische Klinik A
der Universität
Moorenstrasse 5
D-4000 Düsseldorf

Pneumonologie Suppl. 1976, 201-203

A Modified Rebreathing Technique for Estimating Pulmonary O_2 Diffusing Capacity in Man During Exercise

M. Meyer and H. Magnussen

Max-Planck-Institut für experimentelle Medizin, Abteilung Physiologie, Göttingen

---

A b s t r a c t . The rebreathing method that has previously been used to determine lung DO_2 has been modified for application during exercise. This modification allows the subject to breathe normoxic mixture till the onset of rebreathing. Results in healthy subjects show a threefold increase in DO_2 when compared with resting values which conforms with earlier findings.

K e y   w o r d s : Exercise - Pulmonary blood flow - Pulmonary DO_2 - Rebreathing.

From the kinetics of alveolar-capillary equilibration of respiratory and inert gases during rebreathing several basic parameters of pulmonary gas exchange may be determined including cardiac output, $\dot{Q}$, and pulmonary O_2-diffusing capacity, DO_2.

For quantitative analysis a model is used that consists of two homogeneous compartments, lung and rebreathing container. During rebreathing the partial pressures of gases in the closed system approach the partial pressure of mixed venous blood according to a biexponential function, the kinetics being determined by the following parameters: volume of rebreathing bag, lung volume, effective ventilation between bag and lung, effective solubility of a gas species in blood (comprising physical solubility and chemical binding in the case of O_2 and CO_2), pulmonary capillary blood flow, and pulmonary diffusing capacity.

The following differences in the equilibration between various gases are expected due to differences in effective solubility in lung tissue and blood:

(a) P o o r l y   s o l u b l e   i n e r t   g a s e s (e. g., H_2, He, Ar) are not eliminated from the gas phase and therefore become evenly distributed between bag and lung. Thus effective ventilation in the lung-rebreathing container system can be determined from the equilibration kinetics of these gases.

(b) U p t a k e o f h i g h l y   s o l u b l e   i n e r t   g a s e s (e. g., C_2H_2, N_2O) is not limited by membrane diffusion but virtually entirely by pulmonary capillary blood flow. Therefore, the pulmonary blood flow can be calculated from their rate of disappearance from the lung-rebreathing container system, if effective ventilation is determined by poorly soluble gases [see (a)].

(c) The equilibration of oxygen is limited by diffusion, perfusion, and ventilation. If effective ventilation and pulmonary capillary blood flow are determined by rebreathing of He (a) and C_2H_2 (b), respectively, the pulmonary diffusing capacity for oxygen, D_{O_2}, can be estimated from the rate constant of O_2 equilibration between rebreathing gas and mixed venous blood.

The model and the mathematical treatment for the evaluation of D_{O_2} by rebreathing has been basically developed and validated experimentally in isolated dog lungs and in intact animals by Adaro et al. [1, 2] and by Scheid et al. [4].

The feasibility of this technique for estimation of D_{O_2} in resting man has been demonstrated by Cerretelli et al. [3]. The applicability for determination of pulmonary blood flow by using highly soluble inert gases has been verified by Teichmann et al. [5].

However, according to Cerretelli et al. [3] for a bloodless measurement of D_{O_2} in man at rest two separate rebreathing procedures both performed under moderate hypoxic conditions were necessary, one for determination of mixed venous oxygen partial pressure, $P_{\bar{v}O_2}$, a second for evaluation of all other parameters required for calculation of D_{O_2}.

In the present study a modification of the rebreathing method was developed that allows simultaneous determination of all parameters necessary for calculation of D_{O_2} within one single rebreathing maneuver during normoxic exercise. For this purpose the following modifications of the original method [3] have been introduced:

(a) In exercising subjects breathing room air the O_2-dissociation curve between the arterial P_{O_2} and mixed venous P_{O_2} is curved. However, according to the requirements of the method the O_2-dissociation curve should be straight between end capillary P_{O_2} during rebreathing and the mixed venous P_{O_2}. At rest lowering arterial and mixed venous P_{O_2} to the appropriate levels is achieved by having the subject breathe a hypoxic gas mixture (10-12% O_2 in N_2) before rebreathing. Since during exercise $P_{\bar{v}O_2}$ is low it suffices to lower alveolar P_{O_2} during rebreathing only for operating on the linear part of the O_2-dissociation curve. This removes the constraint from the subject of breathing a hypoxic mixture during exercise. In practice starting from open-circuit normoxic breathing during exercise a single breath of an oxygen-free mixture is administered to the subject prior to the onset of rebreathing. By this procedure appropriate initial conditions, e. g., rapid lowering of alveolar P_{O_2} so that arterial P_{O_2} fell on the linear part of the O_2-dissociation curve were achieved without producing discomfort to the subject from prolonged hypoxic breathing.

(b) Mixed venous oxygen partial pressure, $P_{\bar{v}O_2}$, could be calculated from the rate constant of the exponential approach of alveolar P_{O_2} to mixed venous P_{O_2}. Based on the property of exponential curves according to which their asymptote may be defined by three points of the curve, $P_{\bar{v}O_2}$ may be obtained from the rebreathing tracing since $P_{\bar{v}O_2}$ is the asymptotic value of the O_2 equilibration curve.

In two healthy male subjects average D_{O_2} was found to increase from resting values of 35 ml$\cdot$ min$^{-1}\cdot$ torr^{-1} up to 110 ml$\cdot$ min$^{-1}\cdot$ torr^{-1} during exercise on a bicycle ergometer with eightfold increase of oxygen uptake which is consistent with reported data obtained with different methods.

Essentially the advantages of the present method may be summarized as follows:

- the method is noninvasive
- exercise is performed during normoxic breathing
- all parameters are obtained simultaneously from one single rebreathing maneuver.

REFERENCES

1. Adaro, F., Scheid, P., Teichmann, J., Piiper, J.: A rebreathing method for estimating pulmonary D_{O_2}: theory and measurements in dog lungs. Resp. Physiol. 18, 43-63 (1973)
2. Adaro, F., Teichmann, J., Lüdtke-Handjery, A., Scheid, P., Piiper, J.: Comparison of rebreathing and steady state pulmonary D_{O_2} in dogs ventilated by body respirator. Respiration 31, 71-84 (1974)
3. Cerretelli, P., Veicsteinas, A., Teichmann, J., Magnussen, H., Piiper, J.: Estimation by a rebreathing method of pulmonary O_2 diffusing capacity in man. J. Appl. Physiol. 37, 526-532 (1974)
4. Scheid, P., Adaro, F., Teichmann, J., Piiper, J.: Rebreathing and steady state pulmonary D_{O_2} in the dog and inhomogeneous lung models. Resp. Physiol. 18, 256-272 (1973)
5. Teichmann, J., Adaro, F., Veicsteinas, A., Cerretelli, P., Piiper, J.: Determination of pulmonary blood flow by rebreathing of soluble inert gases. Respiration 31, 296-309 (1974)

Dr. M. Meyer
Max-Planck-Institut für
Experimentelle Medizin
Abteilung Physiologie
3400 Göttingen

Pneumonologie Suppl. 1976, 205-212

Adaption der Lungenperfusion an die Okklusion eines Hauptastes der Arteria pulmonalis

R. Goerg und S. Daum

I. Medizinische Klinik und Poliklinik der Technischen Universität München

Adaptation of lung perfusion during unilateral pulmonary artery occlusion

Abstract.   25 patients aged 48 - 80 years (18 of them with a bronchogenic carcinoma and 7 with chronic bronchitis) were investigated by unilateral pulmonary artery occlusion. Increase of mean pulmonary artery pressure by exercise or unilateral occlusion could not be correlated satisfactorily with pressure at rest, and was nearly the same irrespective if occlusion was done at rest or during exercise. Contrary to some other investigations, estimation of pulmonary vascular resistance suggested a decrease by both exercise and unilateral occlusion. We assume that the heterogeneity of our patients with very diverging working capacity did conceal otherwise reported correlations between increase in pulmonary artery pressure during exercise and pressure at rest. Although pulmonary hemodynamics after unilateral occlusion are not identical to those after pneumonectomy, we feel that this investigation does yield valuable information about the risk of pulmonary hypertension after lung resection.

Key words: Lung perfusion - Unilateral occlusion - Lung resection

Zusammenfassung. Bei 25 Patienten im Alter von 48 - 80 Jahren, 18 davon mit Lungentumoren und 7 mit chronischer Bronchitis, wurde die Arteria pulmonalis mit einem Ballonkatheter einseitig okkludiert. Gemessen wurden der Pulmonalis- und der Lungenkapillardruck in Ruhe und bei Belastung, jeweils ohne und mit einseitiger Okklusion. Der Anstieg des Pulmonalismitteldrucks unter Belastung oder unter Okklusion konnte nicht befriedigend zum Ausgangswert korreliert werden. Der Druck in der Arteria pulmonalis stieg während einseitiger Okklusion unter Belastungsbedingungen nicht mehr an als in Ruhe. Im Gegensatz zu anderen Untersuchungen deuten unsere Ergebnisse darauf hin, daß der Lungengefäßwiderstand unter Belastung oder einseitiger Okklusion abnimmt. Daß in der vorliegenden Untersuchung bereits bekannte Korrelationen nicht aufgefunden werden konnten, wird mit

der zu heterogenen Zusammensetzung des Patientenkreises und mit der zu
unterschiedlichen Ergometerbelastung erklärt. Wenn auch durch einseitige
Okklusion der hämodynamische Zustand nach Pneumonektomie nicht simu-
liert werden kann, so können doch Patienten erkannt werden, die durch
eine postoperativ zu erwartende Überlastung des kleinen Kreislaufs besonders gefährdet sind.

EINLEITUNG

Die Ergebnisse der operativen Behandlung des Bronchialkarzinoms sind
insgesamt recht enttäuschend. Die Überlebensquote selbst bei regelmäßig
kontrollierten Personen im Rahmen von prospektiven Studien[8]im Vergleich zu jener von Patienten, die erst bei auftretenden Beschwerden einen
Arzt aufsuchen, scheint kaum den personellen wie materiellen Aufwand
für eine ungezielte Röntgenreihenuntersuchung der Allgemeinbevölkerung zu
rechtfertigen. Bei den geringen Erfolgen dürfte auch die Indikation zu einer
eingreifenden chirurgischen Intervention zurückhaltend zu stellen sein, besonders in jenen Fällen, in denen wegen einer bereits bestehenden pulmonale
Hypertension mit einer nicht tolerierbaren Überlastung des kleinen Kreislaufs nach Lungenresektion gerechnet werden muß. Die Druckmessung in
der Arteria pulmonalis in Ruhe und unter Belastung, evtl. mit einseitiger
Okklusion, bietet sich hier als geeignete präoperative Untersuchungsmethode
an.

PATIENTENKREIS

25 Patienten im Alter von 48 bis 80 Jahre ($\bar{x}$ = 65 Jahre), bis auf eine Ausnahme alle männlichen Geschlechts, wurden wegen Verdachts auf eine pulmonale Hypertension mit einem dreilumigen Ballonkatheter nach Dotter-
Lukas katheterisiert. 18 von diesen 25 Patienten hatten ein Bronchialkarzinom, bei 5 von ihnen (Gruppe 1) waren jedoch sowohl die plethysmographischen Meßwerte nach Amrein et al. [1]wie auch der Druck in der
Arteria pulmonalis und der Lungenkapillardruck in Ruhe und bei Belastung,
jeweils ohne Okklusion, nach den Richtwerten von Tartulier et al. [7]unauf-
fällig. Diese Personen bilden die Vergleichsgruppe. Bei den 13 anderen
Tumorpatienten (Gruppe 2) war entweder eine obstruktive Lungenerkrankung
vorhanden oder die Katheterbefunde waren schon vor Okklusion pathologisch.
Die letzten 7 Patienten (Gruppe 3) hatten eine obstruktive Lungenerkrankung
unterschiedlichen Ausmaßes, aber keinen Tumor.

METHODIK

Die Untersuchungen erfolgten im Liegen und ohne vorherige Sedierung der
Patienten. Die beiden Transducer (Statham P 23 Db) wurden bei normaler
Thoraxkonfiguration in eine Ebene 5 cm unterhalb des angulus Ludovici

gebracht, bei emphysematösem Faßthorax nach Augenmaß in die vermutete Vorhofebene. Das Atemminutenvolumen wurde mit einem Pneumotachometer bestimmt, die Sauerstoffkonzentration in der gesammelten Exspirationsluft mit einer Zirkoniumoxid-Zelle gemessen. Zur Sauerstoffpartialdruckmessung wurde ein Gerät der Fa. Instrumentation Laboratories (Modell No. 313) verwendet und hieraus die Sauerstoffsättigungen ermittelt. Die Herzminutenvolumina wurden nach dem Fickschen Prinzip, die Lungengefäßwiderstände nach dem Ohmschen Gesetz errechnet. - Nach der Einführung des Ballonkatheters von einer präparierten Armvene aus in die Arteria pulmonalis wurde der mittlere Pulmonalisdruck ($\overline{P_{PA}}$) und der Lungenkapillardruck (PCV) in Ruhe gemessen und dann der Ballon des Katheters solange mit Kontrastmittel gefüllt, bis dieser in den zu okkludierenden Ast der Arteria pulmonalis, bei Karzinomträgern der tumorbefallenen Seite, eingekeilt und ein einwandfreier PCV erhalten wurde. Nach 5 Minuten Okklusion wurde der Ballon wieder entleert und der Patient am Fahrradergometer (Fa. Jäger) submaximal oder maximal belastet. Die erreichten Pulsfrequenzen lagen nie über 130/min. In der 5. Belastungsminute wurde die Arteria pulmonalis erneut einseitig okkludiert und die Drücke im kleinen Kreislauf über weitere 5 Belastungsminuten gemessen.

ERGEBNISSE

Die Ergebnisse der Messungen der Pulmonalismitteldrücke ($\overline{P_{PA}}$), der Herzminutenvolumina ($\dot{Q}$) und der Atemminutenvolumina ($\dot{V}$) sind in Tabelle 1 zusammengestellt. Der Anstieg des Pulmonalismitteldrucks unter Okklusion ist in Ruhe mit $P < 0,001$ und unter Belastung mit $P < 0,01$ (einseitiger t-Test) signifikant, jedoch unterscheidet sich der Druckanstieg in Ruhe nicht signifikant von dem unter Belastungsbedingungen, ebenso ist keine Abhängigkeit vom Ausgangswert festzustellen. Dies gilt sowohl für die einzelnen Patientengruppen wie auch für alle Patienten zusammen. Eine Abhängigkeit von plethysmographischen Befunden, insbesondere von der Resistance, kann nicht gefunden werden. Das Atemminutenvolumen nimmt unter Okklusion geringfügig zu, das Herzminutenvolumen bleibt (bis auf die Gruppe der Bronchitiker unter Okklusion) weitgehend konstant. Abb. 1 zeigt ein Beispiel für den Anstieg des systolischen und des diastolischen Pulmonalisdrucks unter Okklusion eines Pulmonalarterienastes; die Amplitude bleibt unverändert. Wegen der Vergrößerung des funktionellen Totraums nimmt die endexspiratorische Kohlensäurekonzentration (im hier vorliegenden Fall extrem) ab. - Der Anstieg des Pulmonalismitteldrucks $\Delta \overline{P_{AA}}$ von Ruhe nach Belastung (ohne Okklusion) kann nicht zur Ausgangshöhe korreliert werden ($P > 0.05$), jedoch findet sich unter Okklusion eine positive Korrelation: $\Delta \overline{P_{AA}} = 0,4 \ \overline{P_{PA}}$ (Ruhe) $+ 6,0$; $r = 0,45$; $P < 0,05$. Abb. 2 gibt das Einzelverhalten aller Patienten wieder.

Tabelle 1. Pulmonalismitteldrücke ($\overline{P_{PA}}$), Herzminutenvolumina ($\dot{Q}$) und Atemminutenvolumina ($\dot{V}$): Mittelwerte $x \pm s$

		RUHE		BELASTUNG	
		vor Okklusion	nach	vor Okklusion	nach
$\overline{P_{PA}}$	Gruppe 1	12,6 ± 4,3	17,0 ± 4,0	22,7 ± 4,0	25,7 ± 2,4
	Gruppe 2	16,9 ± 3,7	22,8 ± 4,6	33,1 ± 6,0	39,4 ± 10,3
	Gruppe 3	21,5 ± 7,7	26,4 ± 8,5	35,4 ± 11,4	41,4 ± 9,5
$\dot{Q}$	Gruppe 1	7,5 ± 1,0	7,2 ± 1,6	13,2 ± 2,8	13,2 ± 1,9
	Gruppe 2	6,9 ± 1,7	7,5 ± 1,9	14,7 ± 5,1	15,0 ± 3,4
	Gruppe 3	6,9 ± 2,6	7,4 ± 1,8	11,9 ± 3,8	13,8 ± 3,6
$\dot{V}$	Gruppe 1	8,7 ± 1,0	10,0 ± 0,8	26,0 ± 4,7	31,3 ± 8,0
	Gruppe 2	9,9 ± 3,7	12,5 ± 3,6	32,0 ± 8,3	42,0 ± 10,3
	Gruppe 3	8,7 ± 2,3	9,3 ± 1,2	24,3 ± 4,9	23,0 ± 1,4

Gruppe 1: 5 Patienten mit Bronchialkarzinom, aber normaler Plethysmographie und normalen Pulmonalismitteldrücken vor Okklusion

Gruppe 2: 10 Patienten mit Bronchialkarzinom und pathol. Plethysmographie und/oder pathol. Pulmonalismitteldrücken vor Okklusion

Gruppe 3: 7 Patienten mit chron. obstrukt. Lungenerkrankung, aber ohne Bronchialkarzinom

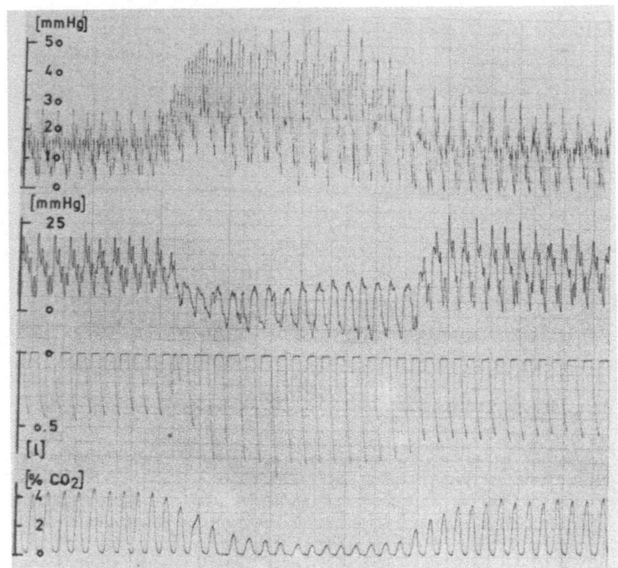

Abb. 1. Okklusion eines Pulmonalarterienastes. Von oben nach unten: Druck proximal des Ballons (P_{PA}), Druck distal des Ballons (P_{PA}/PCV), Atemzugvolumen, Kohlensäurekonzentration der Exspirationsluft. Lockerung der Okklusion bei rigidärer Arterienwand

Abb. 2. Anstieg des Pulmonalismitteldrucks unter Okklusion eines Pulmonalarterienastes in Ruhe und bei Belastung

210

DISKUSSION

Die Bewertung der Druckmessung in der Arteria pulmonalis unter einseitiger Okklusion bereitet Schwierigkeiten, da in der vorliegenden Untersuchung eine Vergleichsgruppe von gesunden Probanden fehlt. Da der
Ballonkatheter wegen seiner Steife schwerer als andere Katheter zu diri-
gieren ist und der Ballon zur Lagekontrolle unter Durchleuchtung gefüllt
werden muß, ergibt sich insgesamt eine Strahlenexposition, die nach
heutiger Auffassung über den Strahlenschutz eine Anwendung dieser Untersuchungsmethode in Fällen ohne gegebene Indikation nicht vertretbar erscheinen läßt. Wenn auch die Patienten unserer Vergleichsgruppe normale
plethysmographische Befunde und normale Pulmonalisdrücke in Ruhe und
unter Belastung (ohne Okklusion) aufwiesen, so bestand bei ihnen immerhin,
vom Tumorleiden abgesehen, klinisch der Verdacht auf eine Einschränkung der pulmonalen Leistungsfähigkeit. Die Ergebnisse innerhalb dieser
Untersuchungsgruppe können deshalb nur mit großen Vorbehalten als
"normal" angesehen werden.
   Der Druckanstieg des pulmonalarteriellen Mitteldrucks von Ruhe nach
Belastung (ohne Okklusion) konnte nicht zur Ausgangshöhe korreliert werden (P>0,05), auch die Aussonderung zweier Patienten mit Anstieg von PCV
auf mehr als 20 Torr unter Belastung erbrachte keine besseren Ergebnisse.
Folgende Erklärungen bieten sich an: 1. Unser eigenes Patientengut war
für die geringe Fallzahl von n=25 zu heterogen (Tumorkranke und Bronchitiker) zusammengesetzt. 2. Die Patienten wurden wegen der Fragestellung
einer Pneumonektomie alle submaximal bis maximal belastet, so daß die
erreichten Wattzahlen und Herzminutenvolumina beträchtlich divergierten.
Eine submaximale oder maximale Belastung wäre somit kein geeignetes
Vergleichsniveau. 3. Die höchsten Pulmonalisdrücke in Ruhe lagen bei
30 Torr. Bei Patienten mit höheren Ausgangswerten stiegen diese entweder
unter Okklusion in Ruhe oder unter Belastung ohne Okklusion so hoch an,
daß eine Belastung unter Okklusionsbedingungen zu risikoreich erschien.
Durch diese Begrenzung des Patientenkreises ist aber das Auffinden einer
Korrelation erheblich erschwert. Auffällig war, daß unter Okklusionsbe-
dingungen kein höherer Druckanstieg gefunden wurde als ohne Okklusion.
Dies kann nur dadurch erklärt werden, daß unter Okklusion eine erhebliche
Vergrößerung der Lungenstrombahn stattfindet. Stanek et al. [6] fanden bei
Ruhe- und Belastungsbedingungen, gleich ob ohne oder mit einseitiger Okklu-
sion, einen unveränderten Gefäßwiderstand der perfundierten Regionen.
Für 36 gesunde Probanden im Alter von 16 - 37 Jahre ergab sich die
Regressionsgerade $\overline{P}_{PA}$ = 0,934 $\dot{Q}$ + 7,71. Bei dem absoluten Glied dürfte
es sich um den wedge pressure handeln, der mit 8,5 $\pm$ 2,5 Torr gemessen
wurde und zur Berechnung des Lungengefäßwiderstandes vom Pulmonalisdruck
abgezogen werden muß, so daß die Gerade dann durch den Koordinatenur-
sprung ginge. Für die Messungen bei 10 gesunden Probanden im Alter von
18 - 26 Jahre gaben diese Autoren bei einseitiger Okklusion die Formel
$\overline{P}_{PA}$ - PCV = 1,22 $\dot{Q}$ + 2,0 an. Nach der multiplen Regressionsformel von
Tartulier et al. [7] hingegen kommt man für einen 20-jährigen Probanden
auf $\overline{P}_{PA}$ - PCV = 0,515 $\dot{Q}$ + 2,91. Die hiernach errechneten Lungengefäß-

widerstände liegen damit deutlich niedriger. Die absoluten Glieder in den
beiden letztgenannten Formeln und jene, die von Lockhart[4]zitiert werden,
müssen nicht unbedingt bedeuten, daß der Lungengefäßwiderstand mit zunehmendem Herzminutenvolumen kontinuierlich abnimmt und damit ein
flexibles System vorliegt, sondern können auch so erklärt werden, daß die
Drücke konstant zu hoch gemessen wurden, wenn, wie z.B. bei Harris
et al. [2],der Referenzpunkt immer in eine Ebene von 10 cm über der
Tischebene und damit bei faßförmigem Thorax zu tief gelegt wird. Die
angegebenen 2 oder 3 Torr entsprechen immerhin nur 2,7 bzw. 4,1 cm
Wassersäule. Die Annahme von Lockhart[4], im Gegensatz zu Gesunden -
bei denen die Gefahr einer falschen Referenzebene nicht so sehr gegeben
ist - müßten die Lungengefäße eines Bronchitikers zwei Strukturen, nämlich ein starres System unter Belastung und ein flexibles unter Okklusion,
aufweisen, dürfte auch morphologisch oder physiologisch schwer zu inter-
pretieren sein.

Lockhart[4]warf die Frage auf, ob es überhaupt statthaft sei, den
Lungengefäßwiderstand nach $R = \Delta P/\dot{Q}$ zu berechnen, da zum einen die
Durchblutung der Lunge erhebliche regionale Unterschiede aufweise, zum
anderen der Flow in den Lungenkapillaren beim Gesunden am Ende einer
Diastole Null, beim Bronchitiker aber auch noch zu diesem Zeitpunkt eine
Pulsation des Kapillardrucks vorhanden sei. Unabhängig von der Frage, ob
der Lungengefäßwiderstand unter einseitiger Okklusion konstant bleibt
oder abnimmt, wurden Zweifel geäußert, daß diese Untersuchungsmethode
geeignet sei, präoperativ die Höhe des Pulmonalisdrucks nach Lungenresektion abzuschätzen. Jezek[3]konnte 7 Patienten, von denen aber nur 4
einer Pneumonektomie unterzogen worden waren, 6 Monate nach Operation
nachuntersuchen. Die Ergebnisse zeigten, daß kein signifikanter Zusammenhang zwischen prä- und postoperativer Untersuchung vorhanden war.
Wilhelm und Widow[9]maßen den Pulmonalisdruck während der Operation,
wobei aber nur summarische Angaben gemacht wurden. Sie fanden, daß
der Pulmonalisdruck nicht unmittelbar nach Unterbindung der Lungengefäße,
sondern erst im Verlauf von mehreren Stunden anstieg und nach 4-6 Stunden
ein Maximum erreichte. Der Endwert stellte sich meist erst nach einer
Woche, nach Pneumonektomie oft sogar erst nach 10 Tagen ein. Nach dieser
Untersuchung wäre anzunehmen, daß sich das Verhalten des Pulmonalisdrucks bei Unterbindung einer Lungenarterie nicht durch Okklusion mit
Ballonkatheter simulieren läßt. Dennoch meinten Jezek[3]wie auch Wilhelm
und Widow[9], daß die Messung des Pulmonalisdrucks unter Okklusion
eine nützliche Information darstellt. Ohlsen et al.[5]konnten durch diese
Untersuchung eindeutig eine Senkung der durch kardio-pulmonale Komp-
likationen bedingten Mortalität erreichen.

LITERATUR

1.   Amrein, R., Keller, R., Joos, H., Herzog, H.: Neue Normalwerte
      für die Lungenfunktionsprüfung mit der Ganzkörperplethysmographie.
      Dtsch. Med. Wschr. 94, 1785-1793 (1969)

2.   Harris, P. , Segel, N. , Bishop, J. M. : The relation between pressure
       and flow in the pulmonary circulation in normal subjects and in patients
       with chronic bronchitis and mitral stenosis. Cardiovasc. Res. $\underline{2}$,
       73-83 (1968)

3.   Jezek, V. : Pulmonary haemodynamics and blood gases during unilat-
       eral pulmonary artery occlusion and after lung resection. Bull.
       Physio-path. resp. $\underline{6}$, 255-264 (1970)

4.   Lockhart, A. : Hémodynamique pulmonaire dans la bronchite chronique.
       Bull. Physio-path. resp. $\underline{9}$, 1069-1099 (1973)

5.   Olsen, G. N. , Blook, A.J. , Swenson, W. , Castle, R. , Wynne, J.W. :
       Pulmonary function evaluation of the lung resection candidate: a
       prospective study. Amer. Rev. Resp. Dis. $\underline{111}$, 379-387 (1975)

6.   Stanek, V. , Jebavy, P. , Hurych, J. , Widimsky, J. : Central haemody-
       namics during supine exercise and pulmonary artery occlusion in
       normal subjects. Bull. Physio-path. resp. $\underline{9}$, 1203-1217 (1973)

7.   Tartulier, M. , Bourret, M. , Deyrieux, F. : Les pressions artérielles
       pulmonaires chez l'homme normal. Effects de l'âge et de l'exercise mus-
       culaire. Bull. Physio-path. resp. $\underline{8}$, 1295-1321 (1972)

8.   Weiss, W. , Seidman, H . , Boucot, K. R. : The Philadelphia pulmonary
       neoplasm research project. Thwarting factors in periodic screening
       for lung cancer. Amer. Rev. Resp. Dis. $\underline{111}$, 289-297 (1975)

9.   Wilhelm, R. , Widow, W. : Der Einfluß der Querschittsänderung
       der Lungenstrombahn auf den Pulmonalarteriendruck beim Menschen.
       Z. Exper. Chirurg. $\underline{7}$, 259-263 (1974)

Dr. R. Goerg
Klinikum rechts der Isar
8000 München - 80

Pneumonologie Suppl. 1976, 213-215

Pulmonaler Gasaustausch nach Ersatz des Luftstickstoffs durch andere inerte Gase

H. Worth, H. Takahashi und J. Piiper

Abteilung Physiologie, Max-Planck-Institut für experimentelle Medizin, Göttingen

Pulmonary gas exchange after replacement of air nitrogen by other inert gases

---

Abstract. The influence of physical properties of the breathing medium on alveolar gas exchange was studied measuring alveolar-arterial partial pressure differences (ΔP) for O_2 and CO_2 in artificially ventilated, anesthetized dogs replacing air nitrogen by helium, argon or sulphur hexafluoride. In both hypoxia and normoxia the ΔP_{O_2} were found to decrease in the sequence He-O_2 >N_2 - O_2 >Ar-O_2 >SF_6-O_2, while ΔP_{CO_2} remained practically unchanged. Additional measurements of pulmonary diffusing capacity for CO (D_{CO}) using the single breath technique revealed no significant differences between the four gas mixtures used. To interpret these results the possible roles played by diffusion limitation (stratification), Taylor dispersion and viscosity-dependent ventilation-perfusion inhomogeneities are discussed.

Key words: Alveolar-arterial P_{O_2} and P_{CO_2} differences CO transfer - Inert gases - Stratification - $\dot{V}_A/\dot{Q}$ distribution

---

Bei Atmung von Zimmerluft beträgt der Anteil des Stickstoffs am Atemgas etwa 80%. Der pulmonale Netto-Austausch von N_2 ist gering bis fehlend, der Stickstoff dient vielmehr als Vehikel für den Transport der respiratorischen Gase O_2 und CO_2. Um den Einfluß physikalischer Eigenschaften des "Trägergases" auf den alveolären Gasaustausch zu analysieren, bietet sich die Möglichkeit, den Luftstickstoff durch andere inerte Gase mit unterschiedlichen physikalischen Eigenschaften (He, Ar, SF_6) zu ersetzen.

Zu diesem Zweck wurden an 10 künstlich beatmeten, narkotisierten Hunden alveolär-arterielle Druckdifferenzen (ΔP) für O_2 und CO_2 bei Atmung von hypoxischen (F_{O_2} = 12%) Inertgasgemischen (He-O_2, N_2-O_2, Ar-O_2 und SF_6-O_2) gemessen. Für die ΔP (torr) ergaben sich folgende Mittelwerte ($\pm$ SE):

214

$$He\text{-}O_2: \quad \Delta P_{O_2} = 9,1 \pm 1,4; \quad \Delta P_{CO_2} = 4,3 \pm 0,7$$

$$N_2\text{-}O_2: \quad \Delta P_{O_2} = 7,8 \pm 0,8; \quad \Delta P_{CO_2} = 3,8 \pm 0,4$$

$$Ar\text{-}O_2: \quad \Delta P_{O_2} = 5,6 \pm .0,7; \quad \Delta P_{CO_2} = 4,2 \pm 0,6$$

$$SF_6\text{-}O_2: \quad \Delta P_{O_2} = 4,7 \pm 0,8; \quad \Delta P_{CO_2} = 3,6 \pm 0,6$$

Zusätzliche Messungen der Diffusionskapazität der Lunge für $CO(D_{CO})$ mit der "single breath" Methode ergaben keine signifikanten Unterschiede bei Atmung der vier Gasgemische.

In einer zweiten Versuchsreihe wurden an 5 Hunden die ΔP_{O_2}, ΔP_{CO_2} und D_{CO} in Normoxie bei Atmung von Zimmerluft und von Gasgemischen gemessen, in denen der Luftstickstoff durch He oder SF_6 ersetzt worden war. Die Ergebnisse zeigten eine ähnliche Tendenz, nämlich eine Abnahme der ΔP_{O_2} mit steigender Dichte der Hintergrundanalyse (He, N_2, SF_6), während ΔP_{CO_2} und D_{CO} keine signifikanten Unterschiede aufwiesen.

Unsere Ergebnisse bezüglich ΔP_{O_2} stimmen mit den Ergebnissen anderer Arbeitsgruppen recht gut überein. So fanden Liese et al. (1970) an lungengesunden Versuchspersonen, daß die alveolär-arteriellen Partialdruckdifferenzen von O_2 bei Atmung des Trägergases He gegenüber N_2 anstiegen. Saltzman et al. (1971) fanden am ruhenden Menschen höhere ΔP_{O_2} bei He-O_2-Atmung als bei N_2-O_2. Nach den Experimenten von Martin et al. (1972) an narkotisierten, künstlich beatmeten Hunden änderten sich die ΔP_{O_2} unter 1 ata Außendruck bei Atmung der Hintergrundgase He, N_2 und SF_6 nicht signifikant, bei 4 ata hingegen lagen die ΔP_{O_2} bei SF_6-O_2-Atmung niedriger als bei Atmung von N_2-O_2. Messungen von ΔP_{CO_2} bei Veränderungen der Atemgasdichte sind uns nicht bekannt.
Für die mit der "single breath" Methode bestimmten Diffusionskapazitäten für CO wurde an gesunden Probanden eine Abnahme in der Sequenz He-O_2> N_2-O_2 >Ar-O_2 beobachtet (Worth, 1975), während Kvale et al. (1975) bei Messungen der CO-Aufnahme unter "steady state" Bedingungen zu entgegengesetzt gerichteten Resultaten kamen. Die bisherigen experimentellen Ergebnisse sind somit recht unterschiedlich.

Die von uns gefundene negative Korrelation zwischen den ΔP_{O_2} und der Dichte der benutzten Gasgemische kann offenbar nicht mit einfachen Stratifikationsmodellen erklärt werden. Sie könnte jedoch auf ein Modell zurückgeführt werden, das auf der Wirksamkeit der sogenannten "Taylor-Dispersion" (die aus dem Strömungsgeschwindigkeitsprofil und der radialen Diffusion resultiert) in den peripheren Atemwegen basiert. Hierbei wäre allerdings für die ΔP_{CO_2} gleich gerichtete und etwa gleich große Änderungen wie bei den ΔP_{O_2} in Abhängigkeit von der Dichte des Atemgasgemisches zu erwarten. Da sich die ΔP_{CO_2} aber nicht signifikant mit steigender Dichte der Hintergrundgase veränderte, wurde versucht, eine von der Viscosität des Trägergases abhängige, ungleichmäßige Verteilung der alveolären Belüftung und des Belüftungs-Durchblutungs-

Verhältnisses zur Erklärung der Versuchsergebnisse heranzuziehen. Solche Verteilungsstörungen würden auf die "single breath" D_{CO} nur einen geringen Einfluß ausüben.

Die vorliegenden Ergebnisse lassen sich durch keinen einzelnen Mechanismus zwanglos erklären. Es ist möglich, daß mehrere Mechanismen in einer komplizierten Weise zusammenwirken oder daß andere, noch nicht berücksichtigte Faktoren im Spiel sind.

LITERATUR

Kvale, P.A., Davis, J., Schroter, R.C.: Effect of gas density and ventilatory pattern on steady-state CO uptake by the lung. Respir. Physiol. 24, 385-398 (1975)

Liese, W., Muyseres, K., Pichotka, J.P.: Die Beeinflussung der alveolär-arteriellen O_2-Druckdifferenzen durch inerte Gase. Pflügers Arch. 321, 316-331 (1970)

Martin, R.R., Zutter, M., Anthonisen, N.R.: Pulmonary gas exchange in dogs breathing SF_6 at 4 ata. J. Appl. Physiol. 33, 86-92 (1972)

Saltzman, H.A., Salzano, J.V., Blenkarn, G.D.; Kylstra, J.A.: Effects of pressure on ventilation and gas exchange in man. J. Appl. Physiol. 30, 443-449 (1971)

Worth, H.: Diffusionskapazität der Lunge für CO bei Atmung von Inertgasgemischen mit unterschiedlichen physikalischen Eigenschaften. Respiration 32, 436-444 (1975)

Dr. H. Worth
Max-Planck-Institut
für Experimentelle Medizin
Abteilung Physiologie
3400 Göttingen

Pneumonologie Suppl. 1976, 217-227

Das arterielle Sauerstoffpartialdruckprofil unter Belastung und in der Erholungsphase – fortlaufende Sauerstoffpartialdruck-messungen bei Lungengesunden und bei Bronchitikern

W. Schwarz und H. Fabel

Abteilung Pulmonologie der Medizinischen Hochschule Hannover

The arterial profile of oxygen tension during work load and recovery - continous recording of oxygen tensions in human subjects without lung disease and in chronic bronchitis patients.

A b s t r a c t. 20 subjects without heart or lung disease and 13 chronic bronchitis patients were studied on a bicycle ergometer with increasing work loads. The arterial oxygen tensions were continuously recorded during 6 min ergometer work and during recovery for 10 min. Subsequently another ergometer test with stepwise increasing work load after each 2 min was performed in 14 of the normal subjects. In the patients with bronchitis simultaneous records of cardiac output and minute ventilation were analyzed. A typical profile of oxygen tension was observed in all examined groups with an initial negative dip, rise of oxygen tension during work and an overshoot reaction after the end of the work load. The initial drop in oxygen tension is mainly caused by a relative alveolar hypoventilation at the beginning of exercise. On the average the oxygen tensions at the end of exercise were 4 - 8 mm Hg higher than before exercise. A possible source of error for falsely high arterial oxygen tension before exercise (transient hyperventilation) is discussed.

Key words: Arterial oxygen tension - Continous recording - Exercise - Recovery

Z u s a m m e n f a s s u n g : 20 herz-lungengesunde Probanden und 13 Patienten mit einer chronischen Bronchitis wurden mit steigenden Wattstufen ergometrisch belastet. Während der 6-minütigen Ergometerarbeit und in der Erholungsphase von 10 Minuten wurde der arterielle Sauerstoffpartial-druck fortlaufend registriert. Bei 14 Probanden des Normalkollektivs erfolgte anschließend eine erneute Tretkurbelarbeit mit stufenweiser Steigerung der Ergometerbelastung nach jeweils 2 Minuten. Bei den Bronchitikern wurden simultane Messungen von Herzminutenvolumen und Atemzeitvolumen

durchgeführt. In allen Untersuchungsgruppen fand sich ein "typisches"
arterielles Sauerstoffpartialdruckprofil mit einer initialen Senke, Anstieg
des Sauerstoffpartialdruckes noch während der Belastung und überschie-
ßender Reaktion nach Belastungsende. Der initiale Sauerstoffpartialdruckabfall ist hauptsächlich durch eine relative alveoläre Hypoventilation bei
Belastungsbeginn bedingt. Die Sauerstoffpartialdruckwerte am Ende der
Ergometerarbeit lagen im Mittel 4-8 Torr höher als die Vorbelastungswerte. Auf eine mögliche Fehlerquelle zu hoch bestimmter arterieller
Sauerstoffpartialdruckwerte vor Belastungsbeginn (kurzfristige Hyperventilation) wird hingewiesen.

Eine pulmonal bedingte Leistungsminderung läßt sich nach Ansicht einiger
Autoren [3, 5, 6, 18] bereits aus dem Belastungsverhalten des arteriellen
Sauerstoffpartialdruckes erkennen, und gerade für gutachterliche Fragen
wurde von Hertz [12] eine blutgasanalytisch ermittelte "respiratorische
Leistungsgrenze" angegeben.

Die Annahme einer drohenden respiratorischen Insuffizienz aufgrund
des Belastungsabfalles der arteriellen Sauerstoffspannung wird bei Berücksichtigung der unterschiedlichen Angaben über das Sauerstoffpartial-
druckverhalten unter Ergometerbelastung allerdings zweifelhaft. Bei
meist Zweipunktmessungen des arteriellen Sauerstoffpartialdruckes in
Ruhe und unter Belastung wurde häufig gerade bei Jugendlichen und Sportlern ein Abfall [8, 10, 11, 13, 16, 24, 25, 31], bei jüngeren und älteren Probanden seltener ein unterschiedliches Verhalten [1, 7, 22, 26, 29, 30] oder
auch nur ein Anstieg unter Ergometerarbeit beobachtet [2, 20]. Zum Teil
zeigten insbesondere die älteren untersuchten Personen einen Belastungsanstieg des P_{aO_2} [22]. Eine Lösung der geschilderten Problematik ist
unseres Erachtens nur durch eine fortlaufende Messung des arteriellen
Sauerstoffpartialdruckes unter Ergometerarbeit möglich.

METHODIK

Bei 20 Probanden (14 Männer, 6 Frauen) im Alter von im Mittel 38
(SD ± 11) Jahren ohne Zeichen einer Herz-Lungenerkrankung (Klinik,
Röntgen, EKG, Bodyplethysmographie) wurde eine kontinuierliche Messung
des arteriellen Sauerstoffpartialdruckes (P_{aO_2}) während jeweils 6-minütiger
Belastung und anschließender Erholungsphase von 10 Minuten durchgeführt.
Belastet wurde liegend auf einem drehzahlunabhängigen Fahrradergometer
(Ergometer EM; Fa. Elema Schönander, Schweden) bei "rechteckförmiger
Belastung" in 25-Wattschritten. 19 der 20 Probanden erreichten hierbei
noch die 100 Watt-Belastung; 12 konnten zusätzlich mit 125 Watt (2 mit
150 Watt) belastet werden. Auf eine erschöpfende Ergometerbelastung
wurde verzichtet.

Bei 14 Probanden dieses Normalkollektivs erfolgte anschließend eine
erneute Tretkurbelarbeit, beginnend mit 25 Watt bis 100 Watt (n = 7) bzw.
125 Watt (n = 7) - entsprechend den Höchstbelastungsstufen der vorausge-

gangenen 6-Minutenbelastungen - wobei alle 2 Minuten ohne zwischenzeitliche Erholungsphase und ohne erneutes Kommando auf die nächsthöhere Wattstufe in 25-Wattschritten umgeschaltet wurde.

Im Rahmen einer weiteren Untersuchungsreihe wurden bei 13 Patienten im Durchschnittsalter von 50 (SD ± 12) Jahren mit einer mittelschweren obstruktiven Ventilationsstörung bei chronischer Bronchitis ohne Hypoxämie und Hyperkapnie Rechtsherzkatheteruntersuchungen und ergospirometrische Messungen bei 6-minütiger Belastung mit 50 Watt (13 Patienten) und 75 Watt (10 Patienten) durchgeführt. Bodyplethysmographisch ergaben sich bei diesen Patienten im Mittel folgende Werte: Vitalkapazität: 3000 ml ± 650 ml = 63% der Soll-VK; Rt: 8,09 ± 4,25 cm $H_2O/l/s$. Neben zahlreichen weiteren Parametern [23] wurden das Atemzeitvolumen ($\dot{V}_E$) in 15-Sekundenintervallen pneumotachographisch, das Herzzeitvolumen ($\dot{Q}$) über die Impedance-Kardiographie [14, 15] ermittelt (IFM/Minnesota Impedance-Cardiograph 304 A; Instrumentation for Medicine Inc., Greenwich; Connecticut). Der P_{aO_2} wurde bei allen Untersuchungen über eine arteria radialis mit der von Fabel [9] angegebenen Durchflußelektrode fortlaufend gemessen und anschließend in 15-Sekundenintervallen ausgewertet. Um Sauerstoffpartialdruck, Ventilation und Perfusion auch zeitgerecht korrelieren zu können, wurde bei der graphischen Darstellung der Sauerstoffpartialdruckkurven die mittlere Zirkulationszeit des Blutes zwischen Lunge und arteria radialis [4] mit berücksichtigt.

ERGEBNISSE

Zeitlich-dynamisches Verhalten sowie Ausmaß der Änderungen des Sauerstoffpartialdruckes bei den 20 herz-lungengesunden Probanden unter 6-minütiger Ergometerarbeit kommen in Abb. 1 deutlich zum Ausdruck.

Bei annähernd gleichen mittleren Ruhewerten vor den verschieden hohen Ergometerbelastungen fiel der arterielle Sauerstoffpartialdruck bei Belastungsbeginn um so rascher ab, je schwerer die Tretkurbelarbeit war und erreichte seinen tiefsten Wert bei der 25 Watt-Belastung nach etwa 90 Sekunden, bei der 125 Watt-Belastung dagegen bereits nach etwa 60 Sekunden.

Das Minimum der initialen Senke der Sauerstoffpartialdruckkurve unter Belastung lag signifikant um so tiefer, je höher die Belastung war (p < 0,020). Je höher im Einzelfall der Ruhe-Ausgangswert war, desto höher lag auch der Minimalwert des Sauerstoffpartialdruckes unter Ergometerbelastung innerhalb der jeweiligen Belastungsgruppe (für alle Belastungsstufen bis 125 Watt; p < 0,001). Bis zum Belastungsende kam es dann in fast allen Fällen zu einem erneuten Sauerstoffdruckanstieg auf Mittelwerte zwischen 4-8 Torr über die mittleren Ruhewerte (bei allerdings nur schwacher Signifikanz: p < 0,220). Die Vorbelastungswerte wurden meist gegen Ende der 2. Belastungsminute bei allen Wattstufen wieder erreicht und überschritten.

Nach Belastungsende kam es immer zu einem überschießenden Sauerstoffpartialdruckanstieg, wobei das Maximum mit Zunahme der Belastungs-

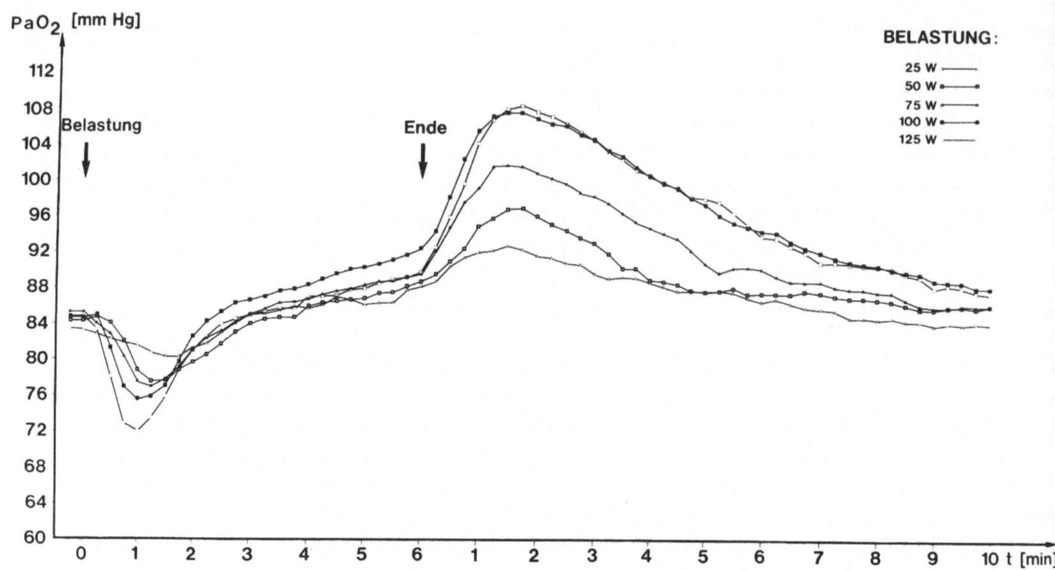

Abb. 1. Fortlaufende arterielle Sauerstoffpartialdruckmessungen bei 20
herz-lungengesunden Probanden unter 6-minütiger Ergometerbelastung mit
25 Watt (n = 15), 50 Watt (n = 17), 75 Watt (n = 18), 100 Watt (n = 19)
und 125 Watt (n = 12) sowie in den 10-minütigen Erholungsphasen

höhe der vorausgegangenen Ergometerarbeit in der Regel etwas früher erreicht wurde und deutlich höher lag. Der Sauerstoffpartialdruckabfall nach
dem meist kurzen Gipfelplateau erfolgte dann langsam. Die Ruhewerte des
Sauerstoffpartialdruckes vor Belastungsbeginn wurden während der 10-minü-
tigen Erholungsphase, besonders bei den höheren Ergometerbelastungen,
noch nicht wieder erreicht. Die Standardabweichungen der 5 Mittelwerts-
kurven des Sauerstoffpartialdruckes lagen meist im gesamten Kurvenverlauf gleichbleibend zwischen 8 und 12 mm Hg.

Auffälligster Unterschied der stufenförmigen 2-Minutenbelastungen
gegenüber den 6-Minutenbelastungen (Abb. 2) war der nur sehr langsame
Anstieg des Sauerstoffpartialdruckes im Anschluß an die initiale Senke.
Nach jeder Umschaltung auf eine höhere Belastungsstufe kam es meist
zu einem erneuten, kurzfristigen Abfall des P_{aO_2}, so daß die Vorbelastungswerte bei der 100 Watt-Belastung erst 5' 45", bei der hier graphisch
wiedergegebenen 125 Watt-Belastungsgruppe sogar erst 7' 30" nach Belastungsbeginn erreicht wurden.

Der kontinuierlich registrierte Sauerstoffpartialdruck der 13 Bronchitiker (Abb. 3) glich formal im gesamten Kurvenverlauf dem Sauerstoffpartialdruckprofil des Normalkollektivs. Das Belastungsminimum wurde
bei der höheren Belastung früher erreicht (1' statt 1' 30"), lag um knapp
1 Torr niedriger und war insgesamt etwas kürzer als bei der 50-Watt-Be-
lastung. Die Vorbelastungswerte wurden im Mittel nach ca. 3 Minuten

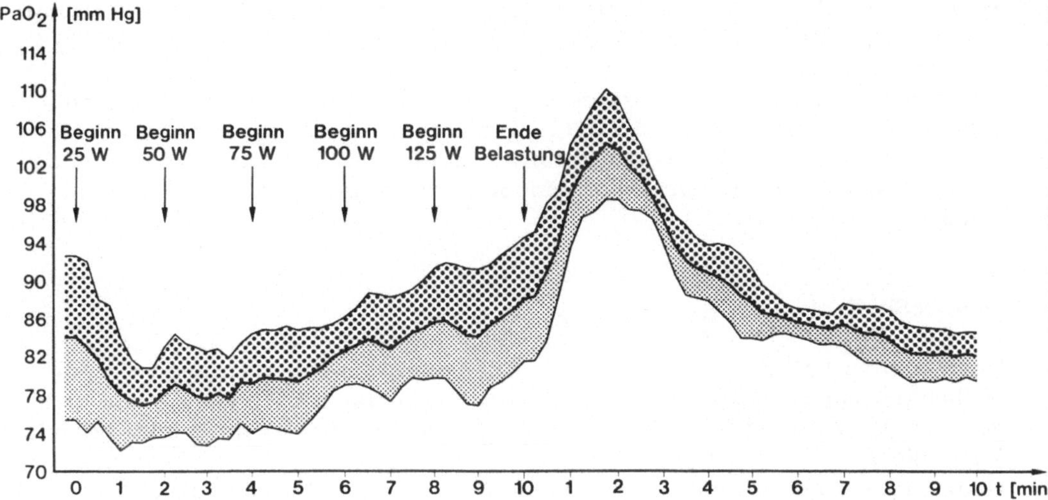

Abb. 2. Fortlaufende arterielle Sauerstoffpartialdruckmessungen bei 7 herz-lungengesunden Probanden unter stufenförmiger Ergometerbelastung bis 125 Watt und in der Erholungsphase von 10 Minuten (Standardabweichung schattiert)

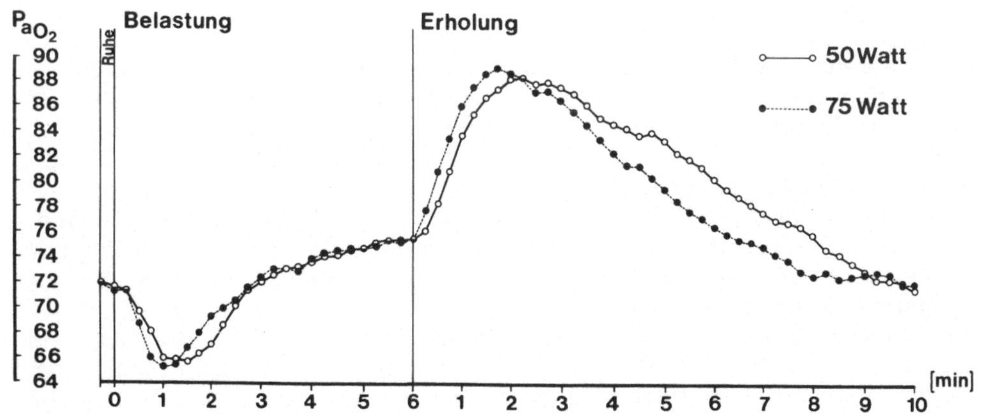

Abb. 3. Fortlaufende arterielle Sauerstoffpartialdruckmessungen bei 13 Bronchitikern unter 6-minütiger Ergometerbelastung mit 50 Watt (n = 13) und 75 Watt (n = 10) und in den 10-minütigen Erholungsphasen

wieder erreicht und überschritten. Am Ende der Tretkurbelarbeit lag der Sauerstoffpartialdruck etwa 4 Torr (nur schwach signifikant : $p < 0,05$) oberhalb der Ruhewerte.

Nach Belastungsende kam es in beiden Gruppen zu einem hochsignifikanten P_{aO_2}-Anstieg ($p < 0,001$), anschließend zu einem langsamen Kurvenabfall, wobei die Ruhe-Sauerstoffpartialdruckwerte bis gegen Ende der Erholungsphase in diesem Patientenkollektiv im Mittel wieder erreicht wurden.

DISKUSSION

Über kontinuierliche Sauerstoffpartialdruckmessungen kleinerer Untersuchungsgruppen unter dosierter Ergometerbelastung wurde bislang erst von wenigen Autoren berichtet [4, 9, 27]. Außer bei Bjurstedt und Wigertz [4], die gleichzeitig fortlaufende Bestimmungen von Atemzugvolumen und Herzfrequenz bei 7 Probanden durchgeführt, erfolgten sonst i. a. keine simultanen Messungen hämodynamischer oder ventilatorischer Parameter.

Ein initialer Belastungsabfall des PaO_2 wurde aufgrund punktueller oder kontinuierlicher Sauerstoffpartialdruckmessungen [4, 9, 24, 27, 30], Berechnung des P_{aO_2} über Sauerstoffsättigungswerte [3, 19, 21] oder über Bestimmungen des endexspiratorischen Sauerstoffpartialdruckes [17] auch von anderen Autoren beschrieben. Da die Herzfrequenz bei Belastungsbeginn wesentlich rascher anstieg als das Atemzugvolumen, nahmen Bjurstedt und Wigertz [4, 28] als Ursache des initialen Sauerstoffpartialdruckabfalls unter Ergometerarbeit eine gegenüber der Perfusion verzögert ansteigende Ventilation an. Dieser Zusammenhang konnte durch unsere Messungen von Herzzeitvolumen ($\dot{Q}$) und Atemminutenvolumen ($\dot{V}_E$) bei den Bronchitikern bestätigt werden (Abb. 4). Die Relativwerte von $\dot{V}_E$ und $\dot{Q}$ (bezogen auf den Vorbelastungswert und den 6-Minutenwert) lassen den steileren Belastungsanstieg der Perfusion gegenüber der Ventilation deutlich werden. Die hierdurch bedingte relative alveoläre Hypoventilation ist daher sicher als wesentliche, allerdings nicht als einzige Ursache des initialen Sauerstoffpartialdruckabfalls anzusehen [23].

Bei stufenförmiger Belastung ohne zwischenzeitliche Erholungsphase erfolgte ein erneuter P_{aO_2}-Anstieg nach dem primären Partialdruckabfall nur sehr verzögert, so daß diese Belastungsform insbesondere für Begutachtungsfragen nicht geeignet erscheint.

Der überschießende Sauerstoffpartialdruckanstieg nach Belastungsende ist durch eine relative Hyperventilation bedingt, wie simultane Messungen von Atemzeitvolumen und Sauerstoffaufnahme zeigten [23]. Ein häufig vorhandener kurzfristiger und nur leichter P_{aO_2}-Anstieg (ca. 1-3 Torr) vor der initialen Senke unter Belastung wurde bei der Auswertung der P_{aO_2}-Kurven in 15-Sekundenintervallen und graphischer Darstellung der Mittelwertkurven nicht mehr beobachtet.

Durch die kontinuierliche Sauerstoffpartialdruckmessung konnte ein stabiler Kurvenverlauf vor Belastungsbeginn abgewartet werden. Sprechen, Hüsteln, unnötige Bewegungen, Schmerzreiz oder Erwartungshaltung

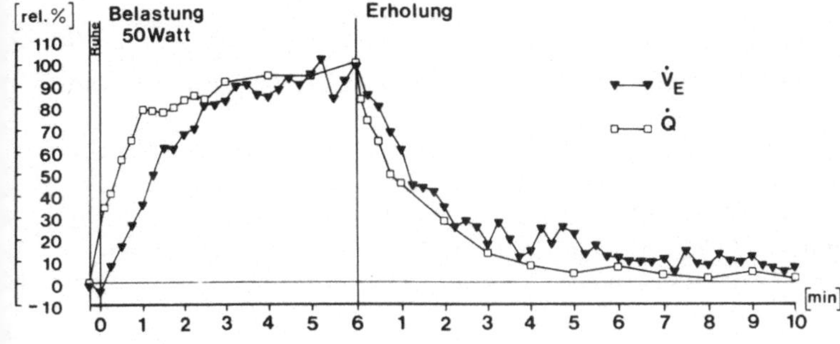

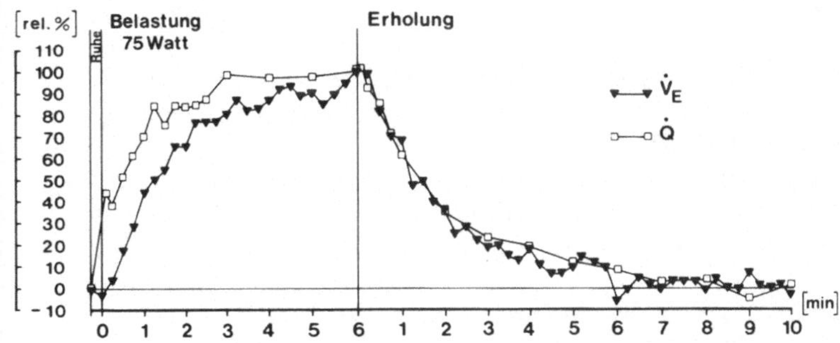

Abb. 4. Relativwerte des Herzminutenvolumens ($\dot{Q}$) und des Atemminutenvolumens ($\dot{V}_E$) von 13 Bronchitikern (bezogen auf den Vorbelastungswert
und den 6-Minuten-Belastungswert) während 6-minütiger Ergometerbelastung mit 50 Watt (n = 13) und 75 Watt (n = 10) sowie in den 10-minütigen
Erholungsphasen

des Patienten vor der Ergometerbelastung können zum Teil erhebliche
Schwankungen des Sauerstoffpartialdruckes verursachen. So bewirkte ein
tiefer Atemzug während der Ruhephase einen maximalen Sauerstoffpartialdruckanstieg von durchschnittlich 15 Torr bei den von uns untersuchten
herz-lungengesunden Probanden. Der von zahlreichen Autoren (s. o.) be-
schriebene Abfall des P_{aO_2} bis zum Belastungsende bei in der Regel Zweipunktmessungen des Sauerstoffpartialdruckes in Ruhe und unter Belastung
dürfte somit häufig durch eine alveoläre Hyperventilation bei der Blutentnahme (nicht zuletzt durch eine meist etwas schmerzhafte Kapillarblutent-
nahme) bedingt sein und hierdurch können die Vorbelastungs-Sauerstoff-
druckwerte im Einzelfall zu hoch bestimmt werden [30]. Die Folge ist
ein "scheinbarer" Sauerstoffpartialdruckabfall durch Normalisierung der
Atmung unter der Belastung [3]. Da eine kurzdauernde Mehratmung zwar
meist zu einem deutlichen Sauerstoffpartialdruckanstieg, jedoch nicht immer

zu einem wesentlichen Kohlensäureabfall führt, kann aufgrund des P_{aCO_2}-Wertes zum Zeitpunkt z. B. einer Ohrblutentnahme nicht in jedem Fall auf eine gleichzeitige oder vorausgegangene Hyperventilation geschlossen werden.

Bei dem herz-lungengesunden Kontrollkollektiv wurden keine simultanen Ventilations- und Perfusionsmessungen durchgeführt. Aufgrund des gleichen typischen Sauerstoffpartialdruckprofils und in Übereinstimmung mit Angaben der Literatur [4, 28] sind jedoch auch hier ähnliche sauerstoffpartialdruckbestimmende Faktoren anzunehmen.

LITERATUR

1. Asmussen, E., Nielsen, M.: Pulmonary ventilation and effect of oxygen breathing in heavy exercise. Acta Physiol. Scand. 43, 365-378 (1958)
2. Bartels, H., Beer, R., Koeppchen, H.-P., Wenner, J., Witt, I.: Messung der alveolär-arteriellen O_2-Druckdifferenz mit verschiedenen Methoden am Menschen bei Ruhe und Arbeit. Pflügers Arch. ges. Physiol. 261, 133-151 (1955)
3. Barr, P.-O., Beckmann, M., Bjurstedt, H., Brismar, J., Hesser, C.M., Matell, G.: Time courses of blood gas changes provoked by light and moderate exercise in man. Acta Physiol. Scand. 60, 1-17 (1964)
4. Bjurstedt, H., Wigertz, O.: Dynamics of arterial oxygen tension in response to sinusoidal work load in man. Acta Physiol. Scand. 82, 236-249 (1971)
5. Bühlmann, A., Scherrer, M., Herzog, H.: Vorschläge zur einheitlichen Beurteilung der Arbeitsfähigkeit durch die Lungenfunktionsprüfung. Schweiz. Med. Wschr. 4, 105-109 (1961)
6. Doll, E., Keul, J.: Blutgase. In: Hertz, C.W.: Begutachtung von Lungenfunktionsstörungen, S. 125-137. Stuttgart: Georg Thieme Verlag 1968
7. Doll, E., Keul, J., Maiwald, Chr., Reindell, H.: Das Verhalten von Sauerstoffdruck, Kohlensäuredruck, pH, Standardbicarbonat und base excess im arteriellen Blut bei verschiedenen Belastungsformen. Int. Z. angew. Physiol. 22, 327-355 (1966)
8. Doll, E., König, K., Reindell, H.: Das Verhalten der arteriellen Sauerstoffspannung und anderer arterieller blutgasanalytischer Daten in Ruhe und während körperlicher Belastung. Pflügers Arch. ges. Physiol. 271, 283-295 (1960)
9. Fabel, H.: Die fortlaufende Messung des arteriellen Sauerstoffdruckes beim Menschen. Methode und Anwendung, sowie Ergebnisse bei Gesunden und Patienten mit gestörter Lungenfunktion. Arch. Kreislaufforschg. 57, 145-189 (1968)
10. Filley. G.F., Gregoire, F., Wright, G.W.: Alveolar and arterial oxygen tensions and the significance of the alveolar-arterial oxygen tension difference in normal men. J. Clin. Invest. 33, 517-529 (1954)

11. Friehoff, F.: Der Gasaustausch bei gesunden Männern unter Ruhebe-
    dingungen und während körperlicher Arbeit. Pflügers Arch. ges.
    Physiol. 270, 431-444 (1960)
12. Hertz, C.W.: Zur Begutachtung von Lungenfunktionsstörungen durch
    den Arbeitsversuch. Dtsch. Med. Wschr. 90, 461-467 (1965)
13. Holmgren, A,, Linderholm, H.: Oxygen and carbon dioxide tensions
    of arterial blood during heavy and exhaustive exercise. Acta Physiol.
    Scand. 44, 203-215 (1958)
14. Kubicek, W.G., Karnegis, J.N., Patterson, R.P., Witsoe, D.A.,
    Mattson, R.H.: Development and evaluation of an impedance cardiac
    output system. Aerosp. Med. 37, 1208-1212 (1966)
15. Kubicek, W.G., Patterson, R.P., Witsoe, D.A.: Impedance cardio-
    graphy as a noninvasive method of monitoring cardiac function and
    other parameters of the cardiovascular system. Ann. NY. Acad. Sci.
    170, 724-732 (1970)
16. Lilienthal, J.L. Jr., Riley, R.L., Proemmel, D.D., Franke, R.E.:
    An experimental analysis in man of the oxygen pressure gradient
    from alveolar air to arterial blood during rest and exercise at sea
    level and at altitude. Amer. J. Physiol. 147, 199-216 (1946)
17. Linnarson, D.: Dynamics of pulmonary gas exchange and heart rate
    changes at start and end of exercise. Acta Physiol. Scand., Suppl.
    415, 1-68 (1974)
18. Marx, H.H., Zühlke, H.E., Schütze, B.: Möglichkeiten und Grenzen
    der Ergometrie für klinische Fragestellungen. Z. Kreislaufforschg.
    54, 1054-1067 (1965)
19. Matell, G.: Time-courses of changes in ventilation and arterial gas
    tensions in man induced by moderate exercise. Acta Physiol. Scand.
    58, Suppl. 206, 1-53 (1963)
20. Mitchell, J.H., Sproule, B.J., Chapman, C.B.: Factors influenc-
    ing respiration during heavy exercise. J. Clin. Invest. 37, 1693-1701
    (1958)
21. Raynaud, J., Boúrdarias, J.P., David, P., Durand, J.: Oxygen
    delivery and oxygen return to the lungs at onset of exercise in man.
    J. appl. Physiol. 35, 259-262 (1973)
22. Scherrer, M., Birchler, A.: Altersabhängigkeit der alveolar-arteriel-
    len O_2-Partialdruckgradienten bei Schwerarbeit in Normoxie, Hypoxie
    und Hyperoxie. Med. Thorac. 24, 99-117 (1967)
23. Schwarz, W.: Habilitationsschrift (in Vorb.)
24. Suskind, M., Bruce, R.A., McDowell, M.E., Lovejoy, F.W.jr.:
    Normal variations in end-tidal air and arterial blood carbon and
    oxygen tensions during moderate exercise. J. appl. Physiol. 3,
    282-290 (1950)
25. Thews, G.: Die Grundlagen der Sauerstoffversorgung der Gewebe,
    insbesondere des Myocards. Beitr. Silikoseforsch. 6, 511 (1965)
26. Ulmer, W.T., Reichel, G.: Untersuchungen über die Altersabhängig-
    keit der alveolären und arteriellen Sauerstoff- und Kohlensäuredrucke.
    Klin. Wschr. 41, 1-6 (1963)

27. Wettengel, R. : Blutgase und zentrale Hämodynamik unter Ergometer-
    belastung bei Gesunden und bei Kranken mit chronisch-obstruktiver
    Bronchitis. Habilitationsschrift, Department Innere Medizin der
    Medizinischen Hochschule Hannover, 1971
28. Wigertz, O. : Dynamics of ventilation and heart rate in response to
    sinusoidal work load in man. J. appl. Physiol. **29**, 208-218 (1970)
29. Woitowitz, H. -J. , Woitowitz, R. H. : Zum Streubereich der arteriellen
    Blutgaswerte lungengesunder, berufstätiger Männer und Frauen vor
    und während dosierter Ergometerbelastung. Med. Klin. **65**, 349-354
    (1970)
30. Woitowitz, H. -J. : Zur Dynamik arterieller Blutgaswerte während
    dosierter Arbeitsbelastung im Hinblick auf die Begutachtung. Klin.
    Wschr. **48**, 402-407 (1970)
31. Worth, G. , Mysers, K. , Siehoff, F. : Zur Problematik der Norm-
    werte der arteriellen O_2- und CO_2-Partialdrucke sowie der alveolo-
    arteriellen O_2- und CO_2-Druckgradienten im Rahmen arbeitsmedizini-
    scher Fragen. Med. Thorac. **20**, 223-234 (1963)

Dr. Wolfgang Schwarz
Prof. Dr. Helmut Fabel
Abteilung Pulmonologie
der Medizinischen Hochschule
Karl Wiechert Allee 9
3000 Hannover

DISKUSSION

F. Schnellbächer , Düsseldorf: Das gezeigte Verhalten des arteriellen
Sauerstoffdruckes unter der Belastung und in der Erholungsphase entspricht
genau dem Verlauf des in unserem Institut routinemäßig fortlaufend massen-
spektrometrisch gemessenen endexspiratorischen O_2-Druckes. Bei den
Schwankungen des arteriellen Sauerstoffdruckes handelt es sich also um die
Folge von Eigentümlichkeiten der Ventilation zu Beginn, während und nach
der Belastung, die auch von Stegemann bei Sportlern beobachtet wurden.
Blutentnahmen für die Bestimmung des arteriellen O_2-Druckes sollten
deshalb nach Möglichkeit stets unter laufender Kontrolle des endexspiratorischen O_2-Druckes (dies wäre auch mit einem schnellen paramagnetischen
Gerät möglich) erfolgen, damit die Punktion erst im steady state der Ventilation vorgenommen wird. Diese Vorgehen erlaubt außerdem die Bestimmung
des endexspirotorisch-arteriellen P_{O_2}-Gradienten.
    Wegen des gezeigten Verlaufes des arteriellen O_2-Druckes unter
a n s t e i g e n d e r   Belastung sollte besonders bei Begutachtungsfällen der
rektangulären Belastung der Vorzug gegeben werden, die 6 Minuten dauert
und bei der die Blutabnahme für die Bestimmung des P_{aO_2} und des P_{aCO_2}
sowie die Messung des arteriellen pH-Wertes in den beiden letzten Belastungsminuten erfolgt.

W. Schwarz, Hannover: Eine fortlaufende Registrierung des endexspiratorischen Sauerstoffdruckes unter einer möglichst 6-minütigen Ergometerbelastung, insbesondere bei Begutachtungsfällen, ist als Kontrolle, ob die
Blutgasentnahmen zumindest im "relativen steady-state" der Ventilation
erfolgten, sicher zu empfehlen.

Ein etwa kurvengleicher Verlauf des endexspiratorischen Sauerstoffdruckes - und übrigens auch des "Lungen RQ" - unter Belastung konnten
u.a. Linnarson (1974) und auch wir bei eigenen Untersuchungen feststellen.
Die endexspiratorisch gemessenen Sauerstoffdruckwerte können allerdings
trotz des ähnlichen Kurvenprofils unter Belastung z.T. erheblich von den
arteriell gemessenen O_2-Druckwerten differieren, wie z.B. aus Untersuchungen von Rosenhamer (1972) bekannt ist.

Die Initialveränderungen des arteriellen Sauerstoffpartialdruckes sind
nicht allein als Folge einer "Eigentümlichkeit der Ventilation zu Belastungsbeginn" anzusehen, sondern sie sind bedingt durch unterschiedliche Einflüsse weiterer Faktoren in der "unsteady-state-Phase" der frühen
Belastungsperiode, auf die im Rahmen dieses Vortrages aus zeitlichen
Gründen nicht weiter eingegangen werden konnte.

Pneumonologie Suppl. 1976, 229-232

A System of Pa_{O_2} Continuously Controlled Ventilation

S. Kunke, V. Schulz, W. Erdmann, and K. H. Schnabel

Pneumologische Abteilung an der II. Medizinische Klinik der
Universität Mainz

Abstract. A newly developed system of Pa_{O_2}-controlled automatic
ventilation is reported on. P_{O_2} microelectrodes (Beckman, IBC) are used
to measure arterial P_{O_2} continuously. In a feedback control system the
inspiratory O_2 concentration of a respirator is adjusted as long as the set
point and actual value of the arterial P_{O_2} correspond. The functional behavior of the feedback control system is described.

Key words: P_{O_2} - catheter electrode - Pa_{O_2}-regulated feedback system

---

Shocked lungs characteristically show strong and rapid changes of functional parameters determining the pulmonary gaseous exchange - the alveolar
ventilation, the pulmonary shunt blood flow, the diffusion capacity, as
well as the distribution inhomogenities of $\dot{V}_A/\dot{Q}$ and $D_L/\dot{Q}$. The nowadays
conventional measuring of the arterial P_{O_2} is characterized by discontinuous sampling of the data. This procedure often does not offer the possibility of detecting the inherent danger for patients in time. Hypoxic and hyper-
oxic periods are often not recognized and corrected. Therefore we developed a system in which arterial P_{O_2} can be measured continuously, and
the following change of inspiratory O_2 concentration is regulated to a constant level.

In the Pa_{O_2}-regulated feedback control system Pa_{O_2} is measured by
means of O_2 microelectrodes (Fig. 1). The electrodes (from Beckman,
IBC) we applied work according to the polarographic measuring method.
The electrodes are inserted in the A. femoralis by means of an arterial
puncture syringe. The 90% adjustment time concerning the Beckman-Elec-
trode amounts to 8 s on average; the IBC electrode shows a 90% adjustment
time on an average of 75 s. The polarographic circuit is equipped with a
P_{O_2} meter especially developed in our department. In this P_{O_2} meter the
polarization voltage is applied to an integrated amplifier that contains a
field-effect transistor. The currents originating in the measuring circuit
belong to the nA range, and are directly proportional to the concentration
of the O_2 molecules at the point of the electrode. The load capacity of the
output voltages ranging from 0 to 10 volts of the P_{O_2} meter corresponds
to the polarographic measuring circuit, that is the arterial O_2 partial
pressure. The corresponding voltages are transmitted as P_{O_2} actual value

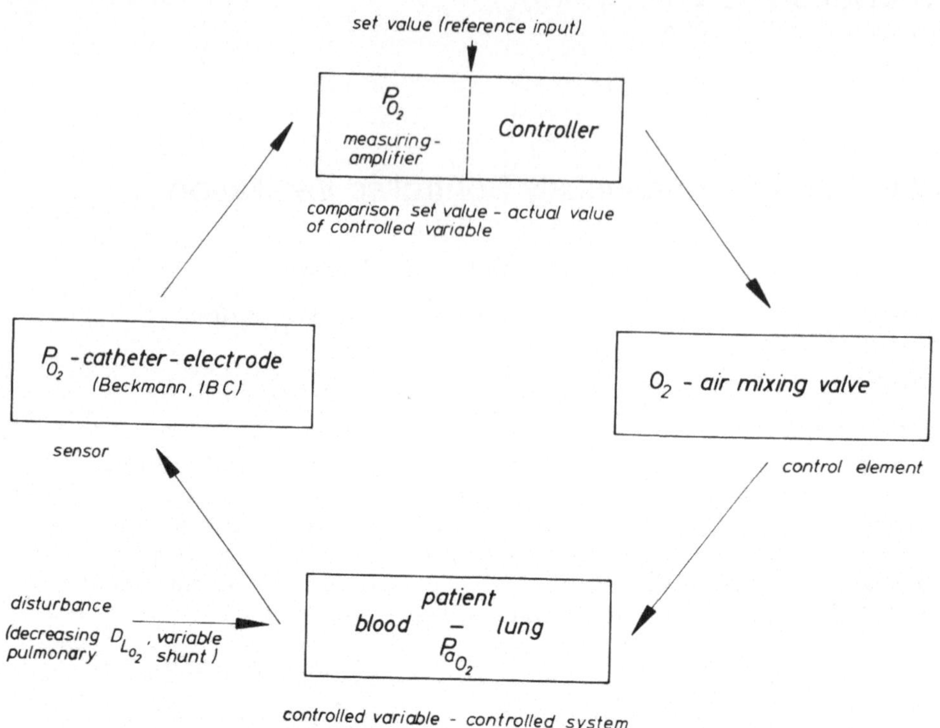

Fig. 1. Diagram of Pa_{O_2}-regulated feedback control system. For details see text

to an electronic amplifier acting as a control unit. During the first step of the mentioned regulator, voltage taken over from the P_{O_2} amplifier is compared to a highly stabilized reference voltage. Now it is possible to choose that adjustable reference voltage as P_{O_2} set point corresponding to the electrode calibration of 40-200 torr. This positive or negative difference between Pa_{O_2} set point and actual value is followed by a network of several integrated amplifiers working as a delay circuit and impedance transformer, as well as four power transistors driving a DC motor. A machine having a gear ratio of 1 : 80000 matches the engine speed with the necessary rate of travel of an O_2 valve defining the respective inspiratory O_2 concentration of the mentioned respirator. An adjustment of the O_2 mixing valve takes place as long as the Pa_{O_2} set point does not correspond to the actual value.

The Pa_{O_2} feedback control system was first proved in a lung model. After the regulation behavior had been optimized in the mentioned way, the control system was applied to man. Fig. 2 shows the transition behavior of the Pa_{O_2} control circuit for a step function input ranging from 70 to 100

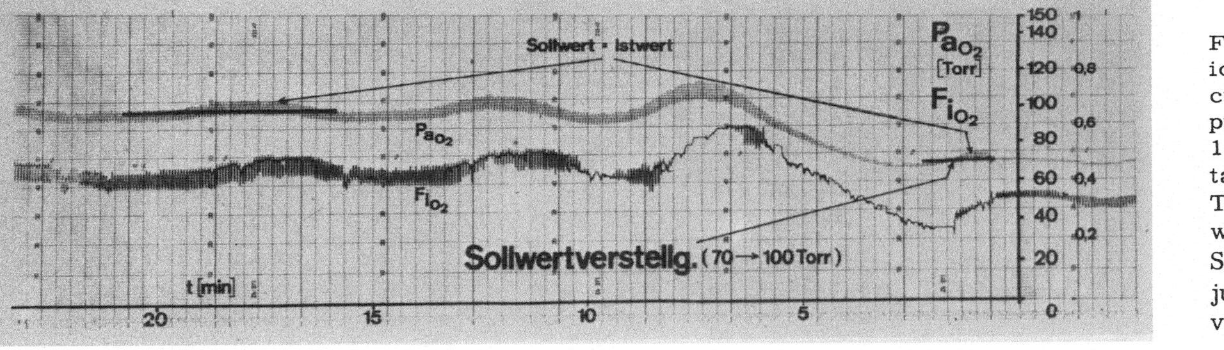

Fig. 2. Transient behavior of Pa_{O_2}-control circuit for step function input ranging from 70 to 100 torr Pa_{O_2}. For details see text. (Sollwert = Theoretical valve; Istwert = Actual valve; Sollwertverstellg. = Adjustment of theoretical valve)

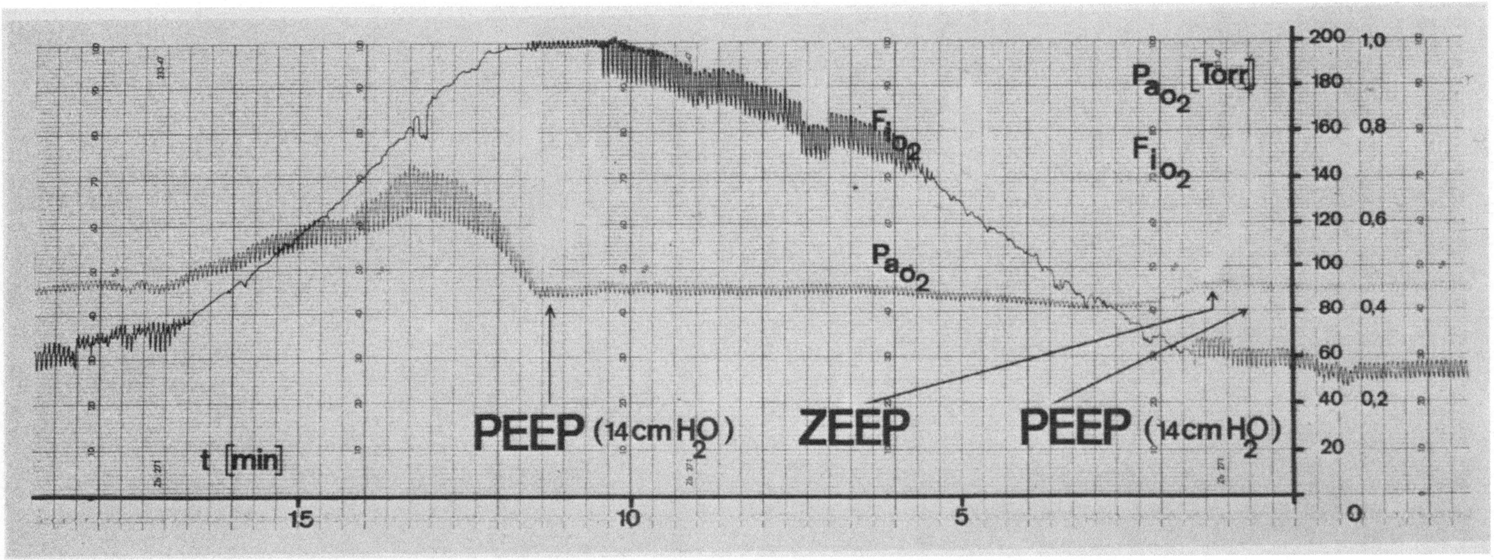

Fig. 3. Dynamic behavior of control circuit-adjustment behavior and control precision at transition from PEEP to ZEEP respiration. For details see text

232

torr Pa_{O_2}. In the form of a PT control system the Pa_{O_2} actual value and inspiratory O_2 fraction F_{IO_2} are adjusted to the set point. The transition takes place in the form of periodic deadbeats. After 15 min the regulation process is finished. For a reference input shift the recovery time is 18.4 ± 4 min on average. The maximum overshoot during the regulatory course did not exceed a value of 11.7 ± 3.2 torr. For proportional control the positional error always present is calculated as small as 3.6 ± 1.5 torr.

The dynamic behavior of the control circuit-adjustment behavior and control precision can be illustrated by a sudden disturbance in the controlled system, that means when under respiration a large restriction of the pulmonary gas-exchange area occurs. Fig. 3 shows the time course of the arterial O_2 partial pressure Pa_{O_2} as well as the course of the inspiratory O_2 concentration F_{IO_2} at the transition from PEEP to ZEEP respiration, and again after the adjustment of a positive end-expiratory pressure. When ZEEP is required the positive end-expiratory pressure adjusted to 14 cm H_2O during the respiration so far is now pushed down to 0 cm H_2O = zero end-expiratory pressure. This is done at the expiration valve. Because of alveolar collapse and following increase of the pulmonary shunt flow the O_2 partial pressure initially adjusted to 90 torr decreases. A further decrease is inhibited, however, because with the help of the control loop the described physiopathologic mechanism is compensated by proper adjustment of the inspiratory O_2 concentration. The inspiratory O_2 concentration increases until the arterial O_2 partial pressure is reset to the set point of 90 torr. When the closing volume is diminished again by repeated PEEP respiration, and when the alveolar space supplied with air is enlarged the inspiratory O_2 concentration is set back. Because of the relatively large time constant of the valve adjustment, the arterializing effect is originally determined by a PEEP-proved O_2 exchange as well as by a simultaneous and high inspiratory O_2 concentration. The arterial O_2 partial pressure rises to an overshoot, and is then adjusted again to the set point of 90 torr. In the overshoot area almost 20 torr differences between in- and expiratory values of the arterial O_2 partial pressure are to be recognized, a phenomenon firstly observed in our laboratories. This phenomenon is to be explained by the pathologic alveolar space properties of a shock lung.

Summing up, one can use the feedback control system to register during a short period of time the effects of various respiration techniques and ventilation adjustments on the arterial P_{O_2}. The optimum adjustment is to be found for each patient separately. Then the control loop provides the possibility to adjust the arterial P_{O_2} to a constant value, even if the function of the lung changes.

Dr. V. Schulz
II. Medizinische Universitätsklinik
Pneumologische Abteilung
6500 Mainz

Pneumonologie Suppl. 1976, 233-239

Über die klinische Anwendbarkeit der Methode des Totluftplateaus zur Messung des anatomischen Totraumes

K. Diether und W. K. R. Barnikol

Physiologisches Institut der Universität Mainz

On the clinical applicability of the method of the dead air plateau for measurement of the anatomical dead space

---

Abstract. The new method of the so-called dead air plateau has been expected to give reliable values of the volume of the anatomical dead space also in case of disturbed lung function. Therefore the new method is compared intraindividually in 6 male patients with different lung diseases to the known method of Bohr and to the determination of the anatomical dead space with the aid of the graphical analysis according to Fowler, using O_2 as test gas. It can be shown that only the dead space volumes measured with the new method are correct, i. e. not increased. In addition the dead space volume has the same correlation to body size which is found in healthy people. The problems to define the socalled alveolar plateau of single breath curves in pathological cases are discussed in connection with the graphical analysis according to Fowler. As examples two PO_2 single breath curves in case of disturbed lung function are given.

Key words: Anatomical dead space - Fast PO_2 electrode - Single breath curves - Dead air plateau - Alveolar plateau

Zusammenfassung: Die neue Methode des sogenannten Totluftplateaus ließ von der Konzeption her erwarten, daß sie auch bei Patienten mit gestörter Lungenfunktion richtige Werte für das anatomische Totraumvolumen liefert. Es wird daher die neue Methode intraindividuell mit der bekannten Methode nach Bohr und der Totraumbestimmung mit Hilfe der graphischen Auswertung nach Fowler (O_2 als Meßgas) an 6 männlichen Patienten mit unterschiedlichen Lungenerkrankungen verglichen. Es zeigt sich, daß nur die neue Methode den anatomischen Totraum richtig, d. h. unvergrößert, mißt. Die gemessenen Volumina zeigen zudem die bei Lungengesunden vorhandene Korrelation zur Körpergröße. Es wird die Schwierigkeit der Definierung des sogenannten alveolären Plateaus für die Fowler'sche graphische Auswertung diskutiert. Hierzu werden 2 Exspirationskurven bei gestörter Lungenfunktion exemplarisch vorgestellt.

Für die Funktionsanalyse der Lunge, insbesondere für die Messung des
Alveolarvolumens und der alveolären Ventilation auch in pathologischen
Fällen, benötigt man eine verläßliche Messung des anatomischen Totraumes.
Bisher wurden im wesentlichen die Methode nach Bohr (1891), eine Mittel-
wertmethode, und die Einatemzugmethode in der Modifikation nach Fowler
(1948) angewandt, die jedoch bekanntermaßen in pathologischen Fällen ver-
sagen. Es wurde daher die Methode des Totluftplateaus entwickelt
(Barnikol, Diether, 1975). Das Prinzip der inzwischen modifizierten
Methode sei nocheinmal kurz erläutert.

Eine PO_2-Gaselektrode mit einer 95%-Einstellzeit von höchstens
15 - 20 ms befindet sich dicht hinter der exspiratorischen Klappe eines
Atemventils. Sie mißt bei Ruheatmung des Patienten im Exspirium die
zeitliche Änderung des PO_2 und dadurch auch das sogenannte Totluftplateau.
Dieses ist im Anstieg durch die Unvollkommenheit der exspiratorischen
Klappe, im Abfall zum Alveolarplateau zusätzlich durch die Strömungs-
und Diffusionsverbreiterung im Respirationstrakt verkürzt. Die Verkür-
zung des Plateaus im Abfall wird korrigiert durch die Simulation der
Strömungs- und Diffusionsverbreiterung mit einem nachgeschalteten Phantom des Respirationstraktes und deren Messung mit einer zweiten PO_2-
Elektrode direkt hinter dem Phantom. Aus der Verschmierung im Anstieg
der zweiten PO_2-Elektrode läßt sich das ungestörte Ende des Totluft-
plateus finden. Voraussetzung für diese experimentelle Korrektur ist, daß
man die Störung der Strömung durch die exspiratorische Klappe und die
Strömungs- und Diffusionsverbreiterung im Respirationstrakt als voneinander unabhängige Vorgänge betrachtet, wodurch sie zeitlich umkehrbar
sind. Das mit einem Pneumotachographen gleichzeitig gemessene, exspirierte Volumen entspricht im Endpunkt des korrigierten Totluftplateaus
dem anatomischen Totraum.

Ein intraindividueller Vergleich der Methode des Totluftplateaus mit
der Meßmethode nach Bohr und der VD-Bestimmung mit Hilfe der graphischen Auswertung des O_2-Plateaus nach Fowler hatte bei Lungengesunden innerhalb der Fehlergrenze die gleichen Totraumvolumina ergeben.
Zusätzlich hatte ein interindividueller Vergleich unserer mit Hilfe der
graphischen Auswertung nach Fowler erhaltenen VD-Volumina mit nach der
klassischen Fowler-Methode gemessenen VD-Volumina von Hart, Cook,
Orzalesi (1963) und Chiang et al. (1973) an großen gesunden Populationen
übereinstimmende Werte gebracht (Diether, Barnikol, 1975). Daraus
leiteten wir die Legitimation ab auch bei Lungenkranken uns auf die
Fowler' sche graphische Auswertung beschränken zu dürfen.

Es sollte nun die Wertigkeit der neuen Methode bei pathologischen Fällen aufgezeigt werden. Es war nämlich von der Konzeption der Methode her
zu erwarten, daß das anatomische Totraumvolumen auch bei Lungenkranken
richtig gemessen wird. Bei 6 Patienten mit isolierten sowie kombinierten
restriktiven und obstruktiven Lungenerkrankungen verschiedenster Genese
und unterschiedlichsten Ausmaßes wurde der anatomische Totraum mit
den 3 Methoden gemessen. Durch diesen intraindividuellen Vergleich er-
hielten wir Meßwerte, die in Abb. 1 zusammengestellt sind.

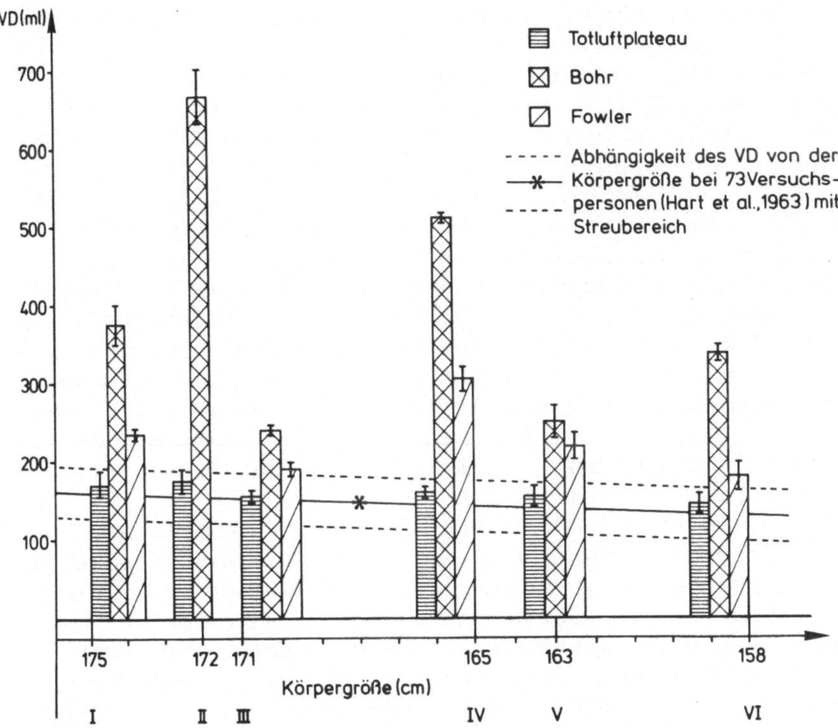

Abb. 1. Intraindividueller Vergleich der Methode des Totluftplateaus mit der Meßmethode nach Bohr und der VD-Bestimmung mit Hilfe der graphischen Auswertung nach Fowler an 6 Patienten mit gestörter Lungenfunktion

Die vergleichenden Meßergebnisse sind von 6 männlichen Patienten mit von links nach rechts abnehmender Körpergröße dargestellt. Die Höhe der Säule repräsentiert jeweils das gemessene Totraumvolumen in ml. Die Standardabweichungen sind zusätzlich eingezeichnet. Die linke Säule stellt jeweils die mit der Methode des Totluftplateaus gefundenen anatomischen Totraumwerte dar. Die rechten schräg schraffierten Säulen beinhalten die Totraumvolumina nach der graphischen Auswertung nach Fowler. Bei Patient II war eine solche Auswertung nicht möglich. Die Gründe dafür werden weiter unten erläutert. Die mittleren Säulen geben die Totraumvolumina wieder, die gesondert mit der bekannten Methode von Bohr gemessen wurden. Diese Totraumvolumina nach Bohr liegen erwartungsgemäß um ein Vielfaches über der Größe des anatomischen Totraumes, da diese Methode bekanntermaßen die alveoläre Totraumventilation mitbestimmt.

Hart, Orzalesi, und Cook bestimmten 1963 mit der Fowler'schen Methode an 73 gesunden Probanden verschiedener Körpergröße den anatomischen Totraum. Sie stellten fest, daß das anatomische Totraumvolumen unter sonst vergleichbaren Bedingungen eng mit der Körpergröße korreliert.

Diese Korrelation zeigt die von links nach rechts abfallende Gerade der Abbildung für den Körpergrößenbereich von 158 - 175 cm. Die gestrichelten Linien begrenzen den interindividuellen Streubereich.

Man erkennt, daß sämtliche mit der Methode des Totluftplateaus gemessenen Totraumvolumina innerhalb des Streubereiches liegen und somit nicht nur größenordnungsmäßig richtig sind, sondern auch diese Korrelation zur Körpergröße zeigen. Die VD-Volumina bestimmt nach der graphischen Auswertung nach Fowler, repräsentiert in den jeweils rechten Säulen, liegen jedoch außerhalb des interindividuellen Streubereiches.

Bei der sogenannten Fowler' schen Methode wird in der exspirierten Luft gleichzeitig das exspirierte Volumen und der Konzentrationsübergang eines Gases vom Totluftniveau zum Alveolarluftniveau gemessen. Zur Festlegung des Übergangspunktes muß ein alveoläres Plateau des betreffenden Meßgases vorhanden sein, wenigstens in Form einer Geraden mit konstanter Steigung. Bekanntermaßen ist diese Forderung bei pathologisch veränderten Lungen nur unzureichend gewährleistet und die Definierung des alveolären Plateaus dadurch sehr willkürlich.

Setzt man den erwähnten, schnellen PO_2-Detektor dicht in den Atemgasstrom unmittelbar hinter die eigens konstruierte exspiratorische Klappe, welche den Atemstrom so wenig wie möglich beeinflußt, so gelangt das Konzentrationsprofil des Atemgasstromes nur minimal gestört an den PO_2-Detektor. Durch diese experimentellen Bedingungen ist es möglich Feinheiten der Exspirationskurven zu erfassen. Bei den so gemessenen Exspirationskurven von lungenkranken Patienten findet man neben dem Endplateau, sogenannte Zwischenplateaus; d. h. das alveoläre Plateau gibt es beim Lungenkranken in der Regel nicht.

Zwei Exspirationskurven von zwei männlichen Patienten mit gestörter Lungenfunktion seien exemplarisch vorgestellt.

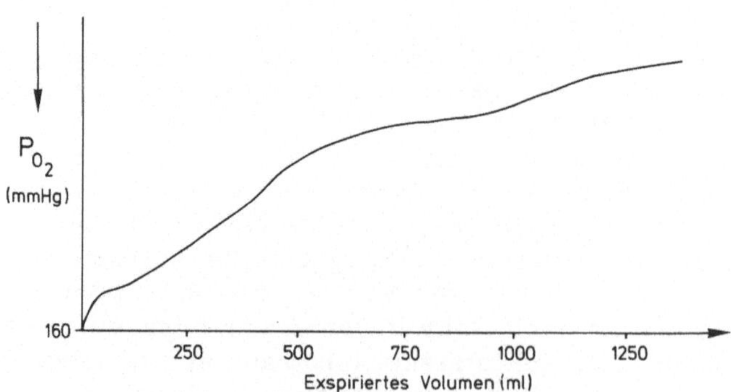

Abb. 2. Beispiel 1 für die PO_2-Änderung in der exspirierten Alveolarluft bei gestörter Lungenfunktion

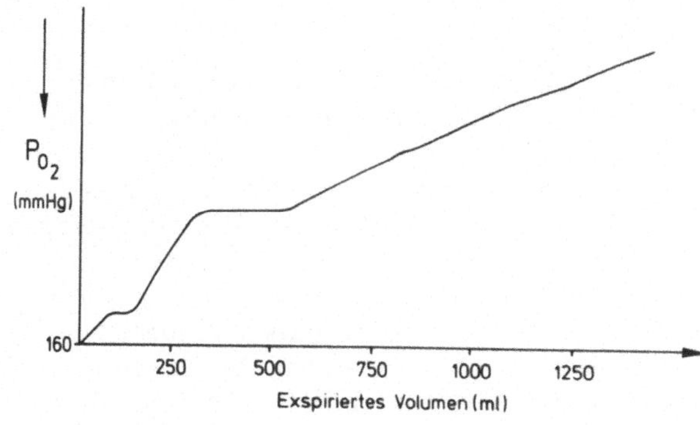

Abb. 3. Beispiel 2 für die PO_2-Änderung in der exspirierten Alveolarluft bei gestörter Lungenfunktion

Auf Abb. 2 ist die PO_2-Abnahme gegen das exspirierte Alveolarvolumen aufgetragen. Die Kurve läßt den normalen S-förmigen Kurvenverlauf des Gesunden nicht einmal mehr im Ansatz erkennen, sondern zeigt einen völlig deformierten Kurvenverlauf. Ursache hierfür sind wahrscheinlich eine ungleichmäßige Verteilung der Inspirationsluft und/oder eine asynchrone Entleerung verschiedner Alveolarbezirke während der Exspiration. Die Exspirationskurve hat neben einem kurzen Endplateau zwei weitere Zwischenplateaus. Es stehen also in diesem Fall zur Bestimmung des Totraumvolumens mit Hilfe der graphischen Auswertung nach Fowler drei Plateaus zur Auswahl. Zieht man zur Auswertung nach Fowler das Endplateau heran, so resultiert in diesem Falle eine Totraumvolumen, das größenordnungsmäßig im Bereich des Bohr'schen Totraums liegt. Wählt man jedoch die Zwischenplateaus, so erhält man Totraumvolumina, die deutlich über bzw. unter dem richtigen anatomischen Totraumvolumen liegen.

Die Abb. 3 zeigt die PO_2-Abnahme in der exspirierten Alveolarluft, die wir beim Patienten II gemessen haben. Die Kurve hat zwei Zwischenplateaus, die besonders deutlich ausgeprägt sind. Eine Bestimmung des anatomischen Totraumvolumens mit Hilfe der Auswertung nach Fowler ist in diesem Fall, wie bereits erwähnt, nicht möglich.

Zusammenfassend bleibt festzustellen, daß durch die geschilderten vergleichenden Meßergebnisse bestätigt wurde, daß mit der Methode des Totluftplateaus auch bei starken Lungenfunktionsstörungen ein richtiges anatomisches Totraumvolumen gemessen wird, wohingegen die beiden bekannten Methoden versagen. Die Methode des Totluftplateaus hat darüber hinaus weitere Vorteile, auch in Hinsicht auf den Patienten: Sie benötigt keine Hilfsgase; bei spontaner Luftatmung liefert jeder Atemzug einen Meßwert für das Totraumvolumen. Die Meßmethode ist wenig zeitraubend; sie erfordert keine besondere Mitarbeit vom Patienten und ist für diesen nicht belastend.

Wir danken Herrn Prof. Thews für die freundliche Unterstützung der Arbeit.

LITERATUR

Barnikol, W.K.R., Döhring, W., Diefenthäler, E.: An extremely fast
   Pt-electrode for O_2-analysis in air. Proc. Int. Union. Physiol. Sci.
   IX, 41 (1971)
Barnikol, W.K.R., Diether, K.: Eine neue Methode zur Messung des
   anatomischen Totraumes mit Hilfe des Totluftplateaus. Pneumonologie
   152, 227-233 (1975)
Diether, K., Barnikol, W.K.R.: The new method of the dead air plateau
   for measurement of the anatomical dead space, intraindividually
   compared to the single breath method of Fowler and to the method
   of Bohr measured in healthy people. Pflügers Arch. Suppl. to Vol.
   355, R 43 (1975)
Döhring, W., Diefenthäler, E., Barnikol, W.K.R.: The production and
   application of 0,2 to 1,0 μ polytetrafluoroethylene membranes to
   continuous polarographic measurement of oxygen tension in the gas
   phase. Oxygen Supply, S. 80-91. München-Berlin-Wien: Urban &
   Schwarzenberg 1973
Fowler, W.S.: Lung function studies II. The respiratory dead space.
   Amer. Physiol. 154, 405-416 (1948)
Hart, M.C., Orzalesi, M.M., Cook, D.C.: Relation between anatomic
   respiratory dead space and body size and lung volume. J. appl.
   Physiol. 18, 519-522 (1963)

Dr.K.Diether
Physiologisches Institut
der Universität Mainz
Saarstrasse 21
6500 Mainz

DISKUSSION

U.Smidt, Moers: Ich stimme Ihnen zu, daß bei lungenkranken Patienten
das Alveolarplateau der exspiratorischen PO_2- und PCO_2-Kurven verloren
geht, aber wir haben niemals solche Zwischenplateaus gesehen, wie Sie sie
gezeigt haben. Wir schreiben diese Kurven ja seit vielen Jahren bei jedem
Patienten gegen die Zeit und gegen das Volumen, aber solche Zwischenplateaus kann ich mir nur als Artefakte erklären.

K. Diether, Mainz: Es könnte auch ein methodischer Artefakt sein, daß man
bisher solche Zwischenplateaus nicht gesehen hat. Ich nehme an, daß ihre
exspiratorischen PO_2 und PCO_2-Kurven in herkömmlicher Art mit dem
Massenspektrometer gemessen worden sind. Üblicherweise haben solche
Geräte eine Verzögerungszeit (Totzeit und Einstellzeit) von etwa 100 ms.
Die von uns gefundenen Schwankungen des PO_2 beim Übergang zum Alveo-
larniveau dauern etwa 200 ms. Zur zeitlichen Auflösung solcher Vorgänge

reicht ein Detektor mit einer Einstellcharakteristik von 100 ms nicht aus-
Die von uns verwendeten PO_2-Elektroden haben hingegen in der Regel eine
Einstellzeit von 15 ms.

Im Übrigen ging es uns in diesem Zusammenhang darum, die Validität
unserer Totraummethode an Lungenkranken aufzuzeigen und nicht darum,
den Beweis für solche Zwischenplateaus zu erbringen. Es handelt sich
lediglich um eine erste Beobachtung. Wir sind auch der Meinung, daß die
Existenz solcher Zwischenplateaus mit weiteren unabhängigen Methoden
bewiesen werden sollte.

Pneumonologie Suppl. 1976, 241-248

Zum Problem der herzsynchronen Partialdruckschwankungen von Atemgasen

M. Reinert, D. Heise, W. Mall und F. Trendelenburg

Medizinische Universitätsklinik, Abteilung Pneumologie, Homburg/Saar

---

Abstract. In 3 patients without severe bronchial disease the expiratory CO_2 and O_2 tensions of lobar and some segmental bronchi have been measured during bronchoscopy. In 2 cases bronchoscopy was done in local anesthesia. There were recorded cardiogenic oscillations of the gas tensions in all parts of the lung, but in the right lung they were only week. Oscillations were more marked during inspiration. The highest oscillations were found during inspiration in the diastole of the heart between the bronchi of the left upper and lower lobe. Furthermore there were differences between the lingula (with the highest oscillations) and the lower lobe (with little oscillations). The findings of the diffuse distribution of oscillations in the whole lung, the concentration differences between right and left lung and left upper to lower lobe may be explained by the conclusion that there exists a functional slow space, anatomically not limited, and the commonly accepted, gravity-dependen regional differences of gas concentrations between upper and lower parts of the lung.

Key words: Mass-spectrometry - Regional expiratory gas concentrations - Bronchoscopy - Cardiogenic oscillations.

Zusammenfassung. Bei 3 Patienten ohne wesentliche Erkrankung der Bronchien wurden während der Bronchoskopie die expiratorischen Atemgase CO_2 und O_2 und die dabei auftretenden kardiogenen Oszillationen in den verschiedenen Lappenbronchien mit einem Massenspektrometer gemessen. Oszillationen fanden sich vor allem links, rechts meistens nur angedeutet. Die höchsten Konzentrationsschwankungen zeigten die Oszillationen diastolisch während der Inspiration im Lingualbronchus, es folgten Oberlappen- und schließlich Unterlappenbronchus. Aus dem Verteilungsmuster der Oszillationen in der gesamten Lunge, aus den unterschiedlichen Konzentrationen zwischen linkem und rechtem Bronchialsystem und den Differenzen zwischen Lingula, Oberlappen einerseits und Unterlappen andererseits wurde geschlossen, daß beim Gesunden ein sogenannter funktioneller slow space besteht, der diffus über die gesamte Lunge verteilt ist. Unabhängig davon bestehen jedoch die bekannten, anatomisch ab-

grenzbaren, schwerkraftabhängigen Verteilungsstörungen zwischen Ober-
und Untergeschossen.

Schlüsselwörter: Massenspektrometer - regionale Atemgasanalyse -
Bronchoskopie - Kardiogene Oszillationen.

Im Alveolarteil expiratorischer Atemgaskurven sieht man gelegentlich
flache Oszillationen. Bei bestimmten Atemmanövern, z.B. dem closing
volume, sind diese Wellen sehr ausgeprägt. 2 Fragen sind dabei von besonderem Interesse: wie entstehen diese Oszillationen und wo entstehen
sie. Untersuchungen über die Herkunft ergaben unterschiedliche Ergebnisse (Dahlstrom, 1954; Langer, 1960; Fowler, 1961 und 1966; Engel,
1973 und 1974; von Nieding, 1975). Da bisher zur Bestimmung der Lokalisation systematisch nur am Mund gemessen wurde, versuchten wir, durch
intrabronchiale Messungen weitere Aufschlüsse zu erhalten.

METHODEN UND PROBANDEN

2 Patienten wurden in Lokal-, 1 Patient wurde in Allgemeinanästhesie
bronchoskopiert. Zur Atemgasanalyse wurde ein Massenspektrometer Varian
MAT (GDM) benutzt mit einem von Heise (1974) konstruierten viskos-viskos
arbeitenden Einlaßsystem. Die Einstellzeiten (10-90%) lagen bei 30 ms,
der Gasverbrauch betrug 30 ml/min. Die expiratorischen Atemgaskurven
(CO_2, O_2) und das EKG wurden synchron auf einem Cardirex-Sechsfach-
schreiber (Siemens) registriert. Mit Hilfe des EKG wurde die Zugehörig-
keit von Teilen der Oszillationen zur Systole und Diastole abgeschätzt. Die
Meßkapillare des Massenspektrometers wurde über das Führungsinstrument
des Bronchoskops in die gewünschten Bronchien und Segmente dirigiert.

ERGEBNISSE

Abb. 1 zeigt die während Allgemeinanästhesie in Apnoephasen registrierten
CO_2-Oszillationen in den verschiedenen Abschnitten des linken Bronchialsystems. Im rechten Bronchialsystem wurden nur flache Ausschläge festgestellt. Diese sind nicht aufgezeichnet. Auffällig sind die Unterschiede
von Konzentration und Form in den verschiedenen Bronchien. Die höchsten

---

Abb. 1. CO_2-Oszillationen während der Apnoephase bei Bronchoskopie in
Allgemeinanästhesie: von oben nach unten im linken Hauptbronchus
(Hpt.-Br.li.), Oberlappenabgang (OL), Lingula, zwischen Oberlappen/
Unterlappensegment (OL/B 6), B 6, Unterlappenbronchus (UL) Unter-
lappensegmentbronchus (UL-Segm.) Ordinate: CO_2 in %, Abszisse: Zeit
in Sekunden

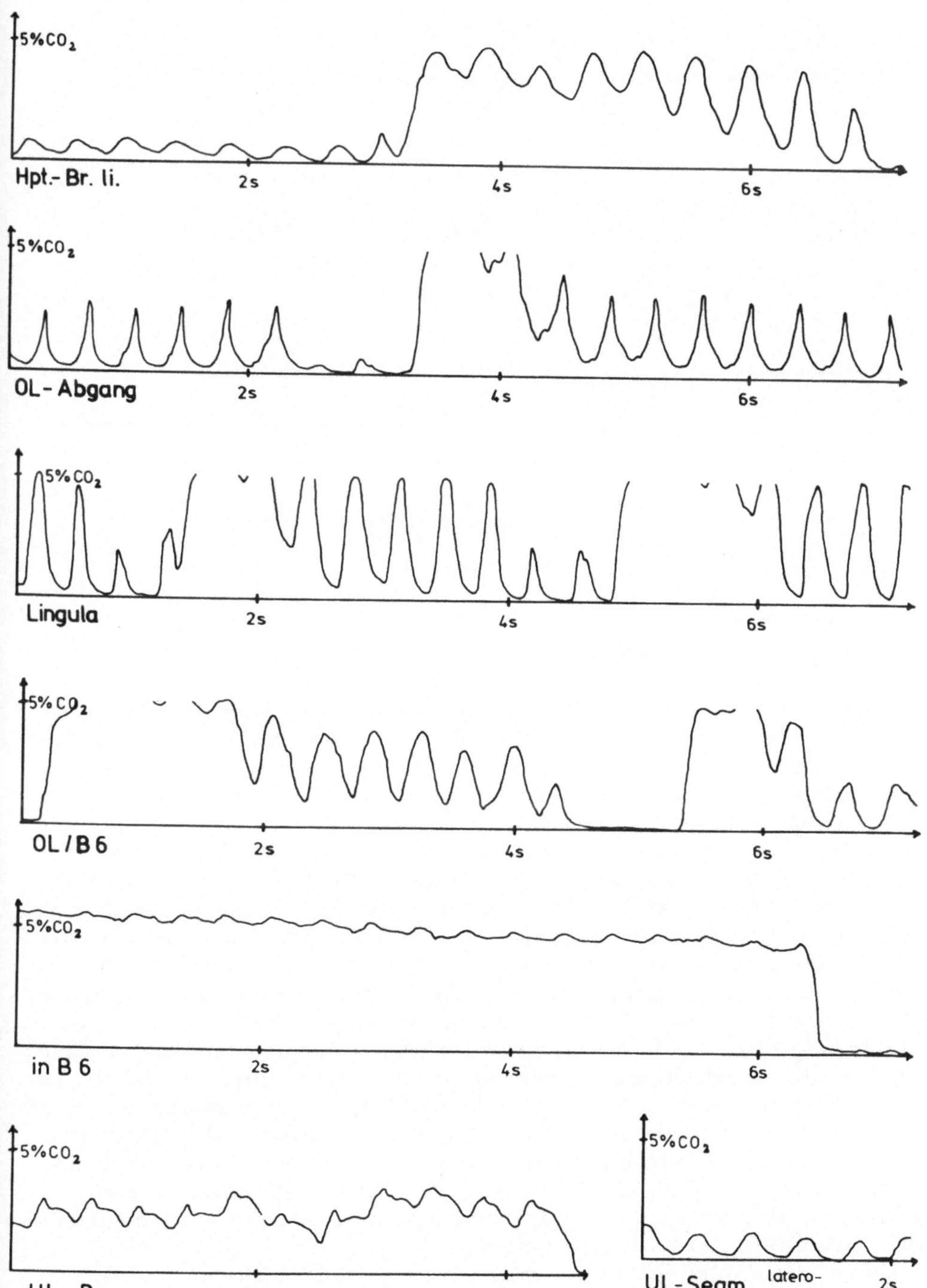

5%CO₂
Hpt.- Br. li.
2s
4s
6s
5%CO₂
OL- Abgang
2s
4s
6s
5%CO₂
Lingula
2s
4s
6s
5%CO₂
OL / B 6
2s
4s
6s
5%CO₂
in B 6
2s
4s
6s
5%CO₂
UL- Br.
2s
4s
5%CO₂
UL- Segm.
latero-basal
2s

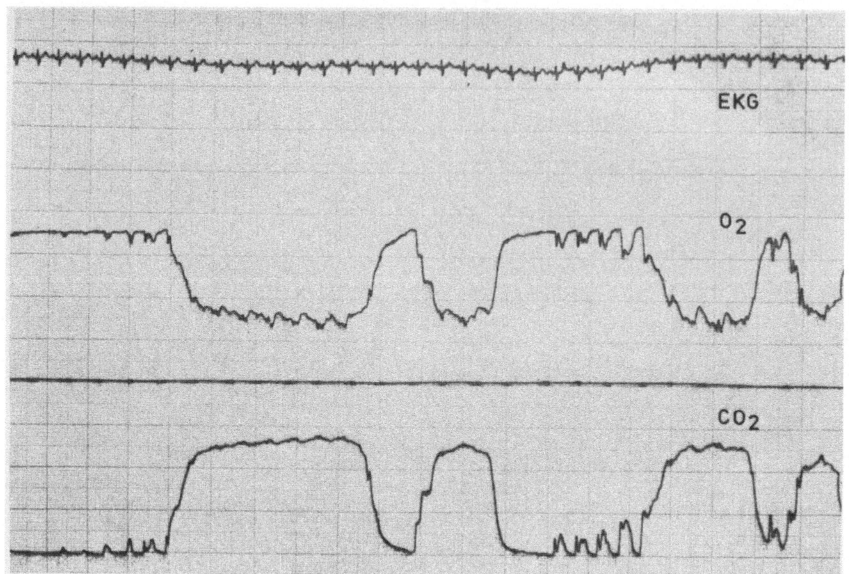

Abb. 2. Bronchoskopie in Lokalanästhesie. Vorschieben der Meßsonde
im linken Hauptbronchus, Zunahme vor allem der inspiratorischen
Oszillationen an den distalen Meßstellen

CO_2-Konzentrationen wurden in der Lingula und im Oberlappen gemessen.
Der Unterlappensegmentbronchus B 6 war in Allgemeinanästhesie offensichtlich unbelüftet, es wurde ein Plateau von etwa 4% CO_2 festgestellt mit auf-
gelagerten kleinen Oszillationen. Die Oszillationen des Unterlappens sind
von der Form her besonders auffällig.

Bei einem spontan atmenden Probanden, bronchoskopiert in Lokalanästhesie, zeigten sich in der Trachea bis zur Bifurkation exspiratorisch
im Alveolarteil flache CO_2 und O_2-Oszillationen. Auffällig sind die unterschiedlichen Konzentrationsänderungen von O_2 und CO_2. Im linken Hauptbronchus (Abb. 2) sieht man mit dem Vorschieben des Katheters eine
Zunahme der Konzentration von CO_2- beziehungsweise einen Konzentrations-
abfall der O_2-Oszillationen. Die absoluten Konzentrationsänderungen be-
tragen für CO_2 etwa 0,8%, für O_2 etwa 1%. Die Oszillationen des CO_2 sind
während der Exspiration fast verschwunden, die Konzentrationsschwankungen der O_2-Oszillationen bleiben sehr deutlich. Am interessantesten sind
die Oszillationen zwischen Abgang des Ober- und zu Beginn des Unterlappenbronchus. Man sieht inspiratorisch ungewöhnlich hohe Konzentrationsänderungen (Abb. 3), CO_2 erreicht 1,5%, O_2 1,8%. Exspiratorisch sind
die CO_2-Oszillationen wiederum fast verschwunden, die O_2-Wellen nur un-
wesentlich schwächer als inspiratorisch.

In beiden Beispielen ist die Form im Bereich des Oberlappen- und
Unterlappenabganges sehr auffällig. Die Zuordnung des Verlaufs der Oszil-
lationen zur Diastole oder Systole (Abb. 3) ergibt inspiratorisch in der
Diastole einen Konzentrationsanstieg von CO_2 und einen Abfall von O_2.

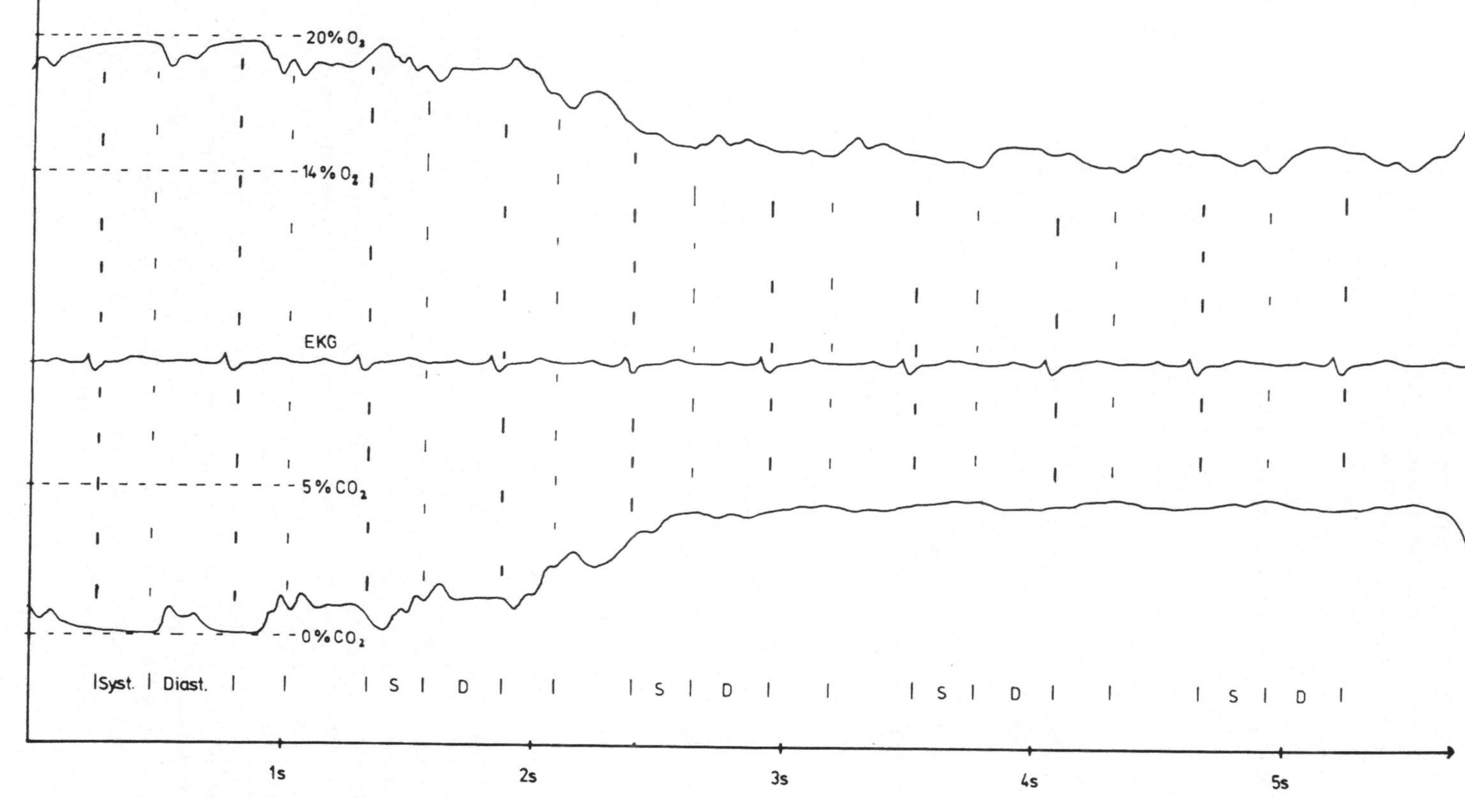

Abb. 3. Bronchoskopie in Lokalanästhesie. Meßstelle zwischen Oberlappen- und Unterlappenbronchus. Inspiratorisch hohe CO_2-Oszillationen, spiegelbildlich die O_2-Oszillationen, synchron das EKG, Zeitverzögerungen zwischen EKG und Massenspektrometer bereits korrigiert. Ordinate: O_2 und CO_2 in %, Abszisse: Zeit in sekunden. S: Systole, D: Diastole

In der Systole tendiert CO_2 zunächst zur Nullinie, steigt aber bereits
prädiastolisch wieder an. Die Sauerstoffkonzentration verhält sich spiegelbildlich. Expiratorisch findet sich ein völlig anderes Verhalten: an derselben Meßstelle sind die CO_2-Oszillationen fast verschwunden, der Sauerstoff fällt während der Systole langsam linear ab, in der Diastole entsteht
ein Peak mit hoher O_2-Konzentration.

Auf der rechten Seite des Bronchialsystems wurden bei allen Broncho-
skopierten ebenfalls Oszillationen gefunden, sie waren jedoch im Gegensatz zu links sehr flach.

DISKUSSION

Die Ergebnisse der intrabronchialen Atemgasanalyse führen zu folgenden
Informationen: Oszillationen sind im gesamten Bronchialsystem nachweisbar, links stärker als rechts. Die Oszillationen wurden bei Normal-
atmung im Liegen nicht nur exspiratorisch sondern noch weitaus stärker
inspiratorisch gefunden. Die höchsten Konzentrationsänderungen wurden
inspiratorisch während der Diastole in Lingula und Oberlappenbronchus gemessen, die komplexeste Form wurde zwischen Abgang des Ober- und
Unterlappens gefunden. Auffällig ist bei der Messung an dieser Stelle auch
das in- und expiratorisch spiegelbildliche Verhalten des Sauerstoffes:
Diastolisch kommt es inspiratorisch zu einem O_2-Abfall, exspiratorisch
dagegen zu einem Anstieg.

Oszillierende Partialdruckschwankungen sind nur unter 2 Voraussetzungen denkbar: Herz und große Gefäße müssen mechanisch die Lunge
in Diastole und Systole beeinflussen, ferner müssen ventilatorische Verteilungsstörungen im Alveolarraum vorhanden sein. Die intrabronchialen
Atemgasanalysen sind für die Frage nach Lokalisation und Herkunft der
Oszillationen sehr aufschlußreich.

1. Die Lokalisation der Oszillationen

Über die Lokalisation der Oszillationen gehen die Meinungen auseinander.
Dahlstrom vermutet schlecht belüftete Alveolen in der Lungenperipherie.
Langer nimmt an, daß die größten ventilatorischen Verteilungsstörungen
in den hilusnahen Lungenbezirken infolge einer dort vorherrschenden
höheren Compliance liegen. Fowler schließlich machte die unterschiedlichen
ventilatorischen Verteilungen zwischen Ober- und Untergeschossen für
die Entstehung der Oszillationen verantwortlich.

Der Nachweis der Oszillationen im gesamten Bronchialsystem bedeutet
jedoch, daß Fehlverteilungen diffus in allen Lungeneinheiten vorkommen.
Der "slow space" des Gesunden ist damit als funktionelle Einheit anzusehen
und nicht streng anatomisch zu lokalisieren. Dagegen weisen die zwischen
Oberlappen und Lingula einerseits und Unterlappen andererseits gefundenen
unterschiedlichen inspiratorischen Konzentrationsschwankungen von CO_2
oder O_2 in der Diastole des Herzens darauf hin, daß neben den diffusen

Fehlverteilungen auch Differenzen zwischen anatomisch abgrenzbaren Ge-
bieten bestehen. Es handelt sich dabei also um Verteilungsstörungen zwischer
Ober- und Untergeschossen, die bereits von Fowler als ursächlich für die
Oszillationen angesehen wurden und die vor allem beim closing-volume-
Manöver zu sehr kräftigen Oszillationen führen. Diese Oszillationen sind
nicht identisch mit den bei Spontanatmung intrabronchial gemessenen Gas-
druckänderungen.

2. Der Entstehungsmechanismus

Sowohl Dahlstrom als auch Langer machten den Pumpeffekt der großen
Lungengefäße für die Entstehung der Oszillationen verantwortlich, Fowler
dagegen den mechanischen Einfluß des Herzens. Die intrabronchialen
Messungen unterstützen die Theorie von Fowler. Dies läßt sich vor allem
an den unterschiedlichen Konzentrationen zwischen rechtem und linkem
Bronchialsystem ablesen. Im rechten Bronchialsystem, also herzfern,
sind wenig und sehr flache Oszillationen feststellbar. Da es unwahrscheinlich ist, daß sich rechte und linke Lunge bezüglich der Ventilation stark
unterscheiden, muß die Ursache in der Nachbarschaft der linken Lunge
zum Herzen, vor allem zur Lingula gesucht werden. Diese Beziehung wirkt
sich vor allem für die Belüftung der Lingula sehr günstig aus: sie ist infolge
ihres anatomischen Aufbaus sehr schlecht belüftbar. Während der Inspiration wird sie im Rhythmus des Herzschlages zusätzlich ventiliert. Vermutlich wirkt sich der Herzschlag auch in den Bronchioli zwischen Mischzone
und Alveolen in ähnlicher Weise aus (Engel und Mitarb.).

LITERATUR

Dahlstrom, H., Murphy, J., Roos, A.: Cardiogenic Oscillations in Com-
position of Expired Gas. The "Pneumocardiogram". J. Appl. Physiol.
7, 335 (1954)
Engel, L., Menkes, H., Wood, L., Utz, G., Joubert, J., Macklem, P.:
Gas mixing during breath holding studied by intrapulmonary gas sampling
J. Appl. Physiol. 35, 9 (1973)
Engel, L., Utz, G., Wood, L., Macklem, P.: Ventilation distribution in
anatomical lung units. J. Appl. Physiol. 37, 194 (1974)
Fowler, K., Read, J.: Cardiac oscillations in expired gas tensions, and
regional pulmonary blood flow. J. Appl. Physiol. 16, 863 (1961)
Fowler, K.: The Mass Spectrometer in the Analysis of Regional Lung
Function. Scand. J. Resp. Dis. Suppl. 62, 73 (1966)
Heise, D., Reinert, M., Walisch, W.: Improvements to Inlet Systems with
Special Reference to the Time Constants. Pneumologie 151, 245 (1975)
Langer, G., Bornstein, D., Fishman, A.: Cardiogenic oscillations in
expired nitrogen and regional alveolar hypoventilation. J. Appl. Physiol.
15, 855 (1960)

von Nieding, G. , Löllgen, H. , Krekeler, H. , Smidt, U. : Heart Synchronous Partial Pressure Oscillations in the Alveolar Plateau and Ventilatory Distribution. Pneumologie $\underline{151}$, 277 (1975)

Prof. Dr. M. Reinert
Viktoriastraße 10
6600 Saarbrücken

Prof. Dr. F. Trendelenburg
Direktor der Abt. für
Pneumologie
Medizinische Universitätsklinik
6650 Homburg/Saar

Pneumonologie Suppl. 1976, 249-251

Experimental Studies on Airway Smooth Muscle Responses[*]

Arend Bouhuys

Yale University Lung Research Center and John B. Pierce Foundation,
New Haven, Connecticut, U.S.A.

Abstract. Airway smooth muscle in vivo is exposed to stimuli from
chemical mediators, neurotransmitters, prostaglandins and exogenous
drugs. Contractile responses of airway smooth muscle, in asthma and in
experimental guinea pig anaphylaxis, may depend to a large extent on the
balance between these contractile and relaxant stimuli, and on their inter-
actions.

Key words: Bronchial asthma - Guinea pig anaphylaxis - β-adrenergic
blockade - Cholinergic blockade - Hydrocortisone - Prostaglandins.

Contractile responses of airway smooth muscle to antigens in the IgE-
mediated allergic response, as well as to other physical and chemical
stimuli, are thought to be important in the pathogenesis of bronchial asthma in man. Studies in man have indicated that these responses vary quan-
titatively, with persons with bronchial asthma often but not invariably being more sensitive to different kinds of contractile stimuli than persons
who do not have bronchial asthma. Our studies attempt to learn which factors influence the sensitivity of airway smooth muscle to contractile stimuli in intact guinea pigs as well as in isolated guinea pig tracheal preparations. The results may help to understand at least some of the factors
which determine the outcome of an antigen-antibody reaction or of environmental exposures to inhaled agents, in terms of the degree of airway nar-
rowing that results from smooth muscle contraction.

Airway responses in intact guinea pigs are measured from breath-by-
breath recordings of dynamic lung compliance, tidal volume and other
parameters of lung function, recorded in the spontaneously breathing animal by suitable transducers and an analog computer (Douglas et al., 1972).
Early results showed that the sensitivity of guinea pigs to inhaled histamine (in terms of the aerosol dose required to decrease dynamic compli-

---

[*] Supported in part by a Specialized Center of Research grant (HE-14179)
from the National Heart and Lung Institute, National Institutes of Health,
Bethesda, Maryland, U.S.A.

ance by 50%) varied about 100-fold among individual animals, with a log-normal distribution (Douglas et al. , 1972). Later, Popa et al. (1974) showed that, in guinea pigs sensitized to egg albumen, the response to antigen correlated with each individual animal's sensitivity to histamine. Thus, the severity of the anaphylactic response in guinea pigs appears to depend, at least in part, upon the responsiveness of the effector tissue, airway smooth muscle, to the chemical mediator, histamine.

We have studied the influence of several autonomic drugs on the guinea pig's airway-constrictor response to inhaled histamine. In these experiments, β-adrenergic blocking drugs (e. g. , propranolol) often increased the animal's response to histamine, while a cholinergic-blocking drug, atropine, always decreased the response. In addition, physostigmine, a cholinesterase-inhibiting drug, increased the response to histamine. The results with these and other drugs could be interpreted by assuming that the response of guinea pig airway smooth muscle to inhaled histamine is determined, to a large extent, by the balance between β-adrenergic and cholinergic stimuli which impinge on airway smooth muscle. β-adrenergic stimuli decrease the response, while cholinergic stimuli have the opposite effect. Hence, β-adrenergic blocking drugs increase the response, while atropine inhibits it (Douglas et al. , 1973). In recent work, we have found that hydrocortisone also inhibits the response to histamine in guinea pigs, and that this effect of hydrocortisone is abolished by propranolol (Brink et al. , 1975). Hence, the protective action of hydrocortisone may depend on increased effectiveness of endogenous β-adrenergic stimuli, perhaps through interference of hydrocortisone with extraneuronal uptake of catecholamines.

Recently, prostaglandins, as well as their precursors and metabolites, have received much attention as substances which may be involved in the pathogenesis of human asthma. Their role is as yet not clear, but it may be of interest that several contractile agonists (histamine, acetylcholine, serotonin, barium and potassium) may release prostaglandins from the isolated guinea-pig tracheal preparation (Orehek et al. , 1973, 1975). This release has been demonstrated directly for histamine and for acetylcholine, and indirectly (by examining the action of prostaglandin-synthesis-inhibiting drugs) for the other agonists. The release of prostaglandins is probably a consequence of the mechanical process of contraction and may depend on cell membrane deformation in the mucosa, submucosa or smooth muscle, or in all of these tissues. Release of prostaglandins from the guinea pig trachea can also be elicited by gentle mechanical stimulation of the mucosa but not of the adventitia (Orehek et al. , 1975).

The released prostaglandins are probably important in the maintenance of the basal tone of airway smooth muscle in the guinea pig. They also influence the degree of contraction elicited by histamine, acetylcholine, serotonin, barium and potassium. When synthesis of prostaglandins is inhibited by drugs such as indomethacin, responses to low doses of these agonists are decreased, while responses to high agonist doses are potentiated. After indomethacin has been washed out of the organ bath, the original responses to contractile agonists can be restored by addition of arachidonic acid, a prostaglandin-precursor substance, to the bath (Orehek et al. , 1975). As yet there is no clear evidence that prostaglandins play a role in contractile airway responses in vivo. This may indicate that their role is of minor, if any, importance, or it might merely indicate our inability to clearly separate the different humoral factors that influence airway smooth muscle responses in in vivo experiments.

The present results can explain certain observations made previously in patients with bronchial asthma, for instance, the inhibitory effect of hexamethonium bromide on responses to inhaled histamine (Bouhuys et al., 1960). They may also offer a basis for hypotheses concerning airway hyper-responsiveness in asthma. Perhaps most importantly, they suggest that airway smooth muscle in vivo is subject to a large variety of humoral stimuli - chemical mediators, neurotransmitters, prostaglandins and exogenous drugs. The study of the interaction between these diverse stimuli may be rewarding in future work on the pathogenesis of bronchial asthma.

REFERENCES

Bouhuys, A., Jönsson, R., Lichtneckert, S., Lindell, S. E., Lundgren, C., Lundin, G., Ringquist, T.: Effect of histamine on pulmonary ventilation in man. Clin. Sci. 19, 79-94 (1960)

Brink, C., Ridgway, P., Douglas, J. S., Bouhuys, A.: Anti-inflammatory drugs and airway responses in the guinea pig. Fed. Proc. 34, 798 (1975) (Abs.)

Douglas, J. S., Dennis, M. W., Ridgway, P., Bouhuys, A.: Airway dilatation and constriction in spontaneously breathing guinea pigs. J. Pharmacol. Exp. Ther. 180, 98-109 (1972)

Douglas, J. S., Dennis, M. W., Ridgway, P., Bouhuys, A.: Airway constriction in guinea pigs: interaction of histamine and autonomic drugs. J. Pharmacol. Exp. Ther. 184, 169-179 (1973)

Orehek, J., Douglas, J. S., Lewis, A. J., Bouhuys, A.: Prostaglandin regulation of airway smooth muscle tone. Nature New Biol. 245, 84-85 (1973)

Orehek, J., Douglas, J. S., Bouhuys, A.: Contractile responses of the guinea pig trachea in vitro: modification by prostaglandin-synthesis inhibiting drugs. J. Pharmacol. Exp. Ther. 194, 554-564 (1975)

Popa, V., Douglas, J. S., Bouhuys, A.: Airway responses to histamine, acetylcholine, and antigen in sensitized guinea pigs. J. Lab. Clin. Med. 84, 225-234 (1974)

Prof. Dr. Arend Bouhuys
Lung Research Center
Yale University
333 Cedar Street
New Haven, Connecticut 06510
U. S. A.

Pneumonologie Suppl. 1976, 253-258

Reflektorische und lokal-irridativ induzierte Bronchokonstriktion

K. Lanser, E. Kaukel und V. Sill

Aus der I. Medizinischen Klinik des Universitätskrankenhauses
Hamburg-Eppendorf

Abstract. Respiratory parameters of 42 spontaneously breathing rabbits
during intratraceal administration of 0,9% NaCl, solution of histamine and
acetylcholine 3% before and after bilateral vagotomy are reported.

The airway resistance is significantly elevated following the application
of isotonic saline (204%), histamine (299%) and acetylcholine (484%) compared
with a unexposed controllgroup.

The NaCl-induced bronchialconstriction was of short duration, whereas
histamine and acetylcholine were effective during a longer period.

Immediately after vagotomy isotonic saline was ineffective in producing
a bronchial constriction, the acetylcholine effect was reduced to 137%, that
of histamine to 204%.

NaCL application did not alter the bloodgassituation, whereas acetylcholine and histamine caused a marked hypoxemia of approximetely 60 mm
Hg.

These findings may indicate that bronchial reaction following the application of isotonic saline or acetylcholine is mediated by reflex mechanism,
the action of histamine seems to be more a local irritation.

Zusammenfassung. Es wird über das Verhalten atemmechanischer
Parameter und der Blutgase bei 42 spontanatmenden Kaninchen unter intratrachealer Applikation von physiologischer Kochsalzlösung, Histamin und
Acetylcholin vor und nach bilateraler cervikaler Vagotomie gegenüber
einem Vergleichskollektiv berichtet.

Im Vergleich steigt der Atemwegswiderstand nach physiologischer NaCl
(204%), Histamin (299%) und Acetylcholin (484%) deutlich an. Nach Vagotomie
bewirkte NaCl keine Bronchialobstruktion mehr, Acetylcholin jedoch einen
geringen Anstieg des bronchialen Widerstandes von 37% gegenüber Kontroll-
tieren. Der Histamineffekt blieb auch nach Vagotomie weitgehend erhalten
(204%).

NaCl zeigte keine Wirkung auf die arteriellen Blutgase, während Histamin-
und Acetylcholinprovokation zu einer ausgeprägten Hypoxämie sowohl mit

und ohne intaktem Vagusnerven führte.

Es wird geschlossen, daß die Bronchokonstriktion von physiologischen
NaCl und Acetylcholin refektorisch verläuft, die Histaminwirkung ein
überwiegend lokal-irritativer Vorgang ist.

Die Inhalation irritativer Substanzen löst eine Bronchialobstruktion aus
Untersuchungen der letzten Jahre haben die Bedeutung des funktionellen
Zusammenhangs zwischen der Innervation durch das autonome Nervensystem und des Tonus der Tracheobronchialmuskulatur hervorgehoben
[10, 11, 12, 14, 15, 16]. Mediatorenstoffe wie Histamin, Acetylcholin, Serotonin und Prostaglandin $F_{2\alpha}$ lösen eine Bronchialobstruktion aus und führen
durch Induktion einer gesteigerten Emfindlichkeit sensorischer Rezeptoren
auf reflektorischem Weg über den n. vagus zu einer verstärkten Konstriktion der bronchialen Muskulatur [1, 4, 6, 7]. Blockade des vagovagalen
Reflexweges läßt selbst eine durch spezifische Allergene hervorgerufene
Exzitation bronchialer Rezeptoren nicht mehr zur Geltung kommen [2, 17].
Andererseits geht insbesondere aus den bekannten Untersuchungen von
Schild et al. hervor, daß isolierte Bronchialringe - und somit bar jeg-
licher nervaler Kontrolle - bei Kontakt mit Allergenen und Histamin
konstringieren [13].

Im Tierexperiment läßt sich beobachten, daß bei inhalativen Provo-
kationstesten die ausgelöste Bronchokonstriktion durch Vagusblockade oder
Vagotomie nicht vollständig zu verhindern ist [5]. Ein vergleichbares
Ergebnis ist auch bei atemmechanischen Untersuchungen beim Menschen
unter systemischer oder inhalativer Applikation von Atropin oder seiner
Derivate bei Provokationstesten zu finden.

Wir sind daher der Frage nachgegangen, welcher Anteil einer Broncho-
konstriktion reflektorisch ist und ob sich bei Applikation unterschiedlicher
Reizstoffe ein gleichartiges Reflexverhalten und eine gleichartige lokale
Irritation am Bronchialmuskel ableiten läßt.

Untersucht wurden 42 spontanatmende, tracheotomierte Kaninchen in 7
Gruppen (n=6):
Gruppe I: Vor und nach Vagotomie ohne Reizexposition
Gruppe II: 0, 5 ml (22°C) physiologische Kochsalzlösung intratracheal
Gruppe III.   wie II, nach Vagotomie
Gruppe IV: 0, 5 ml (22°C) Histamin 3% intratracheal
Gruppe V: wie IV, nach Vogotomie
Gruppe VI: 0, 5 ml (22°C) Acetylcholin 3% intratracheal
Gruppe VII: wie VI, nach Vagotomie
Die Narkose wurde mit Pentobarbital-Natrium durchgeführt. Gemessen
wurde neben dem Atemzugvolumen (AZV) die pro Atemzug aufgebrachte
oesophagale Druckschwankung mit Hilfe eines flüßigkeitsgefüllten Katheters
in mittlerer Ösophaguslage über einen elektromechanischen Druckwandler
der Firma Statham. Als Maß des bronchialen Widerstandes wurde die
pro 10 ml AZV notwendige Ösophagusdruckschwankung bewertet.

Zur Vagotomie wurde der zervikale Vagusanteil beiderseits freipräpa-
riert und zwei Minuten vor der Bestimmung der Meßwerte durchgeschnitten.

Die Blutgasanalyse erfolgte aus Proben arteriellen Blutes der Aorta thoracalis.

Aus der nachfolgenden Tabelle sind die Mittelwerte der einzelnen Parameter für jede Gruppe zu ersehen.

Gruppe		HF	AF	AZV	AMV	$P_{oes.}$	$\Delta P_{oes.}/$ 10 mlAZV	pO_2	pCO_2	pH
1	GT	250	22	27	594	5,5	2,05	89	41	7,432
	V	254	19	21	399	3,7	1,76	91	39	7,430
2		262	23	36	828	15,0	4,18	75	41	7,411
3		266	21	29	609	6,12	2,11	86	40	7,408
4		298	58	28	1624	17,2	6,13	60	38	7,390
5		284	36	30	1080	12,5	4,18	63	41	7,402
6		308	75	18	1350	17,9	9,92	62	43	7,380
7		298	26	22	572	6,18	2,81	61	42	7,380

GT = Ganztier, V = Vagotomie, HF = Herzfrequenz, AF = Atemfrequenz, AZV = Atemzugvolumen, AMV = Atemminutenvolumen, $P_{oes.}$ = Ösophagusdruck

Die Abb. 1 zeigt die prozentuale Veränderung des $\Delta P_{oes.}$ / 10 ml AZV. Die intratracheale Injektion von physiologischer Kochsalzlösung löst einen Anstieg des bronchialen Widerstandes um 204% gegenüber der Kontrollgruppe I aus. Histamin und Acetylcholin führen zu einer Konstriktion der Bronchialmuskulatur von 299% bzw. 484% gegenüber den Tieren der Gruppe I. Diese Effekte sind im Vergleich zur NaCl-Wirkung deutlich prolongiert.

Die bilaterale zervikale Vagotomie hingegen ist in der Lage, bei intratrachealer Kochsalz-Applikation einen Anstieg des Atemwegswiderstandes vollständig zu verhindern (103%). Der Acetylcholin-Gabe folgt nur eine Konstriktion von 37% gegenüber den Ausgangswerten, während der Histamineffekt mit 204% zum überwiegenden Teil erhalten blieb.

Während der pCO_2 unter den gewählten Versuchsbedingungen keine Veränderung zeigte, fand sich sowohl beim unversehrten Ganztier wie nach Vagotomie unter Histamin und Acetylcholin-Exposition eine nahezu gleiche Hypoxämie. Der geringe pO_2-Abfall nach NaCl ist nicht bedeutsam und nur kurzfristig nachweisbar.

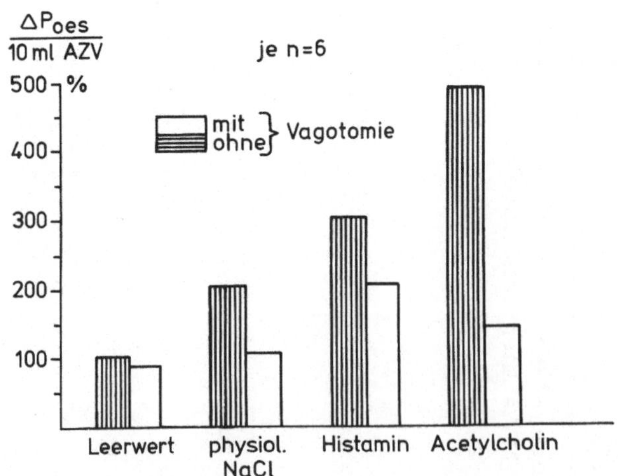

Abb. 1. Prozentualer Anstieg des $\Delta P_{oes.}$ / 10 ml AZV beim Kaninchen vor und nach bilateraler cervicaler Vagotomie infolge intratrachealer Applikation von physiologischer Kochsalzlösung, Histamin und Acetylcholin gegenüber einem nichtprovoziertem Kontrollkollektiv.

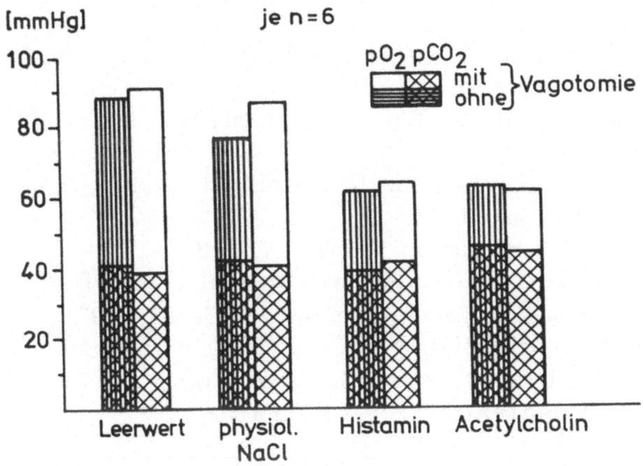

Abb. 2. Verhalten von arteriellem Sauerstoff- und Kohlensäurepartialdruck unter den Versuchsbedingungen der einzelnen Gruppen.

DISKUSSION

Die vorliegenden Ergebnisse bestätigen, daß zwischen einem lokalirritativen und einem reflektorischen Effekt der Mediatoren am Bronchialsystem auch unter in vivo-Bedingungen unterschieden werden kann. Für Histamin war seit langem der direkte wie indirekte (reflektorische) Effekt auf die Bronchialmuskulatur bekannt [4, 13]. Über die bronchokonstriktorische Potenz von 5-Hydrotryptamin und dessen vorwiegende reflektorische Wirkung haben u. a. Islam und Mitarb. berichtet [4, 7]. Bei eigenen Untersuchungen fand sich korrospondierend zu den jetzigen Ergebnissen beim Kaninchen ein lokalwirksamer Effekt von Acetylcholin (37%) nach Vagusblockade im Hundeversuch [5]. Der kurzfristige Anstieg bronchialer Widerstände nach inhalativer Wasserexposition, über die Melville berichtet, dürfte ebenfalls wie die Reaktion auf physiologische Kochsalzlösung als reflexbedingte Antwort am Bronchialmuskel zu erklären sein [9].

Unsere Untersuchungen zeigen im Einklang mit den kürzlich veröffentlichten Ergebnissen von Islam und Mitarb. [8], daß die NaCl- und Acetylcholinwirkung am Bronchialsystem fast ausschließlich einer Reflexbronchokonstriktion entspricht, während bei der Histamprovokation der Atemwege ein vorwiegend lokal-irritativer Vorgang in Betracht zu ziehen ist. Dieses gewinnt durch die zunehmende Verwendung inhalativer Provokationsteste und deren Beurteilung bei der Diagnostik und der Verlaufskontrolle therapeutischer Maßnahmen im Rahmen obstruktiver Atemwegserkrankungen an Bedeutung.

Über die Korrelation biochemischer Untersuchungen von Bronchialsystem und Lunge mit den hier vorgestellten Befunden wird noch berichtet werden.

LITERATUR

1. Dekock, M. A. , Nadel, J. A. , Zwi, S. , Colebatch, H. J. H. ,
   Olsen, C. R. : J. appl. Physiol. $\underline{2}$, 185 (1966)
2. Gold, W. M. , Kessler, G. -K. , Yu, D. Y. C. : J. appl. Physiol. $\underline{33}$,
   719 (1972)
3. Gold, W. M. : in: M. Stein, New Directions in Asthma. Park Ridge,
   Illinois. Amer. Coll. Chest Physic 1974
4. Islam, M. S. , Ulmer, W. T. : Respiration $\underline{30}$, 360 (1973)
5. Islam, M. S. , Lanser, K. , Ulmer, W. T. : Bericht des Silikose-Forschungsinstitutes der Bergbau-Berufsgenossenschaft S. 41 (1973)
6. Islam, M. S. , Ulmer, W. T. : Respiration $\underline{31}$, 332 (1974)
7. Islam, M. S. , Melville, G. N. , Ulmer, W. T. : Respiration $\underline{31}$, 47 (1974)
8. Islam, M. S. , Ulmer, W. T. : Respiration $\underline{32}$, 445 (1975)
9. Melville, G. N. : Respiration $\underline{29}$, 127 (1972)
10. Nadel, J. A. , Salem, H. , Tamplin, B. , Tokiwa, Y. : J. appl. Physiol.
    $\underline{20}$, 164 (1965)
11. Nolte, D. : Verh. Ges. Lungen- und Atmungsforsch. $\underline{1}$, 197 (1967)
12. Paintal, A. S. : Physiol Rev. $\underline{53}$, 159 (1973)
13. Schild, H. O. , Hawkins, D. F. , Mongar, J. L. , Herxheimer, H. :
    Lancet $\underline{1951\ II}$, 376
14. Ulmer, W. T. , Islam, M. S. , Bakran jr. , J. : Dtsch. med. Wschr.
    $\underline{96}$, 1759 (1971)
15. Ulmer, W. T. : Dtsch. med. Wschr. $\underline{100}$, 1575 (1975)
16. Widdicombe, J. G. : Physiol. Rev. $\underline{43}$, 1 (1963)
17. Zimmermann, I. , Islam, M. S. , Lanser, K. , Ulmer, W. T. :
    Respiration (im Druck)

Dr. K. Lanser
I. Medizinische Universitätsklinik
Martinistraße 52
2000 Hamburg - 20

Pneumonologie Suppl. 1976, 259-265

Bronchoconstriction Reflex in Bronchial Asthma

E. Vastag, K. Vass, and L. Nagy

Department of Chest Diseases, Semmelweis University Medical School,
Budapest, Hungary

Abstract. Our results suggest a presumably predominant role of the
parasympathetic nervous system in the mechanism of human bronchial
asthma. Bronchial reaction of the immediate type, induced by a specific
antigen in allergic patients, can be partially but significantly prevented by
a previous parasympathetic efferent blockade. The protective effect of
vagus blockade was nearly complete in 14 out of 22 persons, the increase
of airway flow resistance after antigen stimuli did not exceed 15%. If the
vagus blockade was performed after the antigen stimulus - during the induced bronchospasm - the broncholytic effect was markedly weaker. The
broncholytic effect of selective beta-2-adrenergic stimulation proved to
be faster and stronger in antigen-induced bronchospasm. Vagus blockade
performed by Atrovent® prior to bronchospasm induced by histamine
shows a very weak protective effect.

In spite of the few experimental results an inverse correlation could be
observed between the extent of the protective effect, and the extent of bronchospasm induced by histamine.

Key words: Bronchoconstriction - Cholinergic reflex - Bronchial asthma

Zusammenfassung. Unsere Untersuchungsergebnisse weisen darauf
hin, daß das parasympathische Nervensystem annehmbar eine prädomi-
nante Rolle beim menschlichen Asthma spielt. Bei allergischen Personen
ist die mit spezifischem Antigen induzierte "immediate" Bronchialreak-
tion mittels vorhergehender parasympathischer Efferentblockade teilweise,
jedoch signifikant abzuwehren. Von den 22 Personen war bei 14 eine fast
vollkommene Schutzwirkung der Vagusblockade vorhanden, die Erhöhung
des Strömungswiderstandes übertraf nach Antigenreizung nicht 15%. Wenn
die Vagusblockade erst nach der Antigenreizung verwendet wird, d. h. die
Bronchokonstriktion schon vorhergehend induziert wurde, wird der broncholytische Effekt wesentlich schwächer sein. Die broncholytische Wirkung
der beta-2-Rezeptorenreizung erwies sich als schneller und stärker bei
dem mit Antigen ausgelösten Bronchialspasmus. Bei mit Histamin indu-
zierter Bronchokonstriktion war bei der vorhergehend verabfolgten Vagusblockade - zumindest bei den hier verwendeten Atrovent®-Dosen - eine
verhältnismäßig geringe Schutzwirkung zu beobachten. Trotz der verhält-

nismäßig geringen Zahl der Untersuchungen steht der Grad der Schutzwirkung anscheinend im umgekehrten Verhältnis zu dem mit Histamin indu-
zierten Grad des Bronchialspasmus.

In the last decade our knowledge concerning the pathogenesis of chronic
airway obstruction had been rapidly widened. On the basis of many experimental and clinical examinations the predominant role of the parasympathetic nervous system in the contraction-relaxation cycle of bronchial
smooth muscle can be stressed [2, 12]. This refers to both the maintenance of physiologic resting bronchial tone and the pathologic conditions.
In animals, healthy persons, and patients with chronic obstructive airway
disease various stimuli can induce an acute bronchial spasm by irritation
of the sensoric receptors of a cholinergic reflex mechanism [1, 4, 8, 10, 11,
13].

According to Gold et al. [3] similar mechanisms can be responsible
for airway obstruction provoked by antigenic agents. It has been demonstrated in experimental dog asthma that a previous vagus blockade can pre-
vent the bronchial constriction too which was induced by different antigenic
agents. Examinations on asthmatics are rather scanty up to now, but the
results are in good correlation with the experimental observations [14].

Our examinations were performed on young asthmatic persons. Our
aim was to study the role of the parasympathetic nervous system in bronchial constriction caused by acetylcholine (ach.), histamine, and housedust antigen in asthmatic patients.

MATERIALS AND METHOD

Airway flow resistance (R_t: cmH$_2$O. s. l^{-1}) and intrathoracal gas volume
(IGV ml) were measured by a volume constant plethysmograph (Bodytest,
Fa. E. Jaeger, Würzburg). 0.01% acetylcholine (Acecoline, Laboratoires
Lematte et Boinnott, Paris), 0.005% histamine (Peremin, Chinoin, Budapest), and housedust antigen 150% 0.1 ml = 10^3 PNU (Brentford) solutions
were nebulized by an ultrasonic aerosol instrument (TuR-Usi 2 TuR, Dres-
den). Each aerosol inhalation lasted for 0.5-2 min and the concentration
of the solution was doubled if necessary. The amount of the inhaled substance was determined by volume-backmeasurement supposing a deposi-
tion of 60%. Parasympathetic efferent blockade was produced by a new
derivative of atropine, namely 8-isopropyl-noratropine-methobromide
(Atrovent® Dosier-Aerosol, Boehringer), while for selective stimulation
of the beta-adrenergic receptors p-hydroxyphenyl-orciprenaline (Berotec®
Dosier-Aerosol, Boehringer) was employed.

Examinations were performed on 32 young asthmatics being free of
symptoms or showing perfectly reversible airway obstruction. No drugs
were given to the patients for 24 h prior to the examination. Self-control
data were used. For statistical analysis of results Student "t" test was
employed.

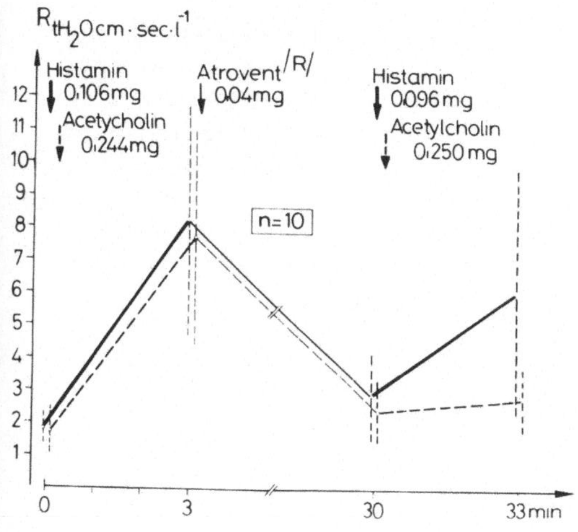

Fig. 1. Protective effect of parasympathetic efferent blockade (0. 04 mg Atrovent® Dosier Aerosol) on bronchospasm induced by acetylcholine and histamine in 10 symptom-free asthmatic patients

RESULTS

The protective effect of the efferent vagus blockade caused by 0. 04 mg Atrovent® inhalation was studied on 10 young symptom-free asthmatics during bronchospasm induced by acetylcholine and histamine administration (Fig. 1).

In Fig. 1 the mean amount of nebulized substances, the mean values of airway flow resistance, and standard deviations can be seen during the examination period. It can be seen that prior to the vagus blockade, inhalation of averagely 0. 244 mg ach. and 0. 106 mg histamine resulted in a marked increase in airway flow resistance (1. 72 $\pm$ 0. 7 - 7. 67 $\pm$ 3. 31 and 1. 79 $\pm$ 0. 46 - 8. 19 $\pm$ 3. 52 $cmH_2O\cdot s. 1^{-1}$ respectively). According to the statistical analysis the effect of both substances proved to be significant in the 3rd min ($\underline{P} < 0. 001$). In the 30th min after the vagus blockade similar doses of ach. and histamine were administered, and determinations were performed prior to and 3 min after the inhalations. Averagely 0. 250 mg acetylcholine administered after the vagus blockade had a nearly negligible effect on airway flow resistance (2. 42 $\pm$ 0. 97 - 2. 77 $\pm$ 0. 99 $cmH_2O. s. 1^{-1}$), but bronchospasm induced by averagely 0. 096 mg histamine could be only partially prevented by the efferent vagus blockade. The increase in airway flow resistance (2. 87 $\pm$ 1. 38 - 6. 10 $\pm$ 3. 84 $cmH_2O. s. 1^{-1}$), proved to be significant ($\underline{P} < 0. 05$).

The protective effect of the efferent vagus blockade on antigen-induced bronchospasm was determined on 15 asthmatics showing a positive cutaneous test against housedust antigen (Fig. 2).

To obtain a perfect efferent vagus blockade, the multiple of the optimal broncholytic dose of Atrovent was administered. In Fig. 2 the mean values of airway flow resistance and standard deviations can be seen at the moments of examination. After inhalation of 2000 PNU Bencard housedust antigen an immediate-type allergic bronchial reaction could be produced in every case. The airway flow resistance markedly increased in the 3rd min, generally accompanied by subjective complaints, and in the 10th min

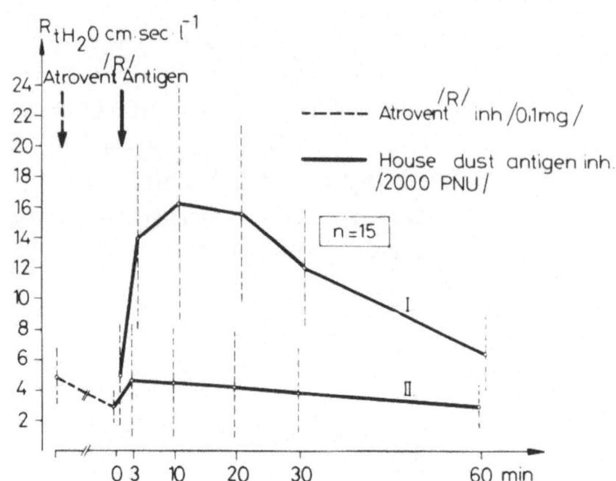

Fig. 2. Bronchospasm induced by housedust antigen (I) and protective effect of previously performed parasympathetic efferent blockade (0. 1 mg Atrovent® Dosier Aerosol) on bronchospasm induced by antigen (II) in 15 asthmatic patients

has reached its maximum level. Even in the 60th min an increased value could be observed. 0. 1 mg Atrovent® administered by inhalation prior to antigenic stimulus caused a decrease in airway flow resistance, and in case of antigen-induced bronchial reaction an intensive, but not perfect protective reaction could be observed.

In Table 1 a significant increase in airway flow resistance can be observed between the 3rd and 30th min after inhalation of 2000 PNU housedust antigen ($\underline{P} < 0.001$). A previous parasympathetic efferent blockade resulted in a significant decrease in flow resistance within 15 min ($\underline{P} < 0.01$) and thereafter the allergen inhalation caused a moderate increase in flow resistance, but statistically this was not significant ($\underline{P} > 0.05$).

The bronchiolytic effect of the vagus blockade and of the selective beta-2-adrenergic stimulation had been determined on seven further asthmatics. Immediate type bronchial reaction was induced by housedust inhalation (Fig. 3). For comparison, vagus blockade had also been performed prior to the antigenic stimuli. The examinations were performed on three consecutive days. In Fig. 3 can be seen, that the broncholytic effect of the vagus blockade is markedly weaker and slower compared to that of beta-2-receptor stimulation. Six minutes after 0. 1 mg Atrovent® inhalation the decrease in airway flow resistance proved to be not significant ($\underline{P} > 0.05$), while after inhalation of 0. 4 mg Berotec® a significant decrease in airway flow resistance could be observed as early as the 3rd min. A significant protective effect could be obtained also in this group if the vagus blockade preceded the antigen stimulus.

DISCUSSION

On the basis of the experimental results the bronchial tree can be divided into two different parts concerning the nervous regulation [7, 8]. The central part supplied by the bronchial arteries ("conductive airways") has a predominant vagus control, while the peripheral part, perfused by the pulmonary circulation, is independent of vagus regulation [8]. Mechanical

Table 1. Bronchospasm induced by housedust antigen (I) and protective effect of previously performed parasympathetic efferent blockade (0.1 mg Atrovent® Dosier Aerosol) on bronchospasm induced by antigen (II) in 15 asthmatic patients

n = 15		0 min	After Atrovent® Dos.-Aer. 0.1 mg 15 min	After 2000 PNU housedust antigen				
				3rd min	10th min	15th min	30th min	60th min
R_t/cmH$_2$O. s. 1^{-1}/	$\overline{X}$	4.94	-	13.90^{xx}	16.10^{xx}	15.53^{xx}	11.96^{xx}	6.42
	S$\pm$	3.41	-	6.22	7.52	5.82	3.87	2.54
/%/ ΔR_t	$\overline{X}$	0	-	+239.9	+291.4	+284.4	+185.0	+45.7
	S$\pm$	0	-	259.1	278.9	271.2	173.4	64.3
IGV /1/	$\overline{X}$	3.63	-	4.61	4.70	4.66	4.54	3.96
	S$\pm$	0.48	-	0.73	0.80	0.88	0.90	0.60
R_t/cmH$_2$O. s. 1^{-1}/	$\overline{X}$	4.82	2.90^{x}	4.55	4.45	4.32	3.86	2.89
	S$\pm$	1.85	1.08	3.84	3.57	3.51	2.80	1.39
/%/ ΔR_t	$\overline{X}$	+67.1	0	+52.2	+48.8	+42.2	+29.4	+0.7
	S$\pm$	47.3	0	112.6	95.3	86.9	73.2	35.8
IGV /1/	$\overline{X}$	3.71	3.35	3.62	3.63	3.61	3.54	3.52
	S$\pm$	0.54	0.42	0.72	0.61	0.53	0.63	0.55

^{x} $\underline{P} < 0.001$ ^{x} $0.001 < \underline{P} < 0.01$

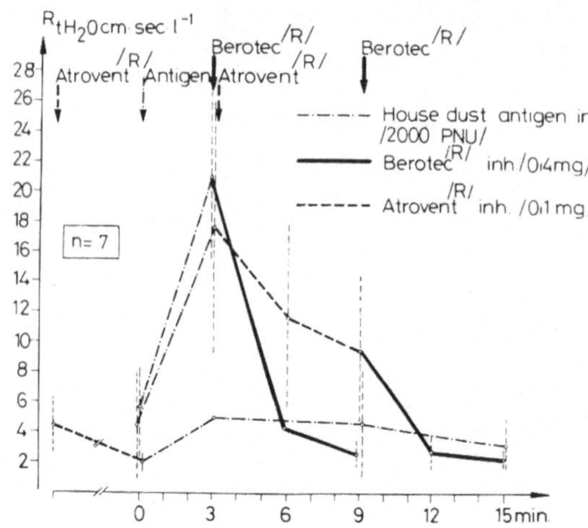

Fig. 3. Broncholytic effect of anticholinergic Atrovent® (0. 1 mg Dosier Aerosol) and beta-2-adrenergic Berotec® (0. 4 mg Dosier Aerosol) on housedust antigen-induced bronchospasm of 7 asthmatic patients

stimuli [9] and changes in the physical characteristics or in chemical composition of inspired air [1, 4, 10, 11, 13] can result in acute broncho-constriction via irritation of the sensoric receptors of airways both in persons and animals. Presumably cholinergic reflex mechanisms play a great role in this process as the induced bronchospasm can be prevented by a previously employed vagus blockade. Various stimuli without antigenic properties can induce bronchoconstriction reflexes in patients with chronic obstructive pulmonary disease [1, 11] as their airways are extremely irritable. Experimental results obtained on animals suggested a double mechanism of action in case of different autacoids such as histamine, serotonin, and acetylcholine [4, 8, 11, 12]. They can induce bronchospasm both directly, through specific receptors of bronchial effectors, and via reflex mechanisms, by stimulation of sensoric receptors.

Experimental results on passively sensitized human lung tissue suggest that in case of in vivo immunologic processes the reflexes mediated by vagus nerves result in acetylcholine release, and this induces the release of further mediators by means of a positive feedback mechanism [5].

Allergen-induced bronchospasm can be prevented by vagus blockade both in experimental dog asthma and in asthmatic patients [3, 14], though such experimental data are rather scanty.

In our series the immediate-type bronchial reaction induced by specific antigen could have been partially but significantly prevented by a previous parasympathetic efferent blockade. In 14 of our 22 patients the protective effect of the vagus blockade was nearly perfect. The increase in airway flow resistance did not exceed 15% after antigen provocation. The broncholytic effect was conspicuously weaker when the antigen stimulus preceded the vagus blockade.

Presumably both adrenergic and cholinergic receptors are present on the mesenchymal target cells having a great role in the release of immunologic mediators and the complex immunologic reaction, and the chemical mediator release can be influenced by their stimulation or inhibition [6].

REFERENCES

1. Booij-Noord, H. , Grobler, N. J. , Orie, N. G. M. , de Vries, K. : Protective action of various drugs on provocation tests with respiratory irritants in patients with chronic non-specific lung disease (CNSLD). Respiration 26, 182 (1969)
2. Cabezas, G. A. , Graf, P. D. , Nadel, J. A. : Sympathetic versus parasympathetic nervous regulation of airways in dogs. J. Appl. Physiol. 31, 651 (1971)
3. Gold, W. M. , Kessler, G. F. , Yu, D. Y. C. : Role of vagus nerves in experimental asthma in allergic dogs. J. Appl. Physiol. 33, 719 (1972)
4. Islam, M. S. , Ulmer, W. T. : Der Wirkungsmechanismus von Serotonin (5-Hydroxytryptamin) und Histamin bei der Atemwegsobstruktion. Respiration 30, 360 (1973)
5. Kaliner, M. , Orange, R. P. , LaRaia, P. J. , Austen, K. F. : Cholinergic enhancement of the immunologic release of histamine and slow-reacting substance of anaphylaxis (SRS-A) from human lung tissue. J. All. Clin. Immunol. 49, 88 (1972)
6. Kaliner, M. , Orange, R. P. , Austen, K. F. : Immunological release of histamine and slow reacting substance of anaphylaxis from human lung. IV. Enhancement by cholinergic and alpha adrenergic stimulation. J. Exp. Med. 136, 556 (1972)
7. De Kock, M. A. , Nadel, J. A. , Zwi, S. : New method perfusing bronchial arteries: histamine bronchoconstriction and apnea. J. Appl. Physiol. 21, 185 (1966)
8. Nadel, J. A. : Structure-function relationships in the airways: Bronchoconstriction mediated via vagus nerves or bronchial arteries; Peripheral lung constriction mediated via pulmonary arteries. Med. thorac. 22, 231 (1965)
9. Nadel, J. A. , Widdicombe, J. G. : Reflex effects of upper airway irritation on total lung resistance and blood pressure. J. Appl. Physiol. 17, 861 (1962)
10. Patel, K. R. : Atropine, sodium cromoglycate and thymoxamine in PGF_2 alfa-induced bronchoconstriction in extrinsic asthma. Brit. med. J. 1975 II, 360
11. Simonsson, B. G. , Jakobs, F. M. , Nadel, J. A. : Role of autonomic nervous system and the cough reflex in the increased responsiveness of airways in patients with obstructive airway disease. J. Clin. Invest. 46, 1812 (1967)
12. Ulmer, W. T. , Islam, M. S. : Die Acetylcholinempfindlichkeit des Bronchialbaumes. Respiration 31, 137 (1974)
13. Widdicombe, J. G. , Kent, D. C. , Nadel, J. A. : Mechanism of bronchoconstriction during inhalation of dust. J. Appl. Physiol. 17, 613 (1962)
14. Yu, D. Y. C. , Galant, S. P. , Gold, W. M. : Inhibition of antigen-induced bronchoconstriction by atropine in asthmatic patients. J. Appl. Physiol. 32, 823 (1972)

Dr. E. Vastag
Semmelweis University Medical School
Department of Chest Diseases
Budapest, Hungary

Pneumonologie Suppl. 1976, 267-273

Mucus Production Influenced by Drugs:
An Electron Microscopic Study

J. Iravani, G. N. Melville, and H. -G. Richter

Lehrstuhl für Anatomie II, Ruhr Universität Bochum

Abstract.   Scanning electron micrographs (SEM) were made of the trachea and bronchi of rats and cats treated with NAB 365 and PGE_1. Both drugs caused an increase in mucus production as is evidenced by the increase in the number of differentiated goblet cells in the trachea and bronchi of both species. PGE_1 appeared to exert a greater influence on mucus production than NAB 365 and under this drug adherence of the cilia tips were observed in rats but not in cats. After PGE_1 administration a complete mucus film is observed in the trachea and bronchi of cats whereas the mucus film is partially complete in rats' trachea. The conclusion is drawn that both NAB 365 and PGE_1 positively influence the mucociliary apparatus.

Key words: Airways - Mucus production - Sympathomimetic drugs - Prostaglandins

---

One of the aims of therapy in chronic obstructive lung diseases is the reduction of any airway obstruction present (Gandevia and Rogers, 1963; Curtis et al. , 1968; Oppenheimer, 1968). This obstruction may be reversible, in which case sympathomimetic or parasympatholytic drugs will alleviate the discomfort (Sheldon and Otis, 1951; Spitzer et al. , 1972; Morton and Turnbull, 1968; Melville and Iravani, 1974) or it may be due to a viscous and stagnant mucus, in which case therapy is aimed at mucus lysis and stimulation of transport (Melville and Iravani, 1974; Hodgkin et al. , 1975).

Several substances are available for achieving the latter purpose and at the same time they stimulate mucus production, a feat that in most cases is linked with increased ciliary beat frequency (Iravani and Melville, 1975). Both these effects facilitate the transport of secretion from the peripheral airways.

In the course of our investigations of bronchodilator drugs, prostaglandin E_1 (Iravani and Melville, 1975) and 4-Amino-α-[(tert. -butylamino) methyl] -3, 5-dichlorobenzyl alcohol hydrochloride (NAB 365) (Iravani and Melville, 1974) were outstanding by their ability to markedly increase mucus production.

The present scanning electron-microscopic study was undertaken to ascertain whether the increased mucus production seen in physiologic studies after administration of PGE_1 and NAB 365 resulted in any demonstrable morphologic changes in the mucus-secreting cells in the trachea and bronchi of rats and cats.

METHODS

Rats and cats were anesthetized with sodium phenobarbital (40 mg/kg i. p.). The airway including the cardiac lobe was isolated and dissected as previously reported (Iravani, 1967). Following dissection, the preparation was slowly heated to 37°C in a bath containing Krebs solution (Krebs and Henseleit, 1932) equilibrated with carbogen (95% O_2, 5% CO_2).

The influence of both NAB 365 and PGE_1 was tested in 4 rats and 4 cats matched for age and weight. After a period of 1 h in the incubating medium, during which time mucus production and mucus transport were stabilized and all of the old mucus transported, one airway preparation each from rats and cats was immediately immersion-fixed in a mixture of 2. 5% glutaraldehyde and 1. 6% formalin in 0. 1N buffer at a pH of 7. 8 (Andres, 1974). The other airway preparations were fixed in a similar manner after exposure to either NAB 365 at a concentration of 10^{-6} g/ml for 30 min or PGE_1 at a concentration of 10^{-11} g/ml for 2 min. The drugs were administered into the Krebs solution. The airways were then washed in buffered solution (0. 22M sucrose in 0. 1M phosphate, pH7. 8). Postfixation was carried out in 4. 5% aqueous OsO_4 and dehydrated in ascending strengths of alcohol. Small pieces of the trachea and bronchi were excised, with care being taken to obtain the identical areas from each animal for examination. The pieces were dried in CO_2 (Anderson, 1951), glued onto copper slides, coated with a uniform layer of evaporated gold, and examined by JEOL scanning microscope U 35.

RESULTS

Following administration of NAB 365 and PGE_1 an increase in the number of differentiated goblet cells was observed in the trachea of both rats and cats (Figs. 1 and 2). The goblet cells appear to be more abundant in the trachea in both species after treatment with either drug. In rats PGE_1 (10^{-11} g/ml) after 2 min seems to stimulate mucus production to a greater extent than NAB 365 and the cilia appear to adhere at their tips. The mucus layer is incomplete and at interval areas goblet cells in various stages of development can be seen protruding.

As a rule cats possess both mucous glands and goblet cells and under normal conditions scattered areas of loose mucus can be seen (Fig. 2a) which increase intensively after PGE_1 (10^{-11} g/ml) to form a homogenous film (Fig. 2b). No adherence of the ciliary tips is seen in cats after the administration of PGE_1. Careful removal of the overlying mucus film to reveal the cilia shows the impressions of the cilia tips on the mucus film

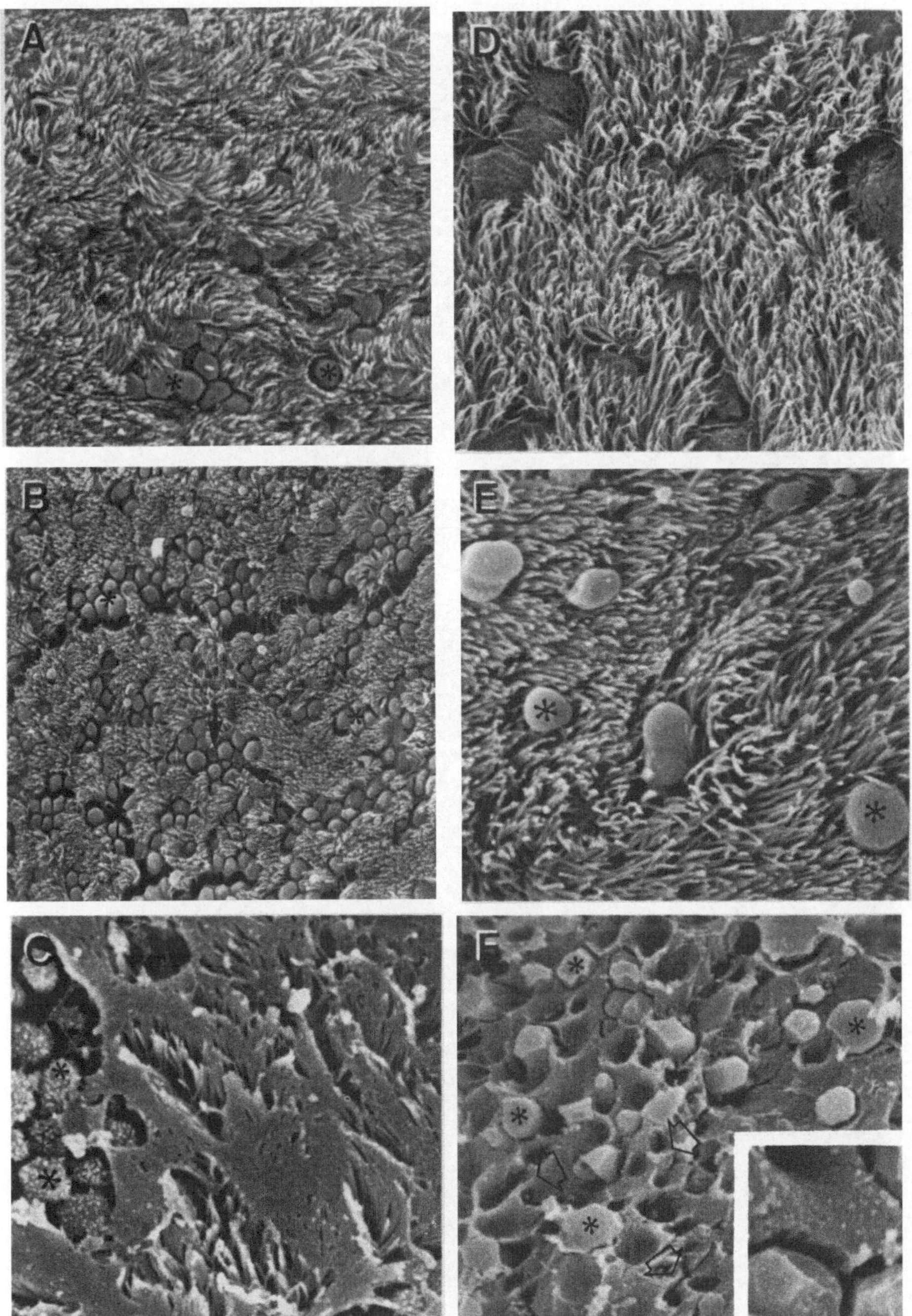

Fig. 1. Scanning electron micrographs of ciliated epithelium of rats. A:
Normal trachea. x 1000; * represents goblet cells in all figures shown. B:
Trachea after administration of NAB 365 (10^{-6} g/ml) for 30 min. Notice
increased differentiation of goblet cells (➤) = brush border cell. x 800. C:
Trachea after PGE_1 (10^{-11} g/ml) for 2 min. Mucus film incomplete especially in regions of protruding goblet cells. x 2200. D: Normal bronchus.
x 1800. E: After NAB 365 (as above). x 2600. F: Bronchus after PGE_1 (as
above). Observe increased number of protruding goblet cells, some of which
have already been extruded thus giving honeycomb structure. (⇨) = adher-
ent cilia tips. x 1200. Inset as in F. x 4600

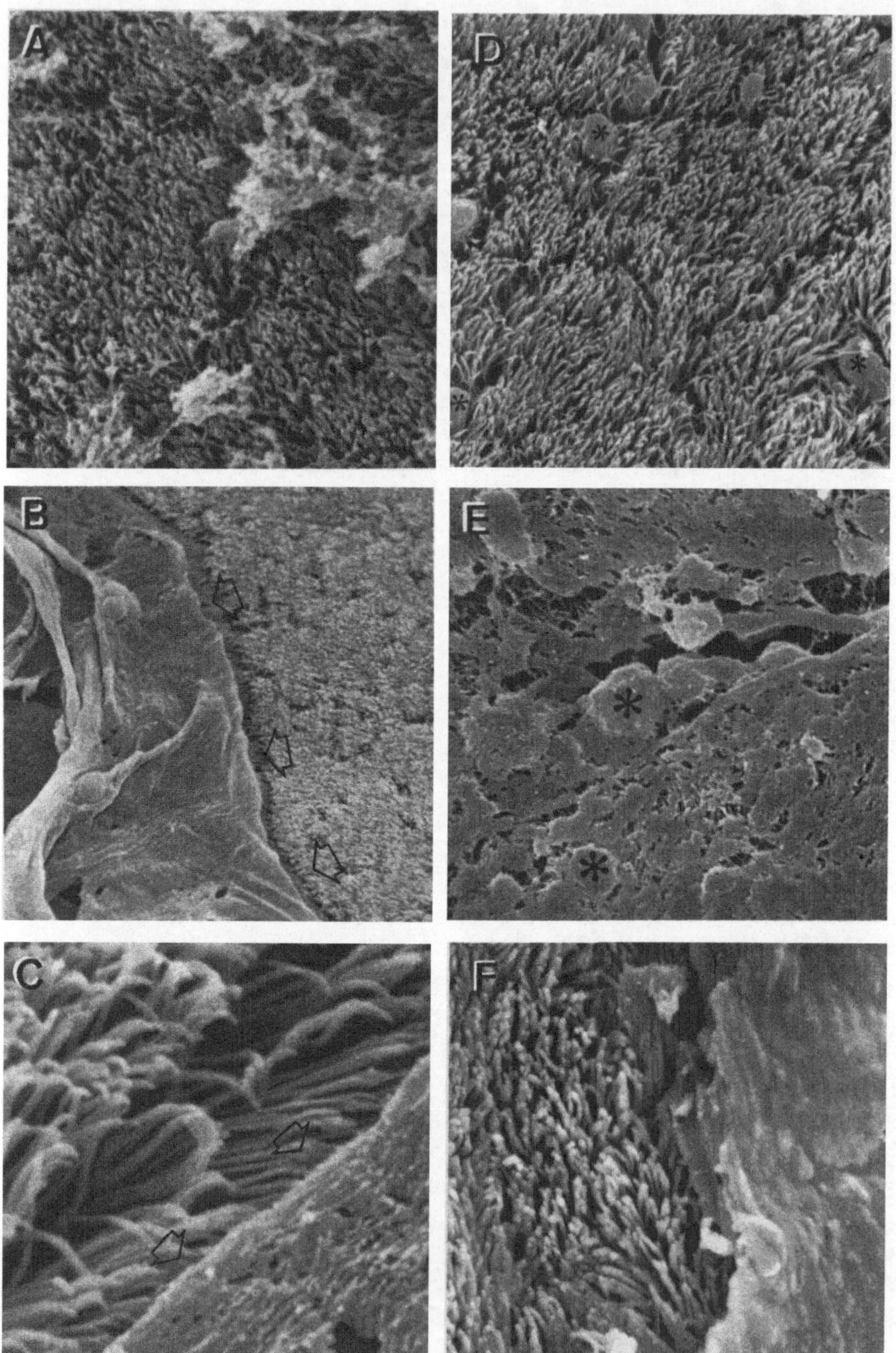

Fig. 2. Scanning electron micrographs of ciliated epithelium of cats. A: Normal trachea. x 1000. B: Trachea after NAB 365 (as in Figure 1). x 700. Notice almost complete and artificially everted mucus film (⇨), which is further magnified in Figure C. x 6500. D: Normal bronchus. x 1900. E: Bronchus after NAB 365 (as above). Observe almost complete mucus film with outlines of goblet cells. x 1800. F: Bronchus after PGE_1 (as in Figure 1). Thick mucus film has been artificially removed to reveal cilia. x 3300

(Fig. 2c) confirming previous suggestions that the mucus lies on the tips of the cilia (Iravani and Melville, 1975). Under higher resolution beadlike structures are seen on the cilia after both PGE_1 and NAB 365.

Increased mucus production was also observed in the bronchi of rats and cats after the administration of NAB 365 (10^{-6} g/ml) and PGE_1 (10^{-11} g/ml). The scanning electron micrographs (Fig. 1e-f) show the strawberry-like profiles of the protruding goblet cells. Transmission electron micrographs confirmed that the outermost pattern of the goblet cells is the un-ripened secretion granules (unpublished data). In the mucus film-free intervals, segmented and attached as well as freely lying granules can be seen on the tips of the cilia. These granules are smaller after the administration of NAB 365 than after PGE_1. Under the latter it appears as though the apical portion of the goblet cell is extruded, thereby giving the typical honeycomb appearance (Fig. 1f).

In the distal bronchi of the treated preparations the overlying mucus film is complete, so that a judgement of the goblet cells from SEM is impossible. In the bronchi of cats treated with NAB 365 (10^{-6} g/ml) an almost complete but loose mucus film is seen through which the apical parts of the goblet cells are visible (Fig. 2e). The goblet cells are less frequent in the untreated bronchi (Fig. 2d).

In cats' bronchi treated with PGE_1 (10^{-11} g/ml) the mucus film is complete and thicker (Fig. 2f). In areas artificially freed of the mucus film, no adhesion of the cilia was observed in contrast to rats' bronchi.

DISCUSSION

In physiologic experiments an increase in mucus production was observed after administration of both NAB 365 (Iravani and Melville, 1974) and PGE_1 (Iravani and Melville, 1975). Morphologic evidence of the pharmacologic effects of drugs is sparse (Horstmann et al., 1975; Melville et al., 1975) and it is at times difficult to explain in physiologic experiments whether the increased mucus production is really the effect of a true mucus elaboration or whether it is an artefact due to altered permeability in the ciliated epithelium for the surrounding medium.

The scanning electron micrographs corroborate previous findings that NAB 365 and PGE_1 positively influence mucus production in mammals (Iravani and Melville, 1974, 1975; Melville et al., 1975).

Rats differ in their response to NAB 365 and PGE_1, in that PGE_1 in addition to its effect on mucus production appears to affect the composition of the interciliary fluid. It is suggested that a change in the composition of the interciliary fluid leads to adhesion of the cilia. In previous studies (Iravani and Melville, 1975) it was difficult to measure ciliary beat frequency under PGE_1 because of the large quantity of secretion. We are of the opinion that the beadlike structures on the cilia are due to the interciliary liquid and that the more viscous this fluid is the greater will be the number of beads formed and the adhesion between the cilia.

Although mucus production in cats treated with PGE_1 was of the same magnitude as in rats, it did not appear to cause the same change in the in-

terciliary fluid and may explain the absence of adherence of the cilia tips
in cats and the decreased number of beadlike structures on the cilia. In
physiologic studies no blurring of the microscopic picture was seen under
NAB 365 in contrast to PGE_1 (Iravani and Melville, 1975). The blurring of
the picture was assumed to be due to the massive increase in interciliary
fluid.

Evidence is provided that the effects of drugs on mucociliary function
can be clearly deduced from morphologic studies. The combination of physiologic and morphologic studies in the evaluation of drug actions on the
respiratory ciliated epithelium is to be recommended.

A suitable drug in respiratory therapy is one that possesses not only
bronchodilator properties but one that also positively influences mucus production, secretolysis, and ciliary beat frequency. Both NAB 365 and PGE_1
satisfy these criteria with the exception of ciliary activity which was not
significantly affected by PGE_1.

REFERENCES

Anderson, T. F. : Techniques for the preservation of three-dimensional
    structure in preparing specimens for the electron microscope. Trans.
    N. Y. Acad. Sci. 13, 130 (1951)

Andres, K. H. : Zur methodischen Perfusionfixierung des Zentralnerven-
    systems von Säugern. Tgg. Niederl. u. Dtsch. Ges. Elektronenmikro-
    scopie, Aachen 1965

Curtis, J. K. , Liska, A. P. , Rasmussen, H. K. : The bronchospastic com-
    ponent in patients with chronic obstructive bronchitis and emphysema.
    J. Amer. Med. Ass. 197, 693 (1966)

Hodgkin, J. E. , Balchum, O. J. , Kass, I. , Glaser, E. M. , Miller, W. F. ,
    Haas, A. , Shaw, D. B. , Kimbel, P. , Petty, T. L. : Chronic obstructive
    airway diseases. Current concepts in diagnosis and comprehensive care.
    J. Amer. Med. Ass. 232, 1243 (1975)

Gandevia, B. , Rogers, N. : Effect of bronchodilator aerosol on ventilatory
    capacity in chronic lung and heart diseases. Brit. Med. J. 1963 II,
    1097

Horstmann, G. , Iravani, J. , Melville, G. N. , Ulmer, W. T. : Physiological
    and electron microscopic investigations of the trachea after pilocarpine.
    Pneumonologie 152, 105 (1975)

Iravani, J. : Flimmerbewegung in den intrapulmonalen Luftwegen der Ratte.
    Pflügers Arch. ges. Physiol. 297, 221 (1967)

Iravani, J. , Melville, G. N. : Mucociliary activity in the respiratory tract
    as influenced by prostaglandin E1. Respiration 32, 305 (1975)

Krebs, A. , Henseleit, K. : Untersuchungen über die Harnstoffbildung im
    Tierkörper. Z. physiol. Chem. 210, 33 (1932)

Melville, G. N. , Horstmann, G. , Iravani, J. : Adrenergic compounds and
    the tracheobronchial tree. Respiration (in press)

Melville, G. N. , Iravani, J. : Resistance and blood gas tensions in bronchi-
    al asthma. Respiration 31, 381 (1974)

Morton, J. W. , Turnbull, K. W. : The reversibility of chronic bronchitis,
    asthma and emphysema. Dis. Chest 53, 126 (1968)

Oppenheimer, E. A. , Rigatto, M. , Fletcher, C. M. : Airways obstruction
   before and after isoprenaline, histamine, and prednisolone in patients
   with chronic obstructive bronchitis. Lancet 1968 I, 552
Sheldon, M. B. , Otis, A. B. : Effects of adrenaline on resistance to gas
   flow in the respiratory tract and on vital capacity of normal and asthmatic subjects. J. Appl. Physiol. 3, 513 (1951)
Spitzer, S. A. , Goldschmidt, Z. , Dubrawsky, C. : The bronchodilator effect
   of salbutamol administered by IPPB to patients with asthma. Chest 62,
   273 (1972)

Dr. J. Iravani
Ruhr Universität Bochum
Lehrstuhl für Anatomie II
4630 Bochum

Pneumonologie Suppl. 1976, 275-277

Theophylline Blood Levels with Theophylline Ethylene Diamine

J. Ahrens

BYK GULDEN Konstanz, Department of Clinical Research

Abstract. Theophylline blood levels following administration of theophylline ethylene diamine, intravenously, orally, and rectally, are compared and correlated with effectiveness of broncholytic action and toxicity. For long-term treatment of patients with airway obstructions the maintenance of constant theophylline plateau concentrations in plasma is desirable. This can be achieved by infusion of the drug at a constant rate after an initial loading dose, by treatment with suppositories due to the slow and limited rectal absorption of aminophylline, and by application of a new retard preparation where the sustained release of the drug determines the rate of gastrointestinal absorption of theophylline. In all three cases the dosage can be adjusted easily to the individually different pharmacokinetic properties of the patients.

Key words: Aminophylline - Blood level - Half-lifes - Long-term treatment

---

The water-soluble theophylline ethylene diamine (Euphyllin®, Aminophyllin®) was synthesized in Germany 70 years ago. First introduced as a diuretic agent, this salt today represents the only intravenous theophylline preparation available. The oral preparations have been used most commonly in the treatment of reversible airway obstructions for more than 40 years. Since Schack and Waxler [4] published a simple spectrophotometric method to determine the concentration of this drug in biological fluids and tissues more than 25 years ago, the pharmacokinetic and pharmacodynamic properties of theophylline are well known.

Following intravenous injection of 120 mg theophylline ethylene diamine, the plasma concentration falls rapidly due to distribution, and then declines more gradually according to the half-life of elimination (Fig. 1). After oral administration of 200 mg aminophylline, the theophylline blood level increases, and thereafter decreases rapidly, reaching a peak 1.5 h after administration. The rectal absorption of a suppository, containing 360 mg Euphyllin, occurs more slowly and seems to be limited. The level is lower in comparison to the same amount of drug administered orally. However, a constant plateau is maintained for several hours, and a significant improvement of the specific airway resistance has been observed in patients with reversible airways diseases [1].

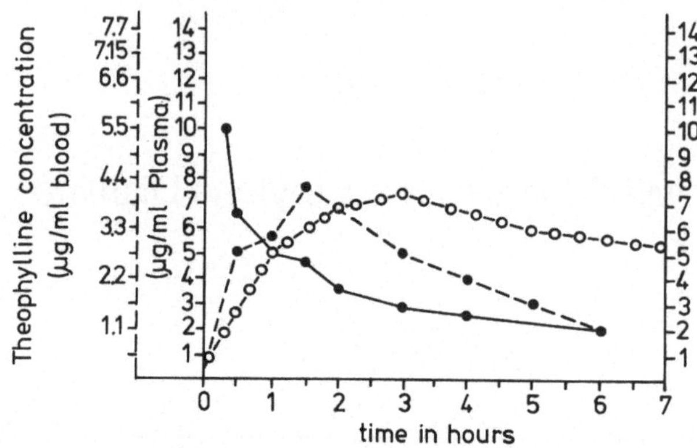

Fig. 1. Comparison of theophylline blood levels following parenteral administration of 120 mg (. -. -.), oral administration of 200 mg (. ---. ---), and rectal application of 360 mg aminophylline (-o-o-o)

The establishment and maintenance of a certain constant theophylline level in a therapeutically effective range and below the toxic region is, indeed, most important for the therapeutic success of long-term treatment.

Serum theophylline concentration correlates directly with the pharmacologic effects and toxicity. A broncholytic effect is observed at theophylline levels above 3. 5 µg/ml plasma. A range between 5 and 12 µg/ml is regarded to be safe and effective. For maximal physiologic reversibility of airway resistance, concentrations between 8 and 20 µg/ml are required. Side effects have been observed above 15, gastrointestinal and central nervous system disturbances are common at 20, cardiac arrhythmia may occur at 40, and convulsions at levels of 60 µg theophylline/ml plasma.

According to these data the concentration curves shown in Figure 1 are in a safe region, with therapeutic activities to be expected for 2, 3, and 6 h, respectively.

Basic studies on theophylline pharmacokinetics, performed by Mitenko and Ogilvie [2, 3], resulted in the rational use of intravenous theophylline in the treatment of status asthmaticus and severe asthma. In order to maintain a constant theophylline level, the amount of drug eliminated in a certain time interval has to be replaced during that time interval. According to the determined plasma clearance rate for a patient of 70 kg body weight the infusion of 62. 5 mg aminophylline per h is required to maintain a theophylline plateau of 10 µg/ml plasma.

For a rapid attainment of this level a loading dose of 400 mg aminophylline, administered intravenously over 15-30 min, is necessary.

The height of the plasma level is directly related to the theophylline half-life. Since the drug is degraded by microsomal enzymes to 90% and the amount and activity of these enzymes may vary strongly, there are large differences in individual theophylline half-lifes. In adults mean values of 4. 5 h (3-9. 5) and in children of 3. 6 (1. 5-9. 5) h have been found. There is strong evidence for enzyme induction. The following theophylline half-lifes have been determined: 3. 6 h for asthma patients, 4. 1 h for heavy smokers, and 7. 2 h for nonsmokers.

Because of the short theophylline half-lifes frequently observed in patients with obstructive airways diseases and due to the rapid gastrointestinal absorption, the constant theophylline plateau desired in long-term therapy can be maintained only by repeated small oral doses administrated in

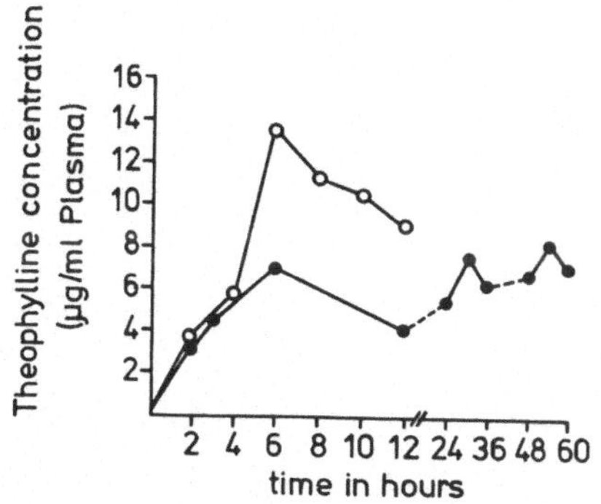

Fig. 2. Theophylline plasma levels after administration of 2 Euphylline retard tablets and after 1 tablet every 12 h

short time intervals, or by retard preparations where the sustained release of the drug determines the rate of absorption.

After oral administration of 1 or 2 Euphyllin retard tablets, each containing 350 mg aminophylline, a slow increase of theophylline plasma concentration occurs for 6 h (Fig. 2). A dosage of 1-2 tablets, at intervals of 8 or 12 h, results in a progressive elevation of drug plasma levels until a steady state is achieved. Thus, a plasma theophylline plateau, which oscillates between a maximum during the interval and a minimum at the time of new administration, is maintained and peak concentrations reaching into the toxic range, which may be observed after oral administration of large doses of conventional aminophylline tablets, are avoided. According to the individually different pharmacokinetic parameters the dosage regimen can be adjusted to the individual needs in order to produce an optimal therapeutic effect. The correlation between theophylline plasma levels and therapeutic response has been demonstrated [5].

REFERENCES

1. Ahrens, J., Krieger, E.: Theophyllin-Blutspiegel und broncholytische Wirkung bei rektaler Applikation. Atemwegs- und Lungenkrankheiten 1, 173 (1975)
2. Mitenko, P.A., Ogilvie, R.I.: Rational intravenous doses of theophylline. New England J. Med. 289, 600 (1973)
3. Mitenko, P.A., Ogilvie, R.I.: Pharmacokinetics of intravenous theophylline. Clin. Pharmacol. Ther. 14, 509 (1973)
4. Schack, J.A., Waxler, S.H.: An ultraviolet spectrophotometric method for determination of theophylline and theobromine in blood and tissues. J. Pharmacol. Ex. Ther. 97, 283 (1949)
5. Wiessman, K.J.: Der Einfluß eines oralen Aminophyllin-Präparates mit Retardwirkung auf die Lungenfunktionsparameter bei obstruktiven Atemwegserkrankungen. Dtsch. med. Wschr. 100, 1781 (1975)

Dr. J. Ahrens
BYK GULDEN Konstanz
Abteilung Klinische Forschung
D-7750 Konstanz

Pneumonologie Suppl. 1976, 279-284

Die Analyse belastungsabhängiger Störungen der Atemmechanik mit Ergo-Bodyplethysmographie*

P. Wyličil, M. Beil und E. Herrmann

Medizinische Klinik des Krankenhauses Nordwest, Frankfurt/Main

The Analysis of Exercise Related Disorders in Mechanics of Breathing by Ergometric Body Plethysmography

Abstract. Ergometric body plethysmography is possible to be applied by connecting the plethysmograph-cabine to a normal bicycle ergometer. No additional equipment of apparatus is required. Resistance and intra-thoracic gas volume (IGV) measurements can be performed well during exercise. Healthy persons show an increase of the total resistance caused by high flow-rates, while the resistance at a flow-rate of 0.5 l/s remains equally or decreases a little. The IGV increases a little by the shift of the endexpiratory volume level. The ergometric body plethysmography is especially useful for determinating the lowest grade of exercise, which induces a bronchial collapse, if this collapse is absent during spontaneous breathing at rest and only detectable by forced exspiratory maneuvers. Following kinds of reactions are possible, when patients with obstructive lung disease are submitted to exercise: bronchial collapse, indifferent response, broncholysis, progressive augmentation of trapped air and exercise induced bronchospasm.

With ergometric body plethysmography therefore it is possible to get new aspects of the mechanics of breathing during exerise.

Key words: Ergometric body plethysmography - Mechanics of breathing Types of exercise reactions - Chronic obstructive lung disease

Zusammenfassung. Die Belastungsganzkörperplethysmographie ist durch Einbau einer Tretkurbel in die Plethysmographenkabine und Koppelung an ein vorhandenes Ergometer ohne großen apparativen Mehraufwand möglich. Resistance- und Verschlußdruckkurven lassen sich unter körperlicher Arbeit gut registrieren. Bei Gesunden kommt es zu einer flow- und turbulenzbedingten Zunahme der Totalresistance, während die R 0,5 gleich bleibt oder gering abnimmt. Das IGV nimmt durch Verschiebung der Atem-

---

* Mit Unterstützung der Deutschen Forschungsgemeinschaft

mittellage leicht zu. Die Domäne der Belastungsganzkörperplethysmographie
liegt in der Ermittlung jener geringsten Belastungsstufe, bei der es zu
einem Bronchialkollaps kommt, wenn dieser in Ruhe noch nicht, sondern
erst bei dem unphysiologischen Manöver des Atemstoßes nachweisbar ist.
Bei Patienten mit obstruktiver Lungenkrankheit sind unter Belastung verschiedene Reaktionsformen möglich: Zunehmender Bronchialkollaps, indifferentes Verhalten, Broncholyse, progrediente Zunahme der trapped
air und Belastungsbronchospasmus.

Die Belastungsganzkörperplethysmographie ist somit in der Lage, neue
Erkenntnisse über die bronchopulmonalen Belastungsreaktionen zu ver-
mitteln.

Für die Beurteilung einer pulmonal bedingten Leistungsbegrenzung ist das
Verhalten des Bronchialwiderstandes und des intrathorakalen Gasvolumens
während körperlicher Arbeit von Bedeutung. Kagawa und Kerr[1] haben
als erste einen Tretkurbelmechanismus in eine Plethysmographenkabine
eingebaut, ihre Messungen aber doch erst unmittelbar nach Belastungsende
und während Hechelatmung durchgeführt. Sie fanden bei vier gesunden Probanden eine Zunahme der spezifischen Conductance. Andere Untersucher
wie Simonsson et al. [3] sowie Schindl [2] haben die Probanden außerhalb
der Kabine belastet und die Messungen ebenfalls unmittelbar nach Belastungs
ende in der Kabine durchgeführt. Sie fanden teils eine Zunahme, teils eine
Abnahme der Resistance je nach Alter und Ausgangswerten.

Unser Anliegen war es nun, direkt während der Belastung und bei Spontanatmung zu registrieren, was durch Einbau einer Tretkurbel in die Kabine eines volumenkonstanten Ganzkörperplethysmographen und Koppelung
dieser Tretkurbel über Kardan und Kegelrad an ein vorhandenes Ergometer
möglich war (Abb. 1). Über methodische Einzelheiten wurde bereits ausführlich berichtet [5]. Zunächst haben wir eine Gruppe gesunder Probanden
untersucht. Dabei zeigte sich ein S-förmiges Abknicken der Totalresistance
während der Belastung, eine bekannte, turbulenzbedingte Erscheinung bei
hohem Flow. Sie ist der Grund dafür, daß die Totalresistance bei den gesunden Probanden mit steigender Wattzahl kontinuierlich und statistisch
signifikant zunahm. Mißt man dagegen nicht die Totalresistance, sondern
den linearen Teil der Kurve, z.B. bei einer Strömungsgeschwindigkeit
von 0,5 l/s, dann ergibt sich während der Belastung keine Zunahme, sondern
eher eine geringfügige Abnahme. Das intrathorakale Gasvolumen nahm bei
den gesunden Probanden innerhalb einer sehr großen Streuung geringfügig
zu, was durch eine leichte Verschiebung der Atemmittellage zur Inspiration
hin ohne weiteres zu erklären ist.

Patienten mit obstruktiver Lungenkrankheit unterschiedlicher Genese
haben wir in dieser ersten Untersuchungsreihe meist nur mit einer Stufe,
nämlich 1/2 Watt/kg belastet. Die Ergebnisse werden besonders deutlich,
wenn man die Ausgangswerte für Resistance und Atemstoß berücksichtigt.

Asthmatiker im beschwerdefreien Intervall mit normaler Resistance
und normalem Atemstoß verhalten sich unter Belastung wie die Gesunden.

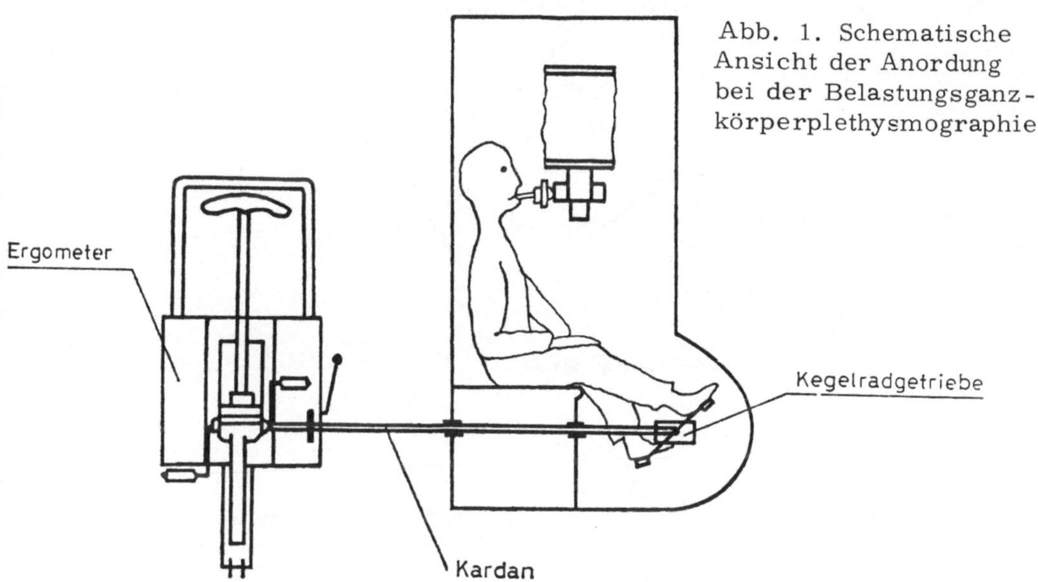

Abb. 1. Schematische Ansicht der Anordung bei der Belastungsganzkörperplethysmographie

Bei Patienten mit normaler Resistance, aber pathologischem Tiffeneau-Wert ist es möglich, d e n Alveolardruck bezw. d i e Belastungsstufe zu ermitteln, bei der es erstmals zum Bronchialkollaps kommt, also Grau-zone zwischen der Ruheatmung und dem unphysiologischen Atemstoßmanö-ver genauer zu untersuchen.

Zwei Einzelfälle mögen dies deutlich machen (Abb. 2): Beide Patienten zeigen normale Resistancewerte bei deutlich pathologischem Atemstoß. Während maximaler, willkürlicher Hyperventilation kommt es bei beiden Probanden zum exspiratorischen Bronchialkollaps. Bei der Belastung von 1/2 Watt/kg zeigt der Patient in der oberen Reihe keine Änderung gegen-über den Ruhewerten. Die Belastung ist ihm daher von dieser Seite zumut-bar. Der Patient der unteren Reihe zeigt dagegen bereits bei dieser Mini-malbelastung einen ausgeprägten Bronchialkollaps. Er brach die Unter-suchung wegen zunehmender Dyspnoe ab.

Will man dieses Verhalten nicht durch die Kurvenform, sondern durch Zahlen ausdrücken, so eignet sich hierfür besonders gut die getrennte An-gabe der inspiratorischen und exspiratorischen Resistance (R_{ti} und R_{te}) nach Ulmer [4].

Eine Tatsache ist besonders wichtig: Die während Belastung auftretenden Veränderungen, insbesondere der Bronchialkollaps, bilden sich unmittelbar nach Belastungsende sofort zurück. Die Registrierung der Kurven direkt nach Belastung vermittelt demnach kein objektives Bild der atemmecha-nischen Veränderungen während Belastung.

Patienten mit bereits in Ruhe pathologischer Resistance zeigen unter Belastung eine Vielfalt von Reaktionen, die sich im Einzelfall überlagern können. Fast immer ist jedoch die eine oder andere Komponente vorherr-schend. In der Reihenfolge der Häufigkeit ihres Auftretens ergaben sich die

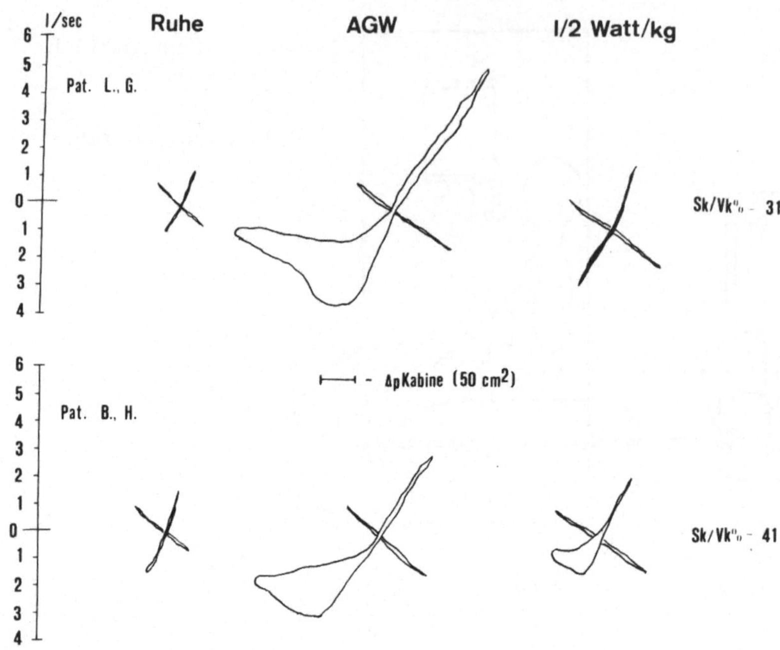

Abb. 2. Resistance- und Verschlußdruckkurven von zwei Patienten mit Lungenemphysem

Tabelle 1. Häufigkeitsverteilung der Reaktionstypen bei 119 Belastungs-GPG-Tests

Gesamtzahl der Fälle	**119**
Gesunde	**19**
Patienten mit obstr. Lungenerkr.	**100**
Bronchialkollaps	40
Indifferenztyp	35
Broncholyse	15
Progr. Air trapping	7
Bronchospasmus	3

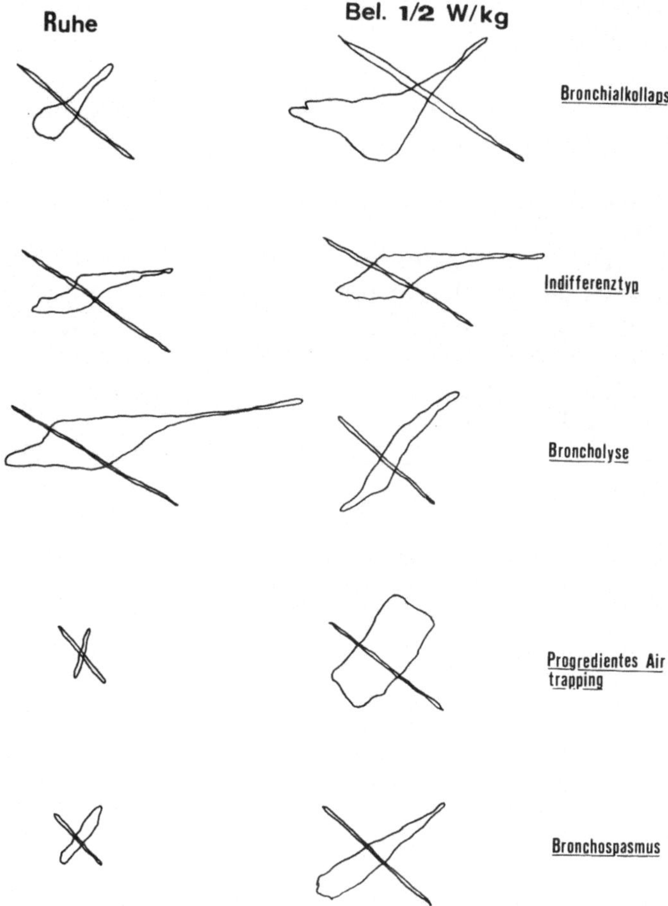

Abb. 3. Verschiedene Belastungstypen bei Patienten mit Bronchialobstruktion

folgenden Belastungstypen (Abb. 3):
1.   Vorwiegender Bronchialkollaps
2.   Indifferentes Verhalten
3.   Broncholytischer Belastungstyp
4.   Überwiegende Zunahme der trapped air
5.   Überwiegender Belastungsbronchospasmus.

Ein unter Belastung auftretender oder sich verstärkender Bronchospasmus war bei den von uns untersuchten Fällen sehr selten. Tabelle 1 zeigt die Häufigkeit der verschiedenen Belastungsreaktionen.

LITERATUR

1. Kagawa, J. , Kerr, H. D. : Effect of brief graded exercise on specific airway conductance in normal subjects. J. Appl. Physiol. $\underline{28}$, 138-144 (1970)
2. Schindl, R. : Belastbarkeit beim obstruktiven Syndrom. Prax. Pneumol. $\underline{26}$, 169-178 (1972)
3. Simonson, B. G. , Skoogh, B. E. , Ekström-Jodal, B. : Exercise-induced airways constriction. Scand. J. Respir. Dis. Suppl. $\underline{77}$, 30 (1973)
4. Ulmer, W. T. , Reif, E. : Die obstruktiven Erkrankungen der Atemwege. Dtsch. med. Wschr. $\underline{90}$, 1803-1809 (1965)
5. Wyličil, P. , Weber, J. M. , Köhlen, K. : Belastungsbodyplethysmographie. Respiration $\underline{30}$, 414-429 (1973)

Dr. Peter Wyličil
Nordwestkrankenhaus
Steinbacher Hohl 2-26
6000 Frankfurt/Main 90

Pneumonologie Suppl. 1976, 285

Importance of Stratificational Inhomogenity for Pulmonary Gas Exchange

J. Piiper and F. Adaro

Abteilung Physiologie, Max-Planck-Institut für experimentelle Medizin, Göttingen

The limiting effects of stratification on the effectiveness of alveolar gas exchange have been calculated using the values for diffusive conductance of distal airways obtained from an analysis of washout kinetics of He and SF_6 by Okubo and Piiper (1974). For the lungs of 10 kg dogs, the stratificational component of the alveolar-arterial P_{O_2} difference is estimated at about 0. 8 torr for resting conditions and at about 3. 5 torr for medium level exercise.

Since the diffusion coefficients of CO_2 and O_2 are of similar magnitude and the alveolar-capillary transfer rates of CO_2 and O_2 are similar, the alveolar-arterial P_{CO_2} and P_{O_2} differences due to stratificational effects should be about equal. In this respect the effect of stratification on alveolar gas exchange closely resembles that of alveolar dead space ventilation.

On the basis of model analysis and experimental data, stratificational effects are expected to be increased with decreased depth of inspiration and increased respiratory rate, and particularly with a combination of these factors (panting, rapid shallow breathing). The alveolar-arterial equilibration deficit due to stratification should be increased with increased O_2 uptake and CO_2 output (combined with high breathing frequency: exercise). In pathologically altered lungs with impaired effective diffusion conditions in airways stratificational effects may be of considerable importance.

(The full-length paper "Limiting role of stratification in alveolar exchange of oxygen", by Adaro and Piiper, has been accepted for publication in Respiration Physiology.)

REFERENCES

1. Okubo, T. , Piiper, J. : Intrapulmonary gas mixing in excised dog lung lobes studied by simultaneous wash-out of two inert gases. Respir. Physiol. 21, 223-239 (1974)

Dr. J. Piiper
Max-Planck-Institut für Experimentelle
Medizin - Abteilung Physiologie
D-3400 Göttingen

Instructions to Authors

Papers should preferably be written in English in order to ensure the widest possible currency. Some editorial assistance with the language may be available to authors writing in English when it is not their mother tongue.

Manuscripts must be typed on one side of the paper only, double-spaced with wide margins. All pages should be numbered consecutively throughout. Tables and legends to figures should be submitted on separate sheets.

Both form and content of the paper should be **carefully checked** to exclude the need for corrections in proof. A charge will be made for changes introduced after the manuscript has been set in type.

The **first page of the manuscript** should comprise:

a) title of the paper (concise but informative); b) name(s) of author(s); c) institute where the work was carried out; d) address to which the proofs should be sent; e) footnotes to the title (marked by asterisks).

Footnotes which do not refer to the heading should be numbered consecutively.

Each paper should be preceded by a brief **abstract** of the essential results (facts); papers not written in English should include an English abstract and an English translation of the title. In addition, each paper should include up to five key words.

The bibliography should include only works referred to in the text. References should be listed at the end of the paper in alphabetical order under the first author's name, more than one reference to the same author or team of authors in chronological order. References to *journal articles* should indicate the names of all authors followed by the initials, full title of the article, abbreviation of the journal according to World Medical Periodicals, number of volume, first and if possible last pages and year of publication. *Books* are cited by authors' names, full title, edition, place of publication, publisher and year, e.g.

Orie, N. G. M.: Die Klinik der gestörten Lungenzirkulation. Beitr. Klin. Tuberk. 141. 62—71 (1969)

Nicholson, J. B., Neuhaus, H., Hasler, M. F.: New spectrometers and accessories for the electron microprobe. In: Vth international congress on X-ray optics and microanalysis, pp. 269—273, G. Möllenstedt and K. H. Gaukler, Eds. Berlin-Heidelberg-New York: Springer 1969

Citations in the text should be by author and year. If an article by two authors is cited, both authors should be mentioned; with three or more authors only the first should be named, followed by "et al.", e.g. (Piiper, 1961; Ulmer et al., 1967; Reichel and Rosenkranz, 1968). Another form of citation uses numbers in square brackets referring to an *alphabetically* ordered bibliography list. Either form is acceptable when used consistently throughout the paper.

Illustrations should be restricted to the minimum needed to clarify the text. Diagrams, schemes, particularly half-tones and X-rays, illustrating findings which could just as well be described in the text will be rejected. If data are fully described in the legend, it is not necessary to repeat this in the text, nor should data be presented in both graph and table form. Coloured and previously published illustrations cannot usually be accepted.

The figures with legends should not extend beyond the print area (12×20 cm). Several figures should be grouped into a plate on one page.

Line drawings: Please submit good quality glossy prints in the desired final size. The inscriptions should be clearly legible: letters 3 mm high are recommended.

Half-tone illustrations: Please submit well-contrasted photographic prints, trimmed at right angles and in the desired final size. Inscriptions should be about 3 mm high.

The original manuscript and art, if returned to the publisher along with the corrected proofs, will be destroyed 3 months after mailing of the issue.